SECOND EDITION

EVIDENCE-BASED TEACHING
IN NURSING

A Foundation for Educators

Edited by

SHARON CANNON, EdD, RN, ANEF
Regional Dean/Professor
Medical Center Hospital Regional Dean Endowed Chair
Co-Director, Center of Excellence in Evidence-Based Practice
Texas Tech University Health Sciences Center
School of Nursing
Odessa, Texas

CAROL BOSWELL, EdD, RN, CNE, ANEF
Professor
James A. "Buddy" Davidson Charitable Foundation
Endowed Chair for Evidence-Based Practice
Co-Director of the Center of Excellence in Evidence-Based Practice
Texas Tech University Health Sciences Center
School of Nursing
Odessa, Texas

JONES & BARTLETT
LEARNING

World Headquarters
Jones & Bartlett Learning
5 Wall Street
Burlington, MA 01803
978-443-5000
info@jblearning.com
www.jblearning.com

Jones & Bartlett Learning books and products are available through most bookstores and online booksellers. To contact Jones & Bartlett Learning directly, call 800-832-0034, fax 978-443-8000, or visit our website, www.jblearning.com.

Substantial discounts on bulk quantities of Jones & Bartlett Learning publications are available to corporations, professional associations, and other qualified organizations. For details and specific discount information, contact the special sales department at Jones & Bartlett Learning via the above contact information or send an email to specialsales@jblearning.com.

Production Credits

VP, Executive Publisher: David Cella
Executive Editor: Amanda Martin
Editorial Assistant: Lauren Vaughn
Production Editor: Keith Henry
Senior Marketing Manager: Jennifer Stiles
VP, Manufacturing and Inventory Control:
  Therese Connell

Manager of Photo Research, Rights & Permissions:
  Lauren Miller
Composition: Cenveo Publisher Services
Cover Design: Kristin E. Parker
Cover Image: (top) © Natali Zakharova/ShutterStock,
  Inc. (bottom) © evv/ShutterStock, Inc.
Printing and Binding: Edwards Brothers Malloy
Cover Printing: Edwards Brothers Malloy

To order this product, use ISBN: 978-1-284-07473-4

Library of Congress Cataloging-in-Publication Data
Cannon, Sharon, 1940- , author.
 Evidence-based teaching in nursing : a foundation for educators / Sharon Cannon and Carol Boswell. — 2nd.
  p. ; cm.
 Includes bibliographical references and index.
 ISBN 978-1-284-04832-2 (pbk.)
 I. Boswell, Carol, author. II. Title.
 [DNLM: 1. Education, Nursing—methods. 2. Teaching—methods. 3. Evidence-Based Nursing—methods. WY 105]
 RT73
 610.73076--dc23
                          2014036941
6048

Printed in the United States of America
18 17 16 15 14 10 9 8 7 6 5 4 3 2 1

Contents

Preface

Evidence-based practice came upon the healthcare scene over 30 years ago. Although it is only within the last 10 to 15 years that evidence-based practice has gained in respect and importance, it has now reached a point of being expected for each and every health skill utilized. Members of the health team and public consumers understand the importance of utilizing healthcare skills and knowledge that are supported by strong evidence. Nursing schools have readily embraced the idea that all components of the program of study must reflect the value and use of evidence-based practice for the novice and expert nurse. If indeed the idea is that all aspects of healthcare provision must reflect evidence-based practice, then of necessity, nursing education should embrace the same level of expertise: evidence-based teaching.

This text assimilates the ideas found within evidence-based practice as it endeavors to confront the initiative of evidence-based teaching. Education is paramount for the development of qualified, competent healthcare providers. The notion that education would not rise to the challenge of confirming the delivery of educational material through the use of evidence-supported principles is unthinkable. The educational field has accepted the idea that everyone "teaches as they were taught." We must move beyond this idea to utilizing teaching techniques and methodologies that are grounded in evidence. Technological advancements, knowledgeable consumers of education, and well-informed clients of health care demand that nursing education keep pace and address our ever-changing world.

Each chapter in this text looks at different aspects of the educational process in light of the evidence. The initial six chapters develop a foundation on which to launch evidence-based teaching. Within these chapters, theories, legal aspects, role development, civility, and definitions are provided for application to the educational environment. Chapter 5 is new to this edition and addresses the thoughts and concerns related to social media and incivility. For each area, the evidence that is currently available is utilized. The next three chapters directly look at the nursing educational settings—classroom, online, and clinical. Within each of these chapters, the evidence for different delivery methodologies is provided. Chapters 10 and 11 round out the discussion of nursing education by considering program evaluation and competency/certification. The final chapter challenges each of us to move evidence-based teaching into the next century. This chapter provides the challenge for every nursing faculty member to consider and embrace.

The contributors to this text are experts in the world of nursing education. It has been a privilege and honor to collaborate with each of them as we take this journey toward evidence-based teaching. It is our resolution and declaration that you will accept the challenge of evidence-based teaching and be invigorated by the potential for advancing the field of nursing education. Though evidence for the different aspects of the educational process is available, research evidence is insufficient. Thus, the other challenge that emerges from this text is the ultimatum that nursing educational research needs to be conducted to confirm or refute the different aspects of the educational process.

Sharon B. Cannon, EdD, RN, ANEF
Texas Tech University Health Sciences Center, School of Nursing
Odessa, Texas

Carol Boswell, EdD, RN, CNE, ANEF
Texas Tech University Health Sciences Center, School of Nursing
Odessa, Texas

Acknowledgments

As opportunities become available and challenges are identified, pathways are found that allow each of us to stretch and grow. We are provided the destiny to step out and look at our environment from different viewpoints. Following the energies put toward evidence-based practice aspects, the natural progression was to apply those same ideas and concepts to the field of nursing education. We would like to take this opportunity to communicate our appreciation to our extraordinary and visionary colleagues who took this trip with us to clarify and refine the idea of evidence-based teaching. In addition to our students who challenge us to be visionary, timely, and real, we express our heartfelt appreciation for the opportunity to begin a journey and to strive for excellence.

Dr. Sharon Cannon and Dr. Carol Boswell

When I started as a young nurse, I never in my wildest dreams imagined that I would or could be where I am today. My parents, Babe and Laurine Cannon, provided the motivation and support for me to continue my education and most of all gave me a love for learning. My brother, Gene Cannon, and his wife, Cathie Cannon, have been and continue to be a source and comfort over the years and, without even being aware, continue to carry on my parents' legacy for education. In addition, my son, Ryan Ganey, and my daughter, Lynn Tischner, and her husband, Joe Tischner, always keep me looking to the future and are always there with encouragement and love. My beautiful grandchildren, Kelly Tischner and Andrew, Shelby, and Shannon Ganey, are the bright stars that will shine for me in the years to come.

My professional life has been blessed by mentors who helped to guide me to seek opportunities that would challenge me and stretch my skills and abilities far beyond the goals I had established. Dr. Shirley Martin and Dr. Martha Welch may not have any idea of the impact they have had on my nursing career. Finally, one mentor, colleague, and friend—Dr. Carol Boswell—is a treasure. She keeps me on the "straight and narrow" and is the sister of my dreams in so many ways. With all of that in mind, I wish for each of you to have the support, love, and encouragement that I have had bestowed upon me in my life. May you seek the evidence and let it take you to newer heights to fulfill your dreams.

Dr. Sharon Cannon

Time is a critical aspect of our lives. The educational community is impacted by it because the majority of our students consider their schedules to be "too full." As a result, every encounter with students needs to be carefully planned and implemented. Having the best methods for providing education allows us to meet the needs of our customers. This text endeavors to provide that "best" evidence to use in the educational environment.

As a parent, the annoyance of hearing the incessant question "WHY?" has resulted in my steadfastness to tackle the "why" query prior to it being solicited, whenever achievable. We all want to appreciate the underlying principle for why we are doing things. As an educator, the enthusiasm to differentiate and acknowledge the rationale and justifications for our teaching methods has led me down this avenue to evidence-based teaching. So to my children (Michael Boswell, Casey Boswell, Jeremy Boswell, and Stephanie Boswell) and my grandchildren (Matthew Boswell, Kobe Boswell, Kayia Howard, and Caleb Boswell), keep stimulating me to respond to the questions of, why are responsibilities required, what is the motivation for taking a path, and where do we go from here? To my husband (Marc E. Boswell) and my mother (Wanda Miller), thank you for your continuing support as I explore new projects and grapple for greater heights. To the nursing students who are engaged and energized about learning, my sincere gratitude makes me form my assignments to better serve you as you strive for excellence in nursing care and to broaden your education. Finally, my friend (Dr. Sharon Cannon) allows me abundant opportunities to brainstorm about innovative and resourceful ideas. Thank you for encouraging me to strive for the stars and hold fast to innovative thoughts. Without the encouragement and determination of my family, friends, and students, I would not be able to endure the challenges of the educational and nursing communities while embracing the authenticity of what is important and indispensable within a person's being.

Dr. Carol Boswell

Contributors

Patricia Allen, EdD, RN, CNE, ANEF, FAAN
Professor and Director, Center for Innovation in Nursing Education
Texas Tech University Health Sciences Center
Lubbock, TX

Linda Caputi, EdD, RN, CNE, ANEF
Professor Emeritus
College of DuPage
Glen Ellyn, IL

Darlene Del Prato, PhD, RN
Professor and Director of Nursing
New England Institute of Technology
East Greenwich, RI

Melinda Mitchell Jones, MSN, JD, RN
Department Chair for Non-Traditional Undergraduate Studies
Associate Professor
Texas Tech University Health Sciences Center
Lubbock, TX

Joyce M. Miller, DNP, RN, WNHP-BC, FNP-BC
Associate Professor
School of Nursing
Texas Tech University Health Sciences Center
Odessa, TX

Beth C. Phillips, MSN, RN, CNE
Assistant Professor
Duke University School of Nursing
Durham, NC

Theresa M. "Terry" Valiga, EdD, RN, CNE, ANEF, FAAN
Director, Institute for Educational Excellence
Clinical Professor
School of Nursing
Duke University
Durham, NC

Chapter 1

Overview of Evidence-Based Practice

Carol Boswell and Sharon Cannon

At the conclusion of this chapter, the learner will be able to:

1. Discuss the differences between evidence-based practice and evidence-based teaching.
2. Identify the evolution of evidence-based practice within health care.
3. Explain key aspects of critical thinking.
4. State the specific steps involved in evidence-based teaching.
5. List the steps needed to conduct a literature review to find evidence related to a teaching/learning topic.

KEY TERMS

- Critical thinking
- Evidence-based practice
- Evidence-based teaching
- PSCOT format

INTRODUCTION

As nursing continues its migration toward professionalism and advancement of the profession, the idea of scholarship becomes increasingly important. The American Association of Colleges of Nursing (AACN) (1999) states that "scholarship in nursing can be defined as those activities that systematically advance the teaching, research, and practice of nursing through rigorous inquiry that (1) is significant to the profession,

(2) is creative, (3) can be documented, (4) can be replicated or elaborated, and (5) can be peer-reviewed through various methods" (para. 5). With the confirmation of **evidence-based practice** (EBP) as a foundational aspect within nursing, the idea of methodically and analytically strengthening the fundamental principles while advancing scholarship to move EBP toward **evidence-based teaching** (EBT) is judicious and appropriate. According to Shultz (2009), nursing education requires work by all the members involved in the provision of the educational experience. This process takes time and energy as the questioning and evaluation of the educational experiences occur. Careful steps and strategies for assimilating the multiplexity of the teaching/learning process require that each of us stay vigilant in asking the right questions. The other side of the coin requires that nursing faculty members stay committed to the lifelong pursuit of knowledge. Kuehn (2010) notes that the Institute of Medicine (IOM) demands that the nursing workforce become a dedicated member at the decision table for health care, which in turn demands that nursing education take on the challenge of preparing the next generation to be successful in this expanded role. While it is imperative that the health care delivered to patients be based on the best evidence, teaching processes used to educate nurses must also be based on best practices.

The healthcare community has embraced, and even has come to expect, EBP. The different activities that are assumed within healthcare delivery are expected to be based upon the best evidence that is available. Can we expect anything less when we move into the area of teaching/learning? Wexler (n.d.) makes an interesting and true statement: "All the rhetoric about passionate teaching, and whether professors care about or value teaching, is meaningless if they are bad or ineffective teachers" (para. 4). Moving away from the idea that anyone can teach and toward the concept that effective and productive teaching must be founded on sound, defensible strategies becomes the desired outcome. No longer can academia accept mediocre teaching. Our overarching goal must be, "Effective teaching results in successful learning." The nursing education community must ensure that the strategies and practices incorporated into the classroom and the learning environment are firmly founded on the best evidence as to what improves the acquisition of knowledge.

Boyer (1990) stated that "we believe the time has come to move beyond the tired old 'teaching versus research' debate and give the familiar and honorable term 'scholarship' a broader, more capacious meaning, one that brings legitimacy to the full scope of academic work" (p. 16). The handiwork of the scholar requires each of us to step back from only encouraging an individual's exploration and move toward networking, constructing connections between theory and practice, and communicating knowledge efficiently to students and others. The process of bringing each of the multiple threads together to form a beautiful tapestry of teaching and learning necessitates the scholar to organize and conceptualize the components based upon the best evidence available. It requires willingness to try new ideas and struggle with the process while keeping an eye on the goal of improving the educational process. Shultz (2009) summarizes the ideas in the statement: "Every faculty member can contribute to the development of the science of nursing education by searching for evidence to support the teaching strategies and evaluation methods to be used in their courses and talking with colleagues about gaps in our knowledge when such evidence is not found" (p. 302). Each and every one of us must accept the responsibility to strive for innovative avenues to engage the student and transfer the knowledge needed to result in competent healthcare providers. In addition to seeing what is currently available in the evidence, we must validate the evidence through research and quality improvement efforts.

HISTORICAL PERSPECTIVES

The nursing process has been at the foundation of nursing practice for well over three decades. Beyea and Slattery (2013) confirm the idea that EBP provides the foundation for clinicians and patients to use for the engagement of shared decision making as it relates to individualized healthcare management. The profession of nursing has begun to look beyond this foundation toward knowledge based upon a firm underpinning of evidence. Malloch and Porter-O'Grady (2009) termed this movement as *disciplined clinical inquiry*. Disciplined clinical inquiry provided nurses with alternatives that allowed learning and engagement with the knowledge available, as it applied to nontraditional settings. The concept of disciplined clinical inquiry evolved into the current term **critical thinking**. As the profession was challenged to base the provision of care on sound knowledge supported by evidence, the inspiration for EBP was born.

EBP was first acknowledged in the 1970s. It was during this time period that different people from different areas realized that the practice of health care needed to be established on facts, rather than just what had been done for years. Dr. Archie Cochrane, a British physician, gained the distinction of being the pioneer and inspiration for the evidence-based medicine movement. As a result of his groundbreaking work in 1972, the

UK Cochrane Centre in Oxford, England, was established in 1992. This effort led to The Cochrane Collaboration being recognized in 1993. The premise for The Cochrane Collaboration was to advance healthcare decision making through the use of systematic reviews concerning the outcome of evidence from healthcare interventions. The Cochrane Collaboration and Centre are international, not-for-profit, independent organizations that are committed to ensuring that state-of-the-art, accurate information concerning the outcomes of healthcare interventions is accessible by the global community.

Following in the footsteps provided by Dr. Cochrane, several nursing leaders transformed the principles to address the profession of nursing. Beyea and Slattery (2013) cite the early efforts of the Western Interstate Commission on Higher Education, the Conduct and Utilization of Research in Nursing, and the Nursing Child Assessment Satellite Training Program. The initial efforts related to EBP were directed toward accessing and the assessment of research findings.

Evidence-based nursing practice models are numerous. Each of the models was formulated to address a key aspect within the nursing practice. The Stetler model was one of the initial prototypes to be established. It was formulated in 1976 as a research utilization model. This version of EBP was initiated as a practitioner-oriented model with a concentration on critical thinking and individual use of the findings. Another well-known international collaboration within EBP and nursing is the Joanna Briggs Institute. This institute was established in 1996 for use by nurses, medical and allied health researchers, clinicians, academicians, and quality managers. The Joanna Briggs Institute is utilized in over 40 countries and on every continent. The centralized impetus for this institute is to establish the usefulness, suitability, meaningfulness, and practicability related to health routine, tradition, and healthcare delivery approaches. A third EBP model, developed in 1999, is the Rosswurm–Larrabee model. This model is based upon the use of theoretical and research literature. It is used to guide practitioners toward the effective utilization of EBP.

In the last 10 years, several nursing EBP models have been showcased to reflect the practical nature of EBP. These initial models are viewed as scholarly in nature. The Iowa Model was established to assist the clinician at the bedside in the acute care setting to utilize a practical EBP organizational model. Within this model, triggers are used to assist the bedside nurse to take the steps to carefully consider the clinical decision-making process as he or she delivers EBP care. The Advancing Research and Clinical Practice Through Close Collaboration (ARCC) model was established to help advance practice nurses to implement EBP successfully. With the ARCC model, the idea of establishing a network of clinicians who are willing to disseminate best evidence and to function as champions for EBP was the foundational support for this model. Another EBP model to consider is called the ACESTAR model. This model originates from the idea of knowledge transformation. It attempts to comprehend the sequences, essence, and characteristics of knowledge. These models are a few of the many EBP models that can be found and used in the clinical provision of health care; furthermore, new models are being developed to address key aspects and applications of EBP.

Though these models are developing and escalating, evidence-based teaching (EBT) models are not found. The concepts and ideas considered in relation to EBT are noted within the literature, but actual models of how to implement EBT are not found. It appears that the accepted attitude leans toward the idea that the models for EBP are enough. With the idea that teaching and learning strategies should be established based on valid and reliable evidence, the application of evidence-based principles directly related to teaching becomes increasingly important. According to Emerson and Records (2008), "The practice of nursing education is that which we do, including teaching didactic and clinical courses, advising students, and designing curricula, as well as our programs of study and the environments in which they are conducted" (p. 359). The teaching/learning environment includes the entire community that comes into play within the teaching/learning experience. The process of EBT must address all of the facets that impact the educational process (**Figure 1–1**). Danielson (2008) presents an important idea that "meaningful conversations about teaching and valid evaluation of teaching must be grounded in a clear definition of practice—a framework for teaching" (para. 1). As we evolve the idea of EBT, a dialogue pertaining to the multifaceted aspects integrated into the acquisition of knowledge within the educational community, will be initiated and followed.

STEPS OF EBP WITH APPLICATION TO EBT

Evidence-based *practice* has been growing in popularity and functionality for many years. As we begin to move this concept into the area of evidence-based *teaching*, several aspects need to be carefully considered. Felver et al. (2010) list several key principles that can help guide the EBT process. For EBT and EBP to be effective, faculty members must embrace and utilize best practices both in teaching and clinical practice. Only when faculty members demonstrate effective decision making and utilization of best

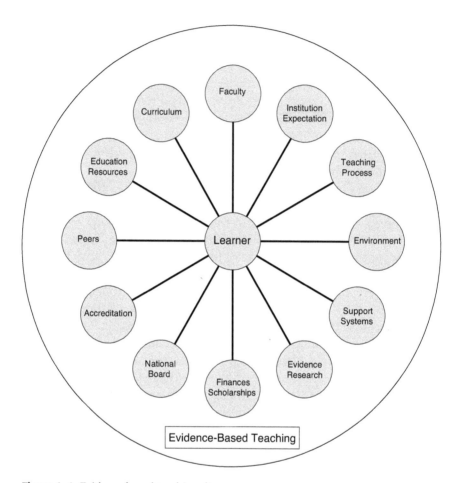

Figure 1–1 Evidence-based teaching diagram

practice can students truly comprehend the usefulness and efficiency of the process.

The definitions of EBP are numerous, so when you then consider EBT, even more problems arise. Is the definition of EBT different from that of EBP? If so, then how? Is finding a unique definition for EBT just splitting hairs? How is EBT different from EBP? In addition to the definition, the process of performing EBT also has unique characteristics that move it beyond the idea of EBP. Whereas EBP works within the clinical realm, EBT resides within a multiplicity of settings, which can include the clinical realm. Teaching is part of the work within the clinical space domain, but it does not take place only within that sphere. Teaching takes many different directions. According to Emerson and Records (2008), "The ultimate imperative facing nursing today is the creation of a culture that values the practice of nursing education and expands evidence-based education through the design, testing, and refinement of education strategies from nursing and other disciplines" (p. 359). The concepts and practices embodied within EBP must be applied to the system of nursing education. The steps and definitions applied to the management of EBP must be tailored to meet the expectations and actions embodied within the delivery of nursing education.

As a person begins to look deeply into the topic of EBP, multiple definitions can be found. Mitchell (2013) characterizes EBP as an organizational, shared, and interdisciplinary effort that resides within the clinical decision-making arena. Care must be given to ensure that EBP and EBT remain a decision-making effort to improve care and that it does not become a cost determination tool. Mitchell (2013) warns that evidence can become a political tool, which can result in voice and power being removed from nursing practice and human care. Evidence must remain a foundation for improving care but not controlling care delivery.

These definitions somewhat address the same areas of concern, but each has a unique focus. According to Boswell and Cannon (2014), the constant characteristics that are found within the multiple definitions relate to the decision-making scheme, clinical application, provider expertise, and client contribution. **Table 1–1** lists several definitions of EBP along with their related characteristics to provide an overview of the challenge in trying to reach a common definition. Bastable (2014) adds one facet for EBT—commitment to the lifelong problem-solving process. This added dimension, which relates to teaching, augments the general aspects of evidence, decision making, patient preference, and clinician expertise that are found in most EBP definitions. The lifelong involvement by individuals in the learning process is key to the process. Only when EBP becomes a key and foundational aspect within our provision of nursing care and nursing education will the *nature* of the process become *natural*. Each of the nursing EBP models seems to have a focal point, such as academia advanced nursing practice, bedside nursing care, and so forth. The definition used for the model is then aimed at addressing the aspects prevailing within that practice arena. Since there is not a common definition for EBP, the likelihood that a universal definition for EBT exists is next to impossible. EBT is just beginning to gain acceptance and support. Prior to this time period, the focus has been, and continues to be, aimed at ensuring that healthcare providers begin to understand and embrace the concepts of EBP. As different groups become increasingly comfortable with the EBP

Table 1-1   Evidence-Based Practice Definitions

Source	Definition	Characteristics Noted
Melnyk & Fineout-Overholt, 2010	A process that permits healthcare providers to achieve the highest standard of care when managing the intricate needs of their patients and families	Quality of care Multifaceted
Rutledge & Grant, 2002	Treatment that assimilates the top scientific data with clinical proficiency, knowledge of pathophysiology, knowledge of psychosocial concerns, and the decision-making processes of the clients	Decision making Clinical focus Evidence Expertise Pathophysiology Psychosocial
Porter-O'Grady, 2010	The assimilation of the paramount research to evidence with clinical proficiency and with client requests	Clinical focus Evidence Expertise Client involvement
Magee, 2005	The meticulous, unambiguous, and prudent utilization of existing preeminent evidence in formulating decisions about the treatment of a particular patient	Decision making Evidence Client involvement
Pravikoff, Tanner, & Pierce, 2005	A methodical tactic of problem solving for healthcare providers exemplified by the employing of top data presently existing for clinical decision making to facilitate reliable and preeminent care to patients	Decision making Clinical focus Evidence Client involvement
Boswell & Cannon, 2014	A method of employing established evidence (research and quality improvement), decision making, and nursing proficiency to regulate the provision of holistic client care	Decision making Clinical focus Evidence Client involvement

foundation, attempts to understand distinctive aspects such as teaching can be explored.

Several definitions for the scholarship of teaching are available for consideration as a definition for EBT is contemplated. According to the AACN (1999), "The scholarship of teaching is conducted through application of knowledge of the discipline or specialty area in the teaching-learning process, the development of innovative teaching and evaluation methods, program development, learning outcome evaluations, and professional role modeling" (para. 12). Each of these areas is viewed as an important theme that must be conscientiously considered as we venture to address teaching as a distinctive coordination of key hallmarks of excellence. The National League for Nursing (NLN) has not communicated a definition for EBT but has developed an Excellence in Nursing Education Model that depicts the different aspects central to the delivery of effective nursing education. The NLN took on the challenge of determining hallmarks of education and establishing academia as a unique discipline within the profession of nursing. This model can be viewed at the NLN website (www.nln.org/excellence/model/index.htm). The model covers the areas of student-centered, interactive, innovative programs and curricula; recognition of expertise; clear program standards and hallmarks that raise expectations; well-prepared faculty; qualified students; well-prepared educational administrators; evidence-based program and teaching/evaluation methods; and adequate, quality resources. For each area, the model further delineates multiple aspects to provide insight into the different foci and facets that reflect the content within those areas.

Definitions for EBT are few in number. Emerson and Records (2008) define EBT practice in nursing as "the validation, generation, application, and perpetuation of those methods that facilitate the preparation of skilled and thoughtful nurses who function in a constantly evolving, global health care environment" (p. 361). It is interesting that within this definition the global aspect of health care is incorporated. Emerson and Records (2008) consider the integration of the responsibility of teaching with the scrutinization within teaching that embraces all of the roles and competencies from administrator to advisor to faculty. This definition reflects the idea that all aspects within the practice and management of the educational environment and process must be embedded in EBT.

Appling, Naumann, and Berk (2001) set forth the requirements subsumed within EBT as "the comprehensive measurement and evaluation of faculty teaching activities, with tools that capture multiple sources of evidence key to the accurate and complete measurement of teaching outcome" (p. 247). Within this definition, the focus of the process appears to be on the faculty and the classroom environment. Other aspects inherent in the academic environment and teaching routine are not evident in this definition. The evidence is intended for confronting the challenges faced within the classroom and learning ecosystem.

As each of these definitions for EBP and EBT is carefully considered and conceptualized, a working definition to be used within this text can be developed. For this text, EBT is a dynamic, holistic system using educational principles validated by evidence to support, maintain, and promote a new level of knowledge for a learner in a variety of settings. The process is viewed within a systems approach, and a system is considered to be a collection of organized, related, and/or mutually dependent components coming together to make a whole that is complex and multifaceted (*Webster's II New College Dictionary*, 1999). Each of the many different components within the EBT diagram (Figure 1–1) supports, interacts, and challenges the other components within the model. The learner is viewed as the center of the process within EBT. Each and every educational session and resource is intended to ensure that the learner is effectively placed in a position to gain the utmost knowledge from the educational environment. Though the individual learner is the focal point of the process, that center can also be represented by a cohort of learners.

The items within the diagram that network with and have effects on the learner during the educational process are faculty, institutional expectations, teaching process, environment, support systems, evidence research, finances/scholarship, national board, accreditation, peers, education resources, and curriculum. When considering each of these items, faculty, curriculum, and peers are familiar aspects within the educational community. Institutional expectations can be viewed as the mission, philosophy, goals, strategic plan, and/or objectives established by the university or school. The aspects subsumed within the teaching processes are those strategies utilized within the educational process to deliver information. Another facet that affects the learner is the environment. The learning environment is a key feature that sets the stage for learning to occur. When the learning environment is stressful, disorganized, or threatening, the learner's ability to assimilate the information is compromised and impeded. Support systems are identified as another feature influencing the learner. Within this diagram, the support systems can include family, consulting services, health services, and other resources provided by the institution, community, or family for the students. On the other side of the diagram, the education resources are those measures such as tutoring services, testing departments, computer services, and so forth that are provided to aid in the delivery of instruction and the facilitation of the instructional process. An additional aspect that should impact the learner is the evidence supported by educational research. Each of these aspects should be founded on supporting evidence related to the feature. One more facet that has a large impact on the learner is the financial cost of acquiring an education. Within this aspect, the idea of scholarships, loans, and grants can play a part, as these different financial resources are used to support the learner's educational experience. The final two aspects are similar but occur at different levels. Accreditation concerns are frequently at the federal level and may be impacted by multiple agencies. National and state boards impact the learning process for several disciplines, nursing being just one.

Though each of these aspects has varying effects on the educational experience, each is viewed as important. Some of the aspects are more readily encountered by the learner, such as the faculty, teaching process, finances, peers, educational resources, and curriculum. Other aspects within the groups are of critical importance but may remain more in the background rather than being readily encountered during the day-to-day practice of the educational process. The holistic educational approach must address all of the aspects that impact the learner, such as peer support, curriculum, accreditation rules, and so forth. This approach is marked by continuous opportunities to evolve through the discovery and application of innovative evidence related to the teaching/learning process. The application of EBT to nursing is a multifaceted process that incorporates key components related to effective methodologies and roles to meet the needs of an ever-changing healthcare environment.

As a definition for EBT is resolved, the process then moves to the activities that are paramount to the successful management of the endeavor. **Figure 1–2** presents a visual depiction of the sequence embedded in the evolution of the process. The posing of the question is the crucial first step in initiating an investigation into the evidence surrounding the educational process. The wording of the question must be clear and concise. By taking care to ensure that the question is effectively developed, the management of the literature review becomes increasingly more attainable. A well-developed question provides the keywords and concepts imperative for identifying and narrowing the selection of the articles. By ascertaining the articles through the literature search driven by the question, the evidence that supports the teaching environment can be discovered. The reviewing of these articles allows for the determination of EBT strategies. Many aspects—such as student values/preferences, student characteristics, academic boundaries, systematic evaluations, and financial/resource boundaries—come to bear on the teaching strategies. Within the synthesis of the evidence, each of these aspects along with other aspects must be carefully and systematically considered as the analysis of the evidence is completed. The evidence used to address the questions may come from faculty or course evaluations.

Within the process of EBP, questions are presented in the PICOT format (**Table 1–2**). The PICOT format structures the question by looking at:

P = Population
I = Intervention(s)

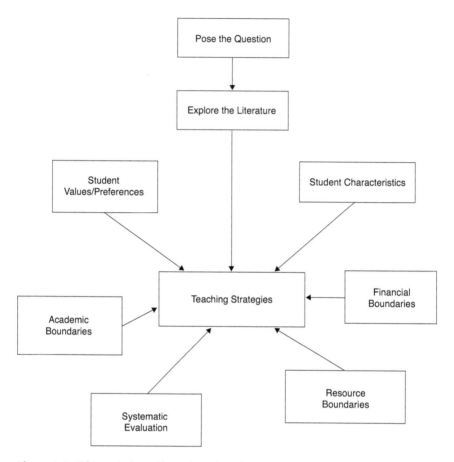

Figure 1-2 Schematic for evidence-based teaching

C = Comparison(s)
O = Outcome(s)
T = Time

By carefully examining each of these aspects, clarity and precision within the question are substantiated. Emerson and Records (2008) suggest the use of the STCO format for EBT questions. The STCO format includes:

S = Student
T = Teaching technique
C = Comparison
O = Outcome

Table 1-2 Comparison of Evidence-Based Practice and Evidence-Based Teaching

Evidence-Based Practice	Evidence-Based Teaching
Pose the clinical question using the PICOT format: P (population), I (intervention), C (comparison), O (outcome), T (time).	Pose the education question using the PSCOT format: P (population), S (strategy), C (comparison), O (outcome), T (time).
Explore the evidence available to determine the best practice using a critical appraisal approach.	Explore the evidence available to determine the best practice using a critical appraisal approach.
Consider individual clinical expertise and client preferences/values as interventions are deliberated.	Integrate teaching expertise with the students' characteristics, preferences, and values in the teaching/learning environment as solutions and ideas are formulated.
Instigate clinical changes as needed within the parameters of the resources and stakeholders.	Initiate educational modifications as needed within the academic, financial, and resource boundaries.
Appraise the change in regard to patient satisfaction, financial considerations, institutional considerations, and professional considerations.	Consider the changes based on key performance criteria identified with the systematic evaluation for the academic setting.

Source: Adapted from Emerson, R. J., & Records, K. (2008). Today's challenge, tomorrow's excellence: The practice of evidence-based education. *Journal of Nursing Education, 47*(8), 359–370.

Although this format places focus on the educational aspects, it limits the population to students only. The educational process is much more than just the students. Many aspects within the educational process need to be founded upon evidence. Modifying the PICOT format to embrace the educational community results in increased continuity within the process of confirming evidence to support best practices. As a result, the use of the **PSCOT format** can address the educational process. PSCOT can be described as follows:

P = Population
S = Strategy
C = Comparison
O = Outcome
T = Time period

As you can see, the "P" continues to be for the population. The population within the educational process can be directed toward students, administrators, faculty, alumni, candidates, preceptors, coaches, and many other groups of individuals who are involved in the educational process. The population can be either the individual or the cohort. Care needs to be given to understanding that within the academic arena, the student body or cohort may be viewed as the population instead of the individual student. As the population is designated, care must be given to narrowing the focus of the designation to allow for a clearer identification of the associates to be investigated. The narrowing of the population can be accomplished by carefully considering such items as the educational level, race/ethnicity, gender, and/or age of the cohort and/or individual. The "S" represents the educational strategy. Educational strategies are any aspect within the educational environment that comes into play for advancing the success of the learning process. Any intervention (strategy) that can affect the population must be carefully investigated to ensure that the overriding evidence is used to manage the learning environment for the betterment of the educational process. The "C" within the format mirrors the "C" within the EBP format. The incorporation of a comparison of educational strategies provides an evaluation of the different avenues for advancing the learning environment. Vigilantly looking at the different strategies within the context of the specific EBT question allows for determination of any divergence between the strategies. The "O" within the format also parallels the inclusion of outcome as used in the EBP format. As the EBT and EBP questions are posed, the identification of the expected outcomes allows the individual to clarify what is believed about the populations and the strategies being considered. The final aspect, the "T," within the question is the incorporation of the time period when applicable. Each and every question does not require the inclusion of the comparison nor a time setting, but it is helpful to clarify the question when used. When all five aspects can be used, locating appropriate articles and evidence becomes easier. The use of all five provides increased clarification for use in discovering the evidence to be considered.

Let's look at some examples of PSCOT questions to see how the different aspects come into play in an EBT setting.

Example 1:

P = first-semester students
S = use of care maps
C = use of care plans
O = improved pathology comprehension
T = (none used)

By looking at these different aspects, the question can be stated as: Do first-semester students who use care maps instead of care plans demonstrate an improved knowledge of the pathological aspect? Another example for consideration is to see how the posing of the question directs the entire EBT process.

Example 2:

P = students in the clinical setting
S = simulation experiences
C = experiences with actual clients
O = improved perception of clinical principles
T = (none used)

As these aspects are composed into a question format, the resulting question emerges: Do students who use simulation experiences in place of clinical experiences with actual clients exhibit improved knowledge of clinical principles within the clinical setting?

A third example of the use of the PSCOT format to determine the best practices available in the learning environment is as follows.

Example 3:

P = students between the ages of 18 and 45
S = delivery of course materials via an online hybrid course-delivery method
C = delivery of course materials via face-to-face active participation course-delivery method
O = increased comprehension of course material
T = (none used)

Taking these components to direct the inquiry into the investigation of the evidence would result in the question: Do students between the ages of 18 and 45 have increased comprehension of course material when the material is delivered by an online hybrid method in comparison to a face-to-face active participation format? A final example of the development of EBT questions is as follows.

Example 4:

P = novice faculty
S = use of designated mentors
C = use of scheduled faculty development sessions
O = increased ease in managing the role
T = following the first year of practice

When using these concepts to formulate a question to investigate, the question could be worded as: Do novice faculty members who have a designated mentor compared to the use of scheduled faculty development sessions during the first year of working as a faculty member have increased ease in performing the faculty role?

Once the question has been determined, the process of EBT continues with the investigation into the evidence (Table 1–2). The exploring of the evidence results from the key concepts and facets identified within the question. Each of the different pieces of the puzzle is used to distinguish the strategic articles and data that can be used to support and/or negate the educational strategy under scrutiny. The discovery and analysis of the articles and data can take many different forms but must address the gaps and/or consistencies within the information available in relation to the teaching strategy.

As the articles and data are summarized to provide a clear and concise picture of the evidence that is accessible related to the topic, the process of EBT necessitates that the students' characteristics, preferences, and values be considered at this point. Though EBT and EBP utilize the evidence as the foundation for practice, the characteristics, preferences, and values of the participants must also be considered as plans for the next phases of the process are considered. Damron-Rodriguez (2008) acknowledged three stages within the "knowledge transfer framework," saying that "knowledge is created and distilled, then it is diffused and disseminated, and finally it is adopted, implemented, and institutionalized" (p. 41). The knowledge transfer framework is supported and utilized by the Agency for Healthcare Research and Quality (AHRQ). Evidence is critical but must be balanced by the individualization of the process for the unique setting in which the teaching strategy is to be used.

After carefully composing the question, investigating the evidence, and considering the uniqueness of the participants, the process of EBT challenges the members involved to integrate academic, financial, and resource boundaries into the plan for utilization of best practices. As opportunities to use the optimum teaching strategy in an educational setting are determined, each of these facets (students, academic environment, finances, and resources) must be conscientiously considered and integrated to ensure that the final outcome is effective. Within the educational environment, it is ill advised to plan changes without considering the financial boundaries, resource availability, student population, and academic environment. Each educational institution is unique and must be considered within the plans to incorporate changes in the learning process based upon the evidence.

The final aspect within EBT is the evaluation of the process. For each question and consideration, key performance criteria must be used to determine if the process and the changes are facilitating the learning within a particular environment. The PSCOT has outcomes listed. These outcomes reflect performance criteria that can be used to further advance the evidence related to the educational strategy under consideration. According to Adams and Valiga (2009), excellence in teaching is the crux of the process by which we understand what it is that we see and understand, although the process of defining the term *excellence* is convoluted and very difficult. Coming to an understanding of how to effectively apply EBP principles to the teaching/learning environment requires succinct and straightforward thinking by leaders in the educational community. Adams and Valiga (2009) further explain that to embrace EBP within teaching, the educational community must integrate high standards for everyone involved in the learning community. Only when each individual accepts the responsibility for these standards, regardless of the challenges or demands to diminish them, can the learning environment obtain the "best practices" within the process of education. Just like nurses had to step up to the plate and accept the principles of EBP, nursing educators must delve into the abyss to organize and establish the concepts and measures imperative for EBT. The advancement of the nursing educational environment requires that each member accept the responsibility of holding fast to high standards. A key approach that will allow the establishment and maintenance of high standards is the confirmation of the teaching/learning aspects through sound and effective evidence.

CRITICAL THINKING

When discussing EBP and EBT definitions and steps, one essential requirement is consideration of the connection of critical thinking to EBP and EBT. Achieving positive patient outcomes requires faculty who think critically about how and what they teach and students who can take content and apply it to practice through critical thinking. Allen (2013) requires nurse educators to establish a process for staying in step and advancing quality care within the fast-paced, ever-changing practice environment. Before going further, perhaps an understanding of critical thinking is necessary.

Paul, Elder, and Bartell (1997) indicate that the origin of critical thinking began 2500 years ago in the time of Socrates and has gained momentum over the years. In 2005, Fitzpatrick suggested nursing, as a discipline, was influenced by David Schron in his classic 1983 work. Ard (2009) also suggested that critical thinking isn't new, and since the 1990s, many publications about critical thinking have emerged. Multiple organizations, such as the AACN, the NLN, and even the IOM, have emphasized the importance of the teaching and application of critical thinking in the provision of patient care. As a result, the subject of critical thinking is a major topic, and "critical thinking" has been listed as a common buzzword in education and practice.

The current emphasis surrounding critical thinking has generated two major controversies related to critical thinking. The first controversy centers on the definition of critical thinking. Thompson (2009), Webber (2008), and Birx (2006) all suggest there is no common standard definition of critical thinking in nursing. The lack of a clear definition leads one to question: If we don't know what it is, then how can we do it? If critical thinking is essential to providing nursing care, how can we translate it into practice? It is beyond the scope of this text to offer all aspects and definitions of critical thinking, but a review of several definitions will provide insight, terms, and an applicable definition for use in EBT.

In 1987, Ennis defined critical thinking as logical and realistic thoughtful judgments that are directed toward clarifying what is true and what is false. Birx (2006) suggests that Paul and Nosich's 1991 definition is more commonly accepted: "Critical thinking is the intellectually disciplined process of actively and skillfully conceptualizing, applying, analyzing, synthesizing, and evaluating information gathered from or generated by observation, experience, reflecting, reasoning, or communication, as a guide to belief or action" (p. 4, p. 300). Paul (2004) suggests that critical thinking is an art that involves analyzing and assessing thinking to get to a better process of thinking.

Terms often associated with critical thinking in nursing include the nursing process, problem solving, rational approach, decision making, reflection, concept mapping, and evidence such as scientific research. The terms have relevance to defining critical thinking. For the purpose of this text, critical thinking will be defined as the art of analyzing and applying information gathered to make decisions regarding nursing care.

The second controversy involves whether or not critical thinking can be taught. Paul (2004) states that studies indicate faculty do not understand the concept of critical thinking. In addition, faculty teach content such as math or biology but not mathematical or biological thinking. At an AACN business meeting in 2009, Bain (2009) indicated that Dewey suggested people don't learn by experience but rather by thinking about experience. Heaslip (2008) goes further to say that a professional nurse must think like a nurse, which is different from the perspective of a doctor or other health professionals concerning how the patient is viewed and the problems associated with providing nursing care. Thus, nurses reason differently than other healthcare providers. Nursing faculty need to teach nursing thinking. Perhaps an example of a clinical learning situation might provide insight into how you would approach critical thinking. Suppose a fourth-semester senior approaches you and says, "My patient is complaining of pain in her arm where I just started an IV. I don't think I hurt her. What should I do?" How would you teach the student to critically think about the situation? Would you tell her what to do? Would you just take care of the problem and then discuss what you did and why? Is your approach a way to teach nursing thinking?

ASSESSING SOURCES OF EVIDENCE-BASED TEACHING

According to Oermann (2009), "Without research and other types of evidence, decisions are often made by the most vocal faculty members, for expediency, or in response to a pressing need" (p. 64). It is unfortunate that nursing education bows to the most vocal faculty members rather than seeking and utilizing an EBT approach. As state-of-the-art teaching/learning strategies become increasingly accepted and expected, the need to access the literature to find the current data becomes of principal importance.

Nursing faculty members must ensure that they are information literate. *Information literacy* is defined by the American Library Association (2006) as "a set of abilities requiring individuals to recognize when information is needed and have the ability to locate, evaluate, and use effectively the needed information" ("What Is Information Literacy," bullet 1). Two key databases that can be used are the Cumulative Index to Nursing and Allied Health Literature (CINAHL; the database of nursing and allied health literature) and PubMed (the National Library of Medicine's bibliographic database). Both of these databases index any published studies related to nursing education. Since EBT is a new area, a further investigation into the educational databases of Education Resources Information Center (ERIC), PsycINFO, and other databases specific to any question posed should be conducted. According to Salmond (2013), effective sources for identifying systematic reviews include the Database of Abstracts of Reviews of Effectiveness (DARE) (www.crd.york.ac.uk/CRDWeb/), The Cochrane Library (www.thecochranelibrary.com), The Campbell Collaboration (www.campbellcollaboration.org), Joanna Briggs Institute for Nursing and Midwifery (www.joannabriggs.edu.au), and several other databases. Systematic reviews are extremely helpful when conducting EBP projects because they can provide summaries, synopses, and syntheses of the key articles related to the topic of interest.

When selecting a database, it is helpful to understand that databases can follow one of two structures. Some databases are set up as bibliographic databases. This type of database provides information about the publication such as author, title, journal name, or publisher. Within a bibliographic database, abstracts and/or synopses are available for review. The second structure for databases is the full-text format. Within this format, the database allows access to the whole article. Thus, an individual can view the text, charts, graphs, references, and so forth.

Another important aspect within information literacy is to understand that databases have languages unique to their materials. A database will either have a specific controlled vocabulary (thesaurus) or use the MeSH headings. The MeSH headings are those headings established by the National Library of Medicine's thesaurus for MEDLINE. The MeSH headings can be accessed through www.nlm.nih.gov/mesh/meshhome.html. By using the MeSH headings to direct the literature review, the number of articles can be streamlined to a more manageable level. These headings and/or other keys derived from the PSCOT help to narrow the focus and get at the appropriate articles within the literature, thus saving time and energy by not accessing ineffective articles.

Only by using healthcare, educational, and other specific databases to query the literature can a full understanding of the current state of a teaching/learning strategy be understood. It is imperative when conducting a literature search that multiple databases be utilized to ensure that the subject has been addressed from multiple directions. By using this approach, the strength of the search is improved.

As articles and evidence are located within the databases and other sites, an evaluation of the information located must be tempered by the nurse educator's specific educational setting. The rating and scoring of evidence related to the applicability is of prime importance. Several organizations have evidence-rating mechanisms available to use within this process. The Cochrane Collaboration, AHRQ, and multiple textbooks provide examples of the different rating mechanisms. Though these rating mechanisms provide a means for evaluating the literature, each instructor must also gauge the literature within the specific context of the educational setting. The instructor must weigh the evidence to determine if it answers the PSCOT question posed and whether it is applicable to the specific setting. The application to a specific setting is unique to the setting. Each faculty member must accept the responsibility of determining if the evidence is relevant in a particular setting. As Oermann (2009) correctly states, "Our problem is not a lack of innovation in nursing education, but instead a lack of evidence about those innovations" (p. 74). Faculty members must take on the challenge of moving the preliminary studies into the next level, where fully developed studies in a larger controlled setting are conducted and disseminated. McCartney and Morin (2005) support this idea by stating that knowledge of the science of education is fundamental to improve the achievements of the individual both as a teacher and as a facilitator of learning for the students.

CRITICALLY APPRAISING KNOWLEDGE FOR TEACHING DECISION MAKING

According to Allen (2013), "The Carnegie Foundation report helped launch a change from viewing students as passive learners to seeing them as active participants" (p. 46). The move toward active learning in place of passive learning requires each member to be responsible for the decisions made. Finding and assessing sources of EBT leads faculty to ask: How do I decide what needs to be taught? Although there may be a paucity of literature on EBT, the current explosion of information, regardless of content for any nursing course, can be overwhelming. Faculty members have a prescribed amount of time to teach a course. As a result, faculty cohorts have to sift through mountains of material and decide what must be taught versus what would be nice or great to teach. Once again, critical thinking must occur, but this time the faculty members aren't teaching critical thinking; instead, they are applying it to the selection of content that will adequately supply knowledge about a given subject. Perhaps using the "see one, do one, teach one" phrase has application to the decisions faculty must make regarding the content to be taught. Through continuing nursing education and formal education programs, faculty members have seen other educators presenting content. Faculty can draw upon those experiences by thinking about how other educators assembled the content to be taught. Having seen items such as outlines, handouts, references, and all the multiple instructional aids, faculty can begin to see how content is selected, organized, and presented. Care must be taken to ensure that the educator is skilled. Another caution at this point is that always teaching the way you were taught may not be EBT.

Once again, faculty members need to turn to the literature. By using the methods for assessing courses as previously discussed, faculty members can then begin to cull through the content to be taught. Other aspects will play a major role in appraising knowledge for making decisions about what to teach. Program, curriculum, and evaluation design; teaching/learning strategies; licensure examinations; and accreditation are just a few considerations that will influence content and will be discussed elsewhere in this text.

SUMMARY THOUGHTS

Evidence-based practice (EBP) and evidence-based teaching (EBT) go hand in hand with critical thinking. Kuehn (2010) reports that nurses must take a greater role in the healthcare system, which requires that enhancements and modifications occur in nursing education. The emergence of EBP and now EBT has provided an educational environment that promotes critical thinking for both faculty and students. The steps of EBP and EBT are foundational to critical thinking about the sources of EBT and the selection of content to be presented. Jones (2013) categorized five items needed by nurses to be successful in implementing EBP—education, access to information, executive/administrative encouragement, mentors, and evidence-based decision making demonstrated by nursing leadership. These same five aspects are critical for nursing faculty members to embrace and demand when accepting and implementing EBT.

SUMMARY POINTS

1. Scholarship in EBT advances the development of the art and science of nursing education.
2. Several models of EBP have emerged since the 1970s.
3. Multiple definitions of EBP exist, but definitions for EBT are few in number.
4. EBT is defined as a dynamic, holistic system using educational principles validated by evidence to support, maintain, and promote a new level of knowledge for a learner in a variety of settings.
5. The steps of EBP have application to EBT.
6. To structure an EBT question, the format should include population, strategy, comparison, outcome, and time (PSCOT).
7. Critical thinking is much discussed, but two major controversies exist: What is critical thinking, and can it be taught?
8. Assessing sources of EBT requires faculty to be informed about literature databases.
9. Critically appraising knowledge for making decisions for teaching involves EBP, EBT, and critical thinking.

TIPS FOR NURSE EDUCATORS

1. Be knowledgeable about EBP and EBT in relation to definitions, steps, similarities, and differences.
2. Explore your own values regarding what critical thinking is and whether you believe it can be taught.
3. Connect with a librarian to obtain current, accurate sources for EBT.
4. Identify how you critically appraise content to be taught.
5. Begin to ask questions about your teaching strategies and educational activities

MULTIPLE CHOICE QUESTIONS

1. The initial EBP method resulted in the development of the:
   A. ARCC.
   B. **Cochrane Centre/Collaboration.**
   C. Joanne Briggs Institute.
   D. Rosswurm-Larrabee model.

   Rationale:
   As a result of Cochrane's pioneering work in 1972, the UK Cochrane Centre in Oxford, England, was established in 1992 and The Cochrane Collaboration was recognized in 1993. The premise for The Cochrane Collaboration is to advance healthcare decision making through the use of systematic reviews concerning the outcome evidence from healthcare interventions. The Cochrane Collaboration and Centre are international, not-for-profit, independent organizations that are committed to ensuring that state-of-the-art, accurate information concerning the outcomes of healthcare interventions is accessible by the global community.

2. One area *not* seen in the characteristics of EBP is:
   A. provider expertise.
   B. client contribution.
   C. **cost.**
   D. decision-making scheme.

   Rationale:
   According to Boswell and Cannon (2014), the constant characteristics that are found within the multiple definitions are the decision-making scheme, clinical application, provider expertise, and client contribution.

3. A systems approach is understood to include:
   A. **interrelated, interacting, and/or interdependent constituents.**
   B. unit-specific constituents.
   C. unilateral, reactive, and/or interdependent constituents.
   D. global, specific constituents.

   Rationale:
   The EBP process is viewed within a systems approach, and a system is a collection of organized, related, and/or mutually dependent components coming together to make a whole that is complex and multifaceted (*Webster's II New College Dictionary*, 1999).

4. The PSCOT format for developing an EBT statement represents:
   A. problem, situation, cost, outcome, time.
   B. problem, strategy, comparison, outcome, time.
   C. population, situation, comparison, outcome, target.
   D. **population, strategy, comparison, outcome, time.**

   Rationale:
   The "P" represents the population. The population within the educational process can be directed toward students, administrators, faculty, alumni, candidates, preceptors, coaches, and many other groups of individuals who are involved in the educational process. The "S" represents the educational strategy. Educational strategies are any aspect within the educational environment that comes into play for advancing the success of the learning process. The "C" within the format mirrors the "C" within the EBP format. The incorporation of a comparison of educational strategies provides an evaluation of the different avenues for advancing the learning environment. The "O" within the format also parallels the inclusion of outcome as used in the EBP format. The final aspect, the "T," is the incorporation of the time period when applicable.

5. In what manner is EBP different from EBT?
   A. **EBP focuses on the clinical setting.**
   B. EBT focuses on the educational setting.
   C. EBP includes only research results.
   D. EBT is no different than EBP.

   Rationale:
   Whereas EBP works within the clinical realm, EBT resides within a multiplicity of settings, which can include the clinical realm.

6. The two key databases for use during the literature review are:
   A. CINAHL and ERIC.
   B. **CINAHL and PubMed.**
   C. PubMed and ERIC.
   D. PubMed and Google.

   Rationale:
   The two key databases are CINAHL (the database of nursing and allied health literature) and PubMed (the National Library of Medicine's bibliographic database).

7. The critical step required to be successful in conducting EBT is:
   A. conducting a thorough literature review.
   B. always including a comparison and intervention.
   C. establishing the student preferences.
   D. **posing an effective question.**

   Rationale:
   Posing the question is the crucial first step for initiating an investigation into the evidence surrounding the educational process. The wording of the question must be clear and concise.

8. The initial step used when conducting a literature review is:
   A. pulling all of the articles that can be located on the topic.
   B. **selecting appropriate terms, such as MeSH terms, related to the topic.**
   C. omitting all articles older than 5 years.
   D. selecting only articles that are research based.

   Rationale:
   A database will either have a specific controlled vocabulary (thesaurus) or use the MeSH headings. The MeSH headings are those headings established by the National Library of Medicine's thesaurus for MEDLINE. By using the MeSH headings to direct the literature review, the number of articles can be streamlined to a more manageable level.

9. Critical thinking in nursing can be defined as:
   A. the science of teaching ways of thinking about nursing care.
   B. **the art of analyzing and applying information gathered to make decisions regarding nursing care.**
   C. a method of making decisions about nursing care.
   D. the systematic process of thinking that results in optimal patient outcomes.

Rationale:

For the purpose of this textbook, critical thinking is defined as the art of analyzing and applying information gathered to make decisions regarding nursing care.

10. The current knowledge explosion in health care:
    A. **impacts what is taught in nursing courses.**
    B. makes selection of course content easier.
    C. allows faculty to quickly decide content to be taught.
    D. is not a problem for determining course content.

Rationale:

As a result of the knowledge explosion, faculty members have to sift through mountains of material and decide what must be taught versus what would be nice or great to teach. Once again, critical thinking must occur, but this time the faculty members aren't teaching critical thinking; instead, they are applying it to the selection of content that will adequately supply knowledge about a given subject.

11. The center of the process within EBT is the:
    A. client.
    B. faculty member.
    C. **student.**
    D. school process.

Rationale:

The learner is viewed as the center of the process within EBT. It is within the learner that each and every educational session and resource intermingles to ensure that the learner is effectively placed in a position to gain the utmost knowledge from the educational environment.

12. A well-developed PSCOT question provides the focus for:
    A. **selecting keywords and concepts used to narrow the determination of the articles.**
    B. selecting articles based on the population and outcomes.
    C. directing the literature search by identifying selected articles.
    D. managing the EBP process outside of the educational focus.

Rationale:

A well-developed question provides the keywords and concepts imperative for identifying and narrowing the selection of the articles. By successfully ascertaining the articles through the literature search driven by the question, evidence that supports the teaching environment can be discovered.

Discussion Questions

1. You have been assigned to teach nursing theories in a 6-week online course. How will you approach the selection of content to be taught?
   Considerations:
   - How many nursing theories exist? Which theories are most commonly used?
   - Determine the reading assignments and coursework students must be able to complete each week.
   - Assign a group or individual students to a theorist to report back on a discussion board.

2. As you begin to mentor a novice faculty member, the individual asks for help in determining the best way to facilitate a fundamental clinical group of 10 students. Formulate a PSCOT question and determine the keywords to use for a literature review as you demonstrate EBT to this individual.
   Considerations:
   - PSCOT—population, strategy, comparison, outcome, time.
   - Key terms should reflect MeSH terms.

3. Identify one example of evidence that is available for each of the following:
   A. A teaching strategy that you are comfortable using.
   B. A teaching strategy that was regularly used when you were a student.
   C. A teaching strategy that you are considering using.

   Considerations:
   - Formulate PSCOT question.
   - Pull keywords using MeSH terms.

References

Adams, M. H., & Valiga, T. M. (2009). *Achieving excellence in nursing education.* New York, NY: National League for Nursing.

Allen, P. (2013). Preparing nurses for tomorrow's healthcare system. *American Nurse Today, 8*(5), 46–50.

American Association of Colleges of Nursing. (1999). Defining scholarship for the discipline of nursing [Position statement]. Retrieved October 18, 2013, from http://www.aacn.nche.edu/Publications/positions/scholar.htm

American Library Association. (2006). Information literacy competency standards for higher education. Retrieved October 18, 2013, from http://www.ala.org/ala/mgrps/divs/acrl/standards/informationliteracycompetency.cfm

Appling, S. E., Naumann, P. L., & Berk, R. A. (2001). Using a faculty evaluation triad to achieve evidence-based teaching. *Nursing & Health Care Perspectives, 22*(5), 247–251.

Ard, N. (2009). Essentials of learning. In C. M. Schultz (Ed.), *Essentials of learning in building a science of nursing education: Foundation for evidence-based teaching–learning.* New York, NY: National League for Nursing.

Bain, K. (2009). Personal communication. American Association of College of Nursing Business meeting, November 1, 2009, Washington, DC.

Bastable, S. B. (2014). *Nurse as educator* (4th ed.). Burlington, MA: Jones & Bartlett Learning.

Beyea, S. C., & Slattery, M. J. (2013). Historical perspectives on evidence-based nursing. *Nursing Science Quarterly, 24*(2), 152–155.

Birx, E. C. (2006). Critical thinking and theory-based practice. In W. K. Cody (Ed.), *Philosophical and theoretical perspectives for advanced nursing practice.* Sudbury, MA: Jones and Bartlett Publishers.

Boswell, C., & Cannon, S. (2014). *Introduction to nursing research: Incorporating evidence-based practice* (3rd ed.). Burlington, MA: Jones & Bartlett Learning.

Boyer, E. L. (1990). *Scholarship reconsidered: Priorities of the professoriate.* New York, NY: The Carnegie Foundation for the Advancement of Teaching.

Damron-Rodriguez, J. (2008). Developing competence for nurses and social workers. *American Journal of Nursing, 108*(9 Supplement), 40–46.

Danielson, C. (2008). *Handbook for enhancing professional practice: Evidence of teaching.* Association for Supervision and Curriculum Development. Retrieved October 18, 2013, from http://www.ascd.org/publications/books/106035/chapters/Evidence-of-Teaching.aspx

Emerson, R. J., & Records, K. (2008). Today's challenge, tomorrow's excellence: The practice of evidence-based education. *Journal of Nursing Education, 47*(8), 359–370.

Ennis, R. H. (1987). A taxonomy of critical thinking dispositions and abilities. In J. B. Baron & R. J. Sternberg (Eds.), *Teaching thinking skills: Theory and practice.* New York, NY: W. H. Fresynk.

Felver, L., Gaines, B., Heims, M., Lasater, K., Laustsen, G., Lynch, M., . . . Tanner, C. (2010). *Best practices in teaching and learning in nursing education.* New York, NY: National League for Nursing.

Fitzpatrick, J. (2005). Critical thinking: How do we know it in nursing education and practice? *Nursing Education Perspectives, 26*(5), 261.

Heaslip, P. (2008). Critical thinking: To think like a nurse. Retrieved October 18, 2013, from http://www.criticalthinking.org/pages/critical-thinking-to-think-like-a-nurse/834

Jones, J. R. (2013). Theory into practice. *Nursing Standard, 27*(19), 61.

Kuehn, B. M. (2010). IOM: Boost nurses' role in health care. *American Medical Association, 304*(21), 2345–2346.

Magee, M. (2005). *Health politics: Power, population, and health.* Bronxville, NY: Spencer Books.

Malloch, K., & Porter-O'Grady. (2009). *Introduction to evidence-based practice in nursing and health care.* (2nd ed.). Burlington, MA: Jones & Bartlett Learning.

McCartney, P. R., & Morin, K. H. (2005). Where is the evidence for teaching methods used in nursing education? *The American Journal of Maternal Child Nursing, 30*(6), 406–412.

Melnyk, B. M., & Fineout-Overholt, E. (2010). *Evidence-based practice in nursing and healthcare: A guide to best practice* (2nd ed.). Philadelphia, PA: Lippincott Williams & Wilkins.

Mitchell, G. J. (2013). Implications of holding ideas of evidence-based practice in nursing. *Nursing Science Quarterly, 26*(2), 143–151.

Oermann, M. H. (2009). Evidence-based programs and teaching/evaluation methods: Needed to achieve excellence in nursing education. In M. H. Adams & T. M. Valiga (Eds.), *Achieving excellence in nursing education* (Chapter 6). New York, NY: National League for Nursing.

Paul, R. (2004). The state of critical thinking today. Retrieved June 9, 2014, from http://www.criticalthinking.org/pages/the-state-of-critical-thinking -today/523

Paul, R., Elder, L., & Bartell, T. (1997). A brief history of the idea of critical thinking. Taken from the California teacher preparation for instruction in critical thinking: Research findings and policy recommendations. State of California, California Commission on Teacher Credentialing, Sacramento, CA. Retrieved June 9, 2014, from http://www.criticalthinking.org/aboutCT/briefHistoryCT .cfm

Porter-O'Grady, T. (2010). A new age for practice: Creating the framework for evidence. In K. Malloch & T. Porter-O'Grady (Eds.), *Introduction to evidence-based practice in nursing and health care.* (2nd ed.). Burlington, MA: Jones & Bartlett Learning.

Pravikoff, D. S., Tanner, A. B., & Pierce, S. T. (2005). Readiness of U.S. nurses for evidence-based practice. *American Journal of Nursing, 105*(9), 40–51.

Rutledge, D. N., & Grant, M. (2002). Introduction. *Seminars in Oncology Nursing, 18*, 1–2.

Salmond, S. W. (2013). Finding the evidence to support evidence-based practice. *Orthopaedic Nursing, 32*(1), 16–22.

Shultz, C. M. (2009). *Building a science of nursing education: Foundation for evidence-based teaching–learning.* New York, NY; National League for Nursing.

Thompson, C. (2009). Teaching-learning in the cognitive domain. In C. M. Schultz (Ed.), *Essentials of learning in building a science of nursing education: Foundation for evidence-based teaching–learning.* New York, NY: National League for Nursing.

Webber, P. B. (2008). Facilitating critical thinking and effective reasoning. In B. K. Penn (Ed.), *Mastering the teaching role: A guide for nurse educators.* Philadelphia, PA: F.A. Davis Company.

Webster's II New College Dictionary. (1999). Orlando, FL: Houghton Mifflin.

Wexler, J. M. (n.d.). Evidence-based teaching at Dartmouth: Students helping teachers. Retrieved October 9, 2009, from http://www.dartmouth.edu/~thepress /read.php?id=1352

Chapter 2

The Role of the Academician

Carol Boswell and Sharon Cannon

CHAPTER OBJECTIVES

At the conclusion of this chapter, the learner will be able to:

1. Discuss generational differences as they apply to the educational experience.
2. Determine a plan for managing generational aspects within the academician's role.
3. Examine curricular issues using an evidence-based teaching approach.
4. Contrast the role of the academician in relation to committee involvement.
5. Compare key issues related to tenure and promotion within the educational experience.
6. Discuss the expectation and value of evidence-based teaching policies and procedures.

KEY TERMS

- Academician
- Baby Boomers
- Committees
- Concept based
- Contextual learning
- Curriculum
- Directive learning
- Generation X
- Generational cohort
- Hard skills
- Inquiry learning
- Item learning
- Millennials
- Mission
- Philosophy
- Policy
- Problem based
- Procedure
- Promotion
- Rational learning

- Soft skills
- Syntactical learning
- Tenure
- Traditionalists/Veterans

INTRODUCTION

As faculty members begin to acknowledge the need for evidence-based teaching (EBT), several concepts related to the academician's role must be carefully considered and incorporated. Never before in history has the workplace been required to engage four distinct generational cohorts. Sherman (2006) defines a **generational cohort** as "a group of people who share birth years, history, and a collective personality as a result of their defining experiences" (p. 2). As with any grouping of individuals, the group members may display many of the same characteristics, but individuals will also have unique characteristics. The information available about generational groups is founded on research evidence as well as opinion evidence. Most of the work has been completed outside of the profession of nursing but is valid when considering the different characteristics of the cohorts. Faculty members must take care that while considering the characteristics for the generational cohort, they do not lose sight that each student and faculty member is also a result of his or her unique heritage. The four cohorts currently present in the workplace are the **Traditionalists/ Veterans**, the **Baby Boomers**, **Generation X**, and the **Millennials** (Hahn, 2009; Wieck, 2008). Hahn (2009) states, "The challenge for the nurse manager is to embrace and respect the multigenerational diversity of the staff while developing and supporting a highly functioning and cohesive nursing team" (p. 8). Though this idea is true for the nurse manager, it is equally true for the educator. The educator frequently represents either the Traditionalists/Veterans or Baby Boomer cohort but must educate the Generation X (Gen X) and Millennial cohorts. We are seeing the Gen X cohort beginning to step up to the plate and assume the educator role. As a result, we have educators potentially from three different cohorts. Although the students may be from numerous generational groups (e.g., Traditionalists/ Veterans, Baby Boomers, Gen X, or Millennials), the student cohorts tend to be primarily from either the Gen X or Millennial groups. The Traditionalist/Veteran Generation is comprised of those individuals who are seen as having years of experience who are approaching or engaged in retirement at this point in their lives. Thus, the faculty cohort may be dealing with the challenge of embracing and respecting these different generational needs within the faculty group in addition to the management of the Gen

Xers and Millennials within the classroom, all while teaching the students about approaches to patients who also represent different generations.

According to Wieck (2008), "Millennial youngsters are the best educated, most affluent and most ethnically diverse of the four generations in the workplace today" (p. 27). This group of individuals values education but not necessarily in the same manner that the Traditionalist/Veteran and Baby Boomer groups do. How each of the generational distinctions comes to bear on the academician's role provides many challenges. The faculty members must carefully engage in productive management of the educational environment based on these different generational characteristics as they address the academic issues of curriculum, committee involvement, tenure and promotion issues, and policy and procedure development. An effective faculty body will use the strengths and manage the weaknesses from each of these generational cohorts to develop and manage an educational program that is visionary and strategically savvy.

GENERATIONAL ASPECTS FOR BOTH FACULTY AND STUDENTS

The majority of the information available within the nursing and healthcare literature concerning the generational differences is directed toward the management of the workplace. Thus, educators must take the information provided and apply it to the educational experience. Hammill (2005) states that "roles today are all over the place and the rules are being rewritten daily" (p. 2). As nursing faculty members, we are called upon to correlate information found in one area with how it applies to another area. Hammill (2005) goes on to state that generational dissimilarities can influence everything from recruiting, retaining, fostering teams, and managing change, in order to encouraging, overseeing, and developing efficiency and output. These same areas are key aspects within the educational environment. Faculty members must develop a sound foundational knowledge about generational strengths and challenges to ensure the success of the educational process while decreasing the frustrations that emerge when conflict and stress are present. Taking the time and energy to consider the different generations and work to meet them somewhere in the middle can and will improve the educational outcomes for a program.

The evidence presented in **Table 2-1** provides a starting point for investigating generational characteristics that can be used to formulate a functional faculty cohort that can effectively work with the differences

Table 2-1 General Generational Characteristics

	Traditionalists/Veterans (born before 1946)	Baby Boomers (born 1946–1964)	Generation X (born 1965–1976)	Millennials (born 1977–1997)
Generational Values	• Hard working • Respect for authority • Disciplined • Accept delayed rewards • Adhere to rules • Conformers • Dedication/sacrifice • Duty before pleasure • Trust in government	• Optimistic • Team players • Strong work effort • Personal gratification • Anything is possible • Want to "make a difference"	• Diverse • Self-reliant • Free agents • Balanced • Informal • Fun • Highly educated • Think globally • Tech literacy	• Globally diverse • Optimistic • Achievement oriented • Flexible • Avid consumers • Civic duty • Extreme fun • Hotly competitive • Street smarts • Realism • Extremely tech savvy
Generational Strengths	• Stable • Detail oriented • Loyal • Hard working • Reliable • Practical • Dedicated • Ethical • Fiscally prudent • Honorable • Task oriented • Follow rules of conduct	• Driven • Team, service, and relationship oriented • Optimistic • Able to handle a crisis • Ambitious • Ethical • Have good communication skills • Live to work • Multitaskers • Politically correct	• Accepting of change • Capable of multitasking • Technologically literate • Self-reliant • Creative • Skeptical • Balanced • Self-starters • Results driven • Self-sufficient • Work to live	• Optimistic • Capable of multitasking • Very technologically savvy • Outcome driven • Determined • Ambitious but not entirely focused • Best educated–confident • Open to new ideas • Focused on self-development • Respect given for competency not title
Other Names	Traditionalists, Silent Generation, Moral Authority, The Forgotten Generation	"Me" Generation, Moral Authority	Gen X, Xers, The Doers, Post Boomers, 13th Generation, Busters, Twenty Somethings	Generation Y, Gen Y, Generation Next, Echo Boomers, Chief Friendship Officers, 24/7 Bridgers, Mosaics, Net Generation

Source: Adapted from Hahn, J. (2009). Effectively manage a multigenerational staff. *Nursing Management, 40*(9), 8–10; and Gaylor, D. (2014). Generational differences. Retrieved June 10, 2014, from http://www.chialpha.com/other-resources/127-generations/file.html.

encountered. Within this table, the values and strengths for each of the four generations are provided for comparison along with the numerous titles that can be used within the literature to depict the different generational divisions. The division within the work environment is depicted to be approximately 5% Traditionalists/Veterans, 45% Baby Boomers, 40% Gen Xers, and 10% Millennials. In an executive dialogue, Scanlan (2013) suggests that combined, Gen Xers and Millennials outnumber Baby Boomers. Several key aspects in regard to their values are evident. The Gen X and Millennial generations are considered to be technologically literate. Since technology is very important to these two generations, the educational environment must embrace and assimilate technology into the classroom and clinical experience. The differences and similarities between each of the generations should be carefully considered. The Baby Boomers are optimistic but desire personal gratification. Gen X, on the other hand, is informal and diverse. The Baby Boomers, though wanting to make a difference, are expecting that their generation will be the group to address the challenges confronting the educational and workplace environment. Gen Xers want to enjoy the world while considering themselves as free agents who are self-reliant. The Millennial generation explodes onto the educational and workplace environments with a fun-loving attitude as well as civic-mindedness. Work is considered to be a requirement by this group but must be confronted in a realistic and ambitious manner. As faculty members consider each of these aspects, one area to conscientiously evaluate is the need to restructure the course delivery to embrace the openness, civic focus, and self-reliant aspects within these groups.

Within **Table 2–2**, the focus for each generation related to engagement with others is presented and reflects the evidence as currently understood. The perception of the Millennial generation concerning education being extremely expensive is cause for concern. Faculty members must remember this perception and ensure that the majority of the educational process is viewed as realistic and meaningful. Since the idea is that education is costly, the practicality of the material presented is imperative. Another dimension important for the faculty to commit to memory is the value for each of the two generations: Gen X looks at the time commitment of the experience whereas the Millennials desire the uniqueness of the experience. So often, the phrase "Tell me what I need to know for the test" is identified as an expectation from students. With the understanding of the focus for these two groups, the rationale for this statement can be better understood. Faculty members must consider the time commitment and the uniqueness of each encounter within the educational process. Clear delineation as to the rationale for each experience needs to be addressed,

Table 2-2 Generational Characteristics and Work-Related Aspects

	Traditionalists/Veterans (born before 1946)	Baby Boomers (born 1946–1964)	Generation X (born 1965–1976)	Millennials (born 1977–1997)
Education	An aspiration	A birthright	A means to progress forward	A staggering expense
Value	Family/community	Achievement	Time	Uniqueness
Focus	Duty	Associations and outcome	Tasks and outcome	International and networked
Interactive Style	Individual	Team player; Revere meetings	Entrepreneur	Participative
View on Respect for Authority	Authority is based on seniority and tenure	Skeptical of authority; Time equals authority	Skeptical of authority figures; Will test authority repetitively	Test authority but seek out authority figures when looking for guidance
Work Ethics That Impact Educational Process	Adhere to rules; Responsibility before fun; Expect everyone to honor commitments; Expect to be respected; Linear; Word is their bond; Value honor, due process, fair play, good attitude, hard work, attendance	Confront authority; Abhor conformity and rules; Loyal to team members; Process oriented; Endeavor to do very best; Willing to take risks; Work efficiently; Demand respect from younger individuals; Value teamwork, personal fulfillment, equality, collaboration	Expect to influence the terms and conditions; Work/family balance important; Like a casual environment; Outcome oriented; Output focused; Prefer diversity, technology, informality, and fun; Want to get in, get the work done, and move on to other things	Believe (due to technology) they can work flexibly anytime, anyplace; Evaluated on work product, not how, when, or where done; High expectations of leaders to mentor them toward attainment of goals; Goal oriented; Mentoring is important; Obsessed with career development; Tolerant; Thrive in a collaborative environment; Seek continuing education to enhance work skills

Source: Adapted from Hahn, J. (2009). Effectively manage a multigenerational staff. *Nursing Management, 40*(9), 8–10; and Gaylor, D. (2014). Generational differences. Retrieved June 10, 2014, from http://www.chialpha.com/other-resources/127-generations/file.html.

thus providing value for the encounter. Another primary area resulting in stress and frustration as the generations come together is the differing views on respect for authority. Both Gen Xers and Millennials expect to test authority repeatedly. Millennials differ in that while testing the authority figure, they continue to seek guidance from that authority. In contrast, the idea held by the Baby Boomers concerning the importance of time in establishment of the authority can result in stress. Baby Boomers perceive that a person with time and experience should be identified as having authority.

Gen Xers and Millennials do not see time involved as a foundation for authority. The amount of time that a person works at a job does not equate to the person having the authority to manage a position per the Gen X and Millennial cohorts. Faculty members must understand that from these generations' viewpoint, being a nurse for multiple years does not mean that the person is, nor can be, an effective teacher. Gen Xers and Millennials seek out individuals who have the experience but also knowledge about how to get a message across. These individuals are the ones that the Gen Xers and Millennial cohorts will embrace as having authority. In addition to the thoughts about authority, an additional difference between the Gen Xers and Millennial cohorts is based on the viewpoint of work ethics. In Table 2–2, some of the different work ethics are listed. Gen Xers are focused on self, whereas Millennials embrace the idea of mentorship. Millennials value involvement with authorities, whereas Gen Xers seem to prefer doing things alone. In regard to work ethics, Gen Xers seem to want to be told what to do by the leader, then the leader needs to step back and let them do it their way. Although the Millennials want to be allowed to do it their way, they seek mentors to help them to work it out. They also want to select their own mentors based on who they perceive as having authority, not by who has a title.

As faculty members strive to engage the different generations in the learning process, several additional ideas need to be considered (**Table 2–3**). The Millennial (Gen Y) cohort treasures the ability to work with bright and energetic individuals. Faculty members coming to the work environment excited about the opportunities and challenges are means for connecting with this generational group. Gen Xers, on the other hand, appreciate freedom to approach problems and challenges in unique ways. Rules are not appreciated by this generation because many regulations are based upon the here and now. Gen Xers view the application of rules and regulations as frequently contingent on the current environment. They view these changing practices as fluid and not set in stone. Thus, freedom to investigate innovative ways to address the challenge and/or problem is a mainstay within the expectations for the Gen X population. Faculty members who

Table 2-3 Generational Work-Related Characteristics

	Traditionalists/Veterans (born before 1946)	Baby Boomers (born 1946–1964)	Generation X (born 1965–1976)	Millennials (born 1977–1997)
Views of Authority	Respectful Endure Honor and respect	Awed Replace them Challenge leaders	Unenthusiastic Ignore leaders	Undisturbed Must feel respected by leaders Choose their own bosses
Role of Career	Means of living	Central focus	Irritant	Always changing
Best Ways to Interact	Know the rules and follow them Reduce the appearance of lack of discipline, respect, logic, and structure Strive to understand their feelings	Value their ideas when possible Work is important to them Silly routines are frustrating Teams Motivated by their responsibilities toward others Responsive to attention and recognition Don't take criticism well Need flexibility, attention, and freedom	Remember they desire independence and informality Allow time to seek other interests Allow time for fun Utilize the most up-to-date technology	Use a team-oriented workplace Get to know their personal goals Treat with respect Nurtured to feel appreciated and very optimistic about self Employ appealing experiences to cultivate transferable skills Provide rationales Supply variety Grow teams and networks with immense attention Reward extra effort and excellence Provide structured, encouraging environment Utilize an interactive environment
Motivated by…	Being respected Security	Being valued, needed Money	Freedom Removal of rules Time off	Working with bright people Time off

Source: Adapted from Hahn, J. (2009). Effectively manage a multigenerational staff. *Nursing Management, 40*(9), 8–10; and Gaylor, D. (2014). Generational differences. Retrieved June 10, 2014, from http://www.chialpha.com/other-resources/127-generations/file.html.

primarily are within the Baby Boomers group desire that their wisdom and experience be valued and accepted when challenges and problems are identified. The tested ways are embraced by the Baby Boomers, whereas an open slate for managing the issues is celebrated by Gen Xers. Baby Boomer faculty members must allow the Gen Xers to try out new approaches while respecting the teamwork orientation found within the Millennials. Gen X individuals do not like teams and groups because singularity is a main principle in their value system. According to Wieck (2008), "The team orientation of the Millennials is in stark contrast to the more independent-minded Gen X" (p. 27). Millennial individuals desire teams and groups to be used to address the challenges presented in the classroom and clinical sites. Wieck (2008) continues with the idea of group engagement with the Millennial generation by stressing the importance that faculty members assign a challenge through establishing goals, forming appropriate teams, providing the teams with the freedom to address the challenge in their own ways, and ending with appropriate feedback and encouragement. One final aspect that is paramount for the Baby Boomer faculty member to realize is the necessity of allowing time off for both the Gen X and Millennial groups. Both groups strongly value free, unrestricted time to embrace the world. Both the Gen Xers and Millennial cohorts expect and demand this time.

Table 2–4 provides the key areas paramount within the educational process. Communication and feedback are critical aspects of the learning process. As one compares the Baby Boomers to the Millennials, several similarities can be noted within the communication aspect. The Baby Boomers communicate with diplomacy and directness. Millennials desire communication that is polite and active in nature. Gen Xers, in contrast, did not develop as many of the networking skills, thus they expect blunt, immediate messages. Both the Gen Xers and the Millennial generations are technologically savvy. Email and voicemail are their primary means of communication. Instant communication is highly valued. Baby Boomers and Traditionalists/Veterans continue to value note writing and personal commitment from handwritten notes. Another interesting communication aspect is that Gen Xers want the messages tied to the outcomes, whereas Millennials value messages that are connected to the goals and aspirations and frequently multitask using technology. Knowledge of this message focus could be very valuable as faculty members strive to communicate with the different members within a class. Messages should be directed toward outcomes and goals/aspirations to gain support for the management of the interaction. While communicating via instant messaging, texting, and emails is of prime importance to these final two generations, it is evident that they are reading less and less.

Table 2-4 Generational Characteristics—Communication and Feedback

	Traditionalists/Veterans (born before 1946)	Baby Boomers (born 1946–1964)	Generation X (born 1965–1976)	Millennials (born 1977–1997)
Communication	Discreet	Diplomatic	Blunt/direct	Polite
	Present in logical manner	In person	Immediate	Positive, respectful, motivational
	Show respect by using titles	Direct style	Straight talk/ present facts	electronic communication styles
	Use formal language	Present options	Use email as primary tool	Use email and voice mail as primary tools
	Don't waste time	Answer questions thoroughly	Talk in short direct phrases	Use action verbs
	Use inclusive language (we, us)	Avoid manipulative/controlling language	Share information immediately	Use visual pictures
	Handwritten notes	Get consensus	Don't micromanage	Be humorous
	More personal interaction	Establish a friendly rapport	Tie the message to outcomes	Tie the message to goals and aspirations
Feedback/Rewards	No news is good news	Like praise and recognition	Freedom is best reward	Need frequent feedback
	Want subtle, private recognition on an individual level	Enjoy having "something for the wall"	Do not want public recognition	Want clear goals and expectations
		Enjoy public recognition	Prefer regular feedback	Communicate frequently
		Appreciate awards for hard work	Need constructive feedback	
Preferred Ways to Learn Soft Skills	On the job	On the job	On the job	On the job
	Discussion groups	Discussion groups	Face-to-face coaching	Peer interaction and feedback
	Peer interaction and feedback	Face-to-face coaching	Assessment and feedback	Discussion groups
	Face-to-face coaching	Classroom instruction live	Discussion group	Face-to-face coaching
Preferred Ways to Learn Hard Skills	Classroom instruction	Classroom instruction	On the job	On the job
	On the job	On the job	Classroom instruction	Classroom instruction
	Workbooks and manuals	Workbooks and manuals	Workbooks and manuals	Workbooks and manuals
	Books and reading	Books and reading	Books and reading	Books and reading

Source: Adapted from Hahn, J. (2009). Effectively manage a multigenerational staff. *Nursing Management, 40*(9), 8–10; Gaylor, D. (2002). Generational differences. Retrieved June 10, 2014, from http://www.chialpha.com/other-resources/127-generations/file.html; and Tolbize, A. (2008). Generational differences in the workplace. In *Research and Training Center on Community Living*. Minneapolis, MN: University of Minnesota Press.

The Millennial generation strives to learn by questioning. The questions are not meant to show disrespect but to gain an understanding of how the previous generations came to the understandings that are being presented (Tolbize, 2008). This generation wants to understand the process, not just learn the facts. Millennials value instant messaging, not the reading of classics and literature. To expect them to read long assignments is beyond the custom for these groups. Another area to consider when dealing with the different generations is that of feedback and rewards. Gen Xers overall do not want public acknowledgement since they tend to be very private individuals. Feedback to this group should be regular and constructive and should allow for freedom. Millennials want frequent feedback that is tied to their focus on goals and expectations. Communication, feedback, and interactions should concentrate on management and attainment of the goals and expectations established. Faculty members would benefit by having a time at the beginning of courses for clarifying and validating the goals and expectations. For the Millennial generation, this clarification and substantiation of the goals and opportunities allows everyone to be working toward the same prize. Baby Boomers, on the other hand, desire praise and recognition. It seems that this generation values external validation, whereas the Gen X group seems to value internal validation.

A final aspect to consider from a faculty member's viewpoint is the preferred routines used by the different generations for learning soft and hard skills. **Soft skills** are those activities that lend themselves to hands-on work. Each generation prefers "on-the-job" experiences when endeavoring to address these types of skills. The change comes when looking at the second way that each generation seeks to further acquire these soft skills. Both of the older generations favor the use of discussion groups as a second means of addressing the soft skills. Whereas Gen X is inclined toward face-to-face coaching as a valued process for acquiring soft skills, the Millennial group looks toward peer interaction and feedback that speaks to group encounters. In contrast, the methods desired for acquiring hard skills take different routes. **Hard skills** are those aspects that are acquired as a result of classroom experiences. Again, the older two generations desire the use of classroom instruction to develop a foundation for the hard skills, whereas both of the younger generations seek the acquisition through on-the-job training. So, basically, for both soft and hard skills, the younger generations desire the provision of the material within the job performance, or hands-on experience. As was stated previously, the younger generations do not want to be expected to read books and work on workbooks and manuals. They want to be involved with the material. O'Connor (2009) provides insight into this desire, describing the following dynamics in regard to the use of technology (p. 9):

- Digital literacy: The younger generations' learners are adept at navigating the Internet for information and are comfortable with a wide variety of technology.
- Connected: Never far from their cell phones, these learners are talking or texting constantly, including at work and in class.
- Immediacy: These learners expect speed and become impatient if they have to wait for a response or to get information.
- Experiential: They learn best by doing as opposed to being told what to do.
- Social team work: They are highly interactive and communicative.

Since these generations seek connectivity, faculty members must strive for ways to engage them via the Web and other immediacy types of teaching opportunities. The movement in nursing education is from the "sage on the stage" to the "guide on the side."

The technological focus embraced by both the Gen Xers and the Millennial groups is significant to the management of the classroom and clinical experience. Even during lecture and classroom activities, these groups want to be able to access the Internet to validate the material being presented and to acquire additional information that they then can share in class. O'Connor (2009) states that "while annoying to the more mature leader and faculty member, this feeling of connectivity is of high importance to this generation" (p. 9). The ability to use technology to search the literature for evidence of clinical, managerial, and educational best practices is a valuable asset that the Gen Xers and Millennial groups bring to the table. This skill of the groups should be capitalized upon within the educational process and further perfected to maximize the ability to locate sound evidence on which to base practice decisions (O'Connor, 2009). The opportunities within technology to engage the students and faculty members are immeasurable when embraced.

Sherman (2006, p. 6) provides these summative recommendations for working with and among the different generations:

- Seek to understand each generational cohort.
- Accommodate generational differences in attitudes, values, and behaviors.
- Develop generationally sensitive styles to effectively coach and motivate all members of the healthcare team.

- Develop the ability to flex a communication style to accommodate generational differences.
- Promote the resolution of generational conflicts so as to build work teams.
- Capitalize on generational differences, using these differences to enhance the work of the entire team.

These simple but complex recommendations basically stem from a need to constantly be assessing our commitment to accept and engage with each generation and culture. Wieck, Dols, and Northam (2009) add to this list of recommendations the following suggestions: actively listen, give opportunities for input, build cohesive environments that are conducive to friendships, promote respectful relationships, and facilitate good communication. Each of these skills attempts to focus on the individual rather than the generational expectations.

Another aspect regarding generational differences requires attention. Traditionalists/Veterans and Baby Boomers may be offended when Millennials multitask (Putre, 2013). For example, a Traditionalist/Veteran may find it rude when a Millennial texts someone while conversing with the Traditionalist faculty. Thus, each generation must know their generational category while being aware of differences among other generations. Conflicting generational norms can occur in both an academic and a clinical workplace, impacting faculty-to-faculty, faculty-to-student, student-to-student, and faculty/student-to-patient relationships. Effective communication and civility skills are necessary regardless of the setting. Interacting with the members of each and every generation with openness and respectfulness establishes a beginning place for the development of a sound working/learning environment. According to Tolbize (2008), "Generational conflict is more likely to arise from errors of attribution and perception, than from valid differences" (p. 13). Expecting to encounter problems with the management of the generations usually results in conflict and stress. As with working with any generation and culture, a sound knowledge of the group does help to understand when and how the group can come to the table to work and/or learn. Embracing these differences and using them to everyone's advantage allows for a "win–win" opportunity. As Wieck (2008) sums it up, "The key to managing this generational mix will be open doors, open minds, and an abundance of patience" (p. 29). As we all strive to address the challenges that confront us within the academic setting, the thoughts and expectations presented by each new generation must be incorporated into our manner of delivery if we are to be successful.

CURRICULUM

Many different definitions can be found for the term **curriculum**. Each definition considers the idea from differing viewpoints. Oliva (1988) suggested the definition of curriculum as "a plan or program for all the experiences which the learner encounters under the direction of the school" (p. 9). Madeus and Stufflebeam (1989) used Tanner's definition, which stated that a curriculum was the premeditated and guided learning encounters using projected learning conclusions that were devised by means of a methodical rebuilding of knowledge and experiences, within an academic setting, resulting in the learners' ongoing and deliberate evolution in personal social competence. Another example of a definition of curriculum is provided by Penn (2008) and addresses the basic components. Penn (2008) lists the components as "the mission and philosophy of the nursing unit, the conceptual framework of the program of study, course sequencing and courses required for the program of study, program objectives, learning activities, outcomes or competencies of the graduate of the program, and a program of evaluation" (p. 153). Each of these definitions implies written documents that are used to direct the learning process. Ironside (2007) takes a slightly different approach to the idea: "The most common agreement seems to be that curriculum is what actually occurs between and among persons in the educational enterprise and not some 'plan' for learning that is reflected in written materials" (p. 78). Curriculum moves from a document into a working process whereby learning can occur. The National League for Nursing (NLN) established the Hallmarks of Excellence in 2004. Within the Hallmarks, the points related to curriculum are presented as follows (Speakman, 2009, pp. 45–48):

- The design and implementation of the program is innovative and seeks to build on traditional approaches to nursing education.
- The curriculum is flexible and reflects current societal and healthcare trends and issues, research findings, and innovative practices, as well as local and global perspectives.
- The curriculum is evidence based.
- The curriculum provides learning experiences that support evidence-based practice, multidisciplinary approaches to care, student achievement of clinical competence, and, as appropriate, expertise in specialty roles.
- The curriculum provides experiential cultural learning activities that enhance students' abilities to think critically, reflect thoughtfully, and provide culturally sensitive, evidence-based nursing care to diverse populations.

- The curriculum provides learning experiences that prepare graduates to assume roles that are essential to quality nursing practice, including but not limited to those of care provider, patient advocate, teacher, communicator, change agent, care coordinator, user of information technology, collaborator, and decision maker.
- The innovativeness of the program helps create a preferred future for nursing.
- Teaching/learning/evaluation strategies used by faculty are evidence based.
- The educational environment empowers students and faculty and promotes collegial dialogue, innovation, change, creativity, values development, and ethical behavior.

Each of these ideas helps to provide an understanding of the functionality of the curriculum. It provides the framework from which the entire learning process should flow.

As faculty members consider the different aspects of curriculum, the types of learning (**Table 2–5**) should be contemplated. The six types of learning have been designated to provide a framework for leveling the learning that is planned within the curriculum. The initial three types of learning (**item**, **directive**, and **rational**) provide a "black-and-white" involvement with materials to be used. These three levels are considered to be at the technical levels of learning. The upper three types of learning (**syntactical**, **contextual**, and **inquiry**) strive to encourage critical thinking and a sense of investigation and analysis. As a curriculum is pulled together, faculty members should wisely consider what level of learning is appropriate at each stage within the learning process.

Once the levels of learning are determined, the curriculum can be fleshed out. Madeus and Stufflebeam (1989) provide four fundamental questions to be used when developing a curriculum:

1. What educational purposes should the school seek to attain?
2. What educational experiences can be provided that are likely to achieve these purposes?
3. How can these educational experiences be effectively organized?
4. How can we determine whether and to what extent these purposes are being attained?

The process of curriculum development must embrace several different levels within the educational process. The institution's **philosophy** of education provides the foundation for the entire educational experience at an institution. From this philosophy, the goals and aims within each designated program can be determined. Once the program has these aspects

Table 2-5 Types of Learning

Type	Description
Item Learning	Focused on learning facts, pieces of information, individual aspects, straightforward associations; involuntary, automatic, and predictable
Directive Learning	Ascertaining of regulations, restrictions, and omissions; systems of direction that provide the "do's" and don'ts" for everyday jobs
Rational Learning	Introduces theory and the "why's" for doing things into the logical management of tasks; beginning of the use of logic to influence judgment and decision making
Syntactical Learning	Investigation into the understanding of the whole; relationships and patterns are sought to guide unique client care; encourages individuals to make intuitive efforts as theory is meshed into practice
Contextual Learning	Inclusion of cultural aspects to frame the provision of care; symbols, political aspects, power, relationships, values, aesthetic aspects, ethical perspectives, and philosophical facets are considered as transition into caring, compassionate, and positive care
Inquiry Learning	Resourcefulness, exploration, theorizing, strategizing, ascertaining, illuminating, and categorizing challenges and approaches to solve aspects of care; striving to find the foundations and questioning the process; demanding validation for aspects provided

Source: Adapted from Ironside, P. M. (Ed.). (2007). *On revolutions and revolutionaries: 25 years of reform and innovation in nursing education.* New York, NY: National League for Nursing.

determined, specific instructional objectives and outcomes can be established that will provide the underpinning for task analysis, content selection, and learning activities.

Penn (2008) said it correctly when stating that "curriculum development is a dynamic process and requires continuous evaluation" (p. 160). The curriculum within schools of nursing is viewed as the responsibility of the faculty. The strengths and/or weaknesses of the learning plan are directly related to the effort put into the curriculum by each faculty member. It becomes imperative that faculty members understand and embrace the development and management of the curriculum within a school. According to Conway and Little (n.d.), "Curriculum content should focus on what nurses do rather than where they work" (p. 3). Each member of the faculty has to appreciate and comprehend the nuances within the curriculum to effectively provide the guidance required within the learning environment. In light of the generational issues and the NLN's Hallmarks of Excellence, Speakman (2009) states, "Our programs and curricula must be student-centered, interactive, and innovative" (p. 44). To work within the boundaries of the learning environment, students must be empowered to learn. Instead of being thought of as pieces of clay or sponges within their seats, students need to be actively involved and central to the learning process. By embracing the idea of "colleagues in learning," each member becomes responsible for different components of the learning process. The responsibility for learning does not fall to one group of individuals. No longer can faculty members play the role of "sage on the stage"; they must be the "guide on the side." The curriculum must incorporate the idea that each participant (administration, faculty members, and students) in the learning environment has an active role in the learning process.

Two approaches have recently gained attention. The first in regard to curriculum design is a **concept-based** approach. Giddens (2010) suggests that concepts are a way to organize knowledge such as categories or themes. An example of concepts used in this context could be health/illness such as oxygenation, infection, pain, or reproduction. Another example could be professional nursing such as critical thinking, leadership, ethics, or safety. Faculty decide which concepts are needed and organize knowledge surrounding those concepts.

Problem-based curriculum design has also emerged and focuses heavily on clinical situations, which may be based in the classroom, in simulation, or both (Ohman, 2010). Case studies/scenarios are presented for students to solve a clinical problem. Students become immersed in the problem and attempt to deep dive for resolution. This approach may occur through debates or group discussions and is often supported through other learning.

Regardless of the curriculum design chosen, the faculty and students are engaged and support interactive learning. Curriculum needs are met in a variety of methodologies to engage all participants in learning.

COMMITTEE INVOLVEMENT

From the previous discussion about generational differences and curriculum, one can quickly see that characteristics of each generation will impact the role of faculty serving on **committees**. Whether faculty members are elected or appointed to committees, they still must be able to accomplish the **mission** and goals of the school. A simple solution to addressing differences would be to put all members of a generation into a single group. Unfortunately, this approach is nearly impossible and would also omit the rich diversity of opinions/perceptions necessary for embracing opportunities to grow and change in the fast-paced health arena. Thus, a mix of generations within faculty committees allows for creativity and innovation that is realistic and necessary for committee decisions and/or recommendations.

Recognizing the need for each generation's contribution to a committee, there are ways to utilize the generational characteristics so the committee can accomplish its goals. Since most committees have a chair to provide leadership, the chair can begin by identifying the generation to which each member belongs. Once the identification has been made, the work of the committee is considered (i.e., curriculum, student affairs, faculty affairs, admissions/progressions, etc.). The chair can then use Tables 2–1 and 2–3 to guide communication, feedback, and decisions for positive outcomes for the committee tasks. This approach allows for each generation of faculty members to participate, yet recognizes the differences inherent in each generation.

TENURE AND PROMOTION

Achieving **tenure** and/or **promotion** is a quest for the majority of faculty members regardless of the type of educational institution. Perhaps at this point, tenure and promotion need to be discussed separately because not all faculty members will seek tenure. However, most faculty members at some point in time will pursue promotion.

Let's begin with the examination of tenure. It is important to keep in mind that, as mentioned, some faculty members do not wish to be on the tenure track. They choose to negotiate their faculty contract on a yearly basis. In addition, tenure is not easily obtained and all schools recognize the need for nontenured faculty. The nontenured faculty members should be recognized for their contributions.

Tenure is highly regarded and respected. It is considered to be both recognition and a reward for individual accomplishments over a designated period of time. Each school establishes the criteria for tenure. Obviously, each generation of faculty will have characteristics and work-related aspects (see Tables 2–1 and 2–2) that will be of advantage to obtaining tenure.

Since tenure is based on specific criteria instituted by the school, the Traditionalist/Veteran generation may achieve tenure more easily than the other generations. The Traditionalists/Veterans are disciplined, accept delayed rewards, and are hard working. Their values, strengths, and work ethics enhance their skills and abilities to obtain tenure.

The Baby Boomers are optimistic, driven, willing to take risks, and work efficiently. However, they believe time equals authority, and they abhor conformity and rules. Since tenure is more than time in a position and requires specific criteria (rules), Baby Boomers may encounter difficulty achieving tenure.

The Gen X group is diverse, creative, self-starting, and output focused. This generation wants to get in, get the job done, and move on. Tenure requires patience and formal structure through specific criteria. Tenure would never be considered casual or fun.

Millennial individuals are realistic, competitive, outcome driven, and goal oriented. Their obsession with career development and desire to enhance work skills through continuing education are assets that assist them through the tenure process.

Much attention has been given in the literature to recruiting faculty to assist in the nursing shortage, but approaches to retaining faculty are needed. Roughton (2013), after surveying faculty perceptions regarding retention of faculty in light of the current faculty shortage, suggests that tenure alternatives will be needed for the future.

Promotion is one aspect of the role of the **academician** that most faculty members will pursue. There are two major reasons that faculty seek promotion. Promotion can be viewed as a career ladder for faculty members that brings recognition to their work and accomplishments. Another reason to seek promotion is financial gain. In most institutions, the only significant increase in salary is through promotion from one rank to the next. Thus, promotion is an honor and a reward for hard work. Again, Tables 2-1, 2-2, and 2-3 point out how each generation is successful in reaching the next highest rank. Traditionalists/Veterans would view promotion more as an honor and a means for moving up in their career. The Baby Boomer lives to work, wants to "make a difference," and views a career as a central focus. Gen Xers want a balanced life, work to live, and view careers as getting in the way of having fun. Millennials are optimistic, want to be evaluated on their work products, and perceive their careers to be always changing.

As a result of these generations' characteristics and work aspects, promotional efforts need to focus on the strengths of each. Promotion is possible for members of each generation but will require adherence to criteria established by individual schools. Again, this may cause stress for some but be motivating for others. For instance, global health/service learning in which students experience providing nursing care in a foreign country may appeal to some but not all.

POLICY AND PROCEDURE

A **policy** can be considered a course of action—a plan. A **procedure** can be considered the means to carry out the action/plan. Policies and procedures are a part of every aspect of the role of faculty in academia. The regents/trustees of the educational institution establish overall policies and procedures to govern the operation of the institution. In accordance with the institution, each school develops policies and procedures for faculty, staff, and students. Faculty members play an important role in the development, recommendations, and implementation of policies and procedures at the school and institutional levels. In the past, policies and procedures were based on "what's always been done." Currently, the emphasis is on evidence-based policies and procedures that allow for accurate, legal, and ethical considerations that are constantly changing as new information, new laws, and ethical situations emerge. Whether recommending, developing, or implementing policies, faculty members must be cognizant of the need for evidence to guide their decisions, and diligent in acquiring this evidence. The importance of that statement cannot be stressed enough. The nurse educator's role is grounded in policies and procedures on a daily basis, regardless of the setting—classroom, simulation lab, or student clinical experience.

SUMMARY THOUGHTS

As we consider engaging the multigenerational groups currently found within the educational system, we should examine new approaches to constructing a healthy work environment. Hahn (2009) proposes several such tactics: completing a self-assessment on a regular basis, pursuing knowledge about the generational differences, embracing the commonalities, and creating and establishing a culture of respect while endeavoring to bridge the generational gap that can exist. Another key aspect discussed in relation to generational differences is that of respect. Whereas the older generations establish respect based on years of experience and commitment to the activity, the younger generations place respect based upon engagement by the individuals and their ability and willingness to listen and mentor (Hahn, 2009; Tolbize, 2008; Wieck, 2008). Respect is earned by doing, not by number of years worked at a site. Conway and Little (n.d.) assert that faculty members must become facilitators, and students must increasingly develop a self-directed learner approach as education moves forward. No longer can students expect to be "spoon-fed" the necessary material. They must step up and take an active role. Faculty members must develop strategies to help the students to make this change in the educational environment.

In regard to curriculum, Speakman (2009) states that "students will need to be engaged in student-centered curricula that are innovative and challenging, a curriculum both in the classroom and clinical setting that inspires a student to challenge assumptions, examine multiple methodologies of care and utilize current literature to frame their practice" (p. 46). Each faculty member must develop skills and commitment to embrace a student-centered curriculum that will challenge individuals to take an active part in the learning process. Students cannot be relegated to passively learning healthcare fundamentals at this time. Active involvement and commitment to learning on a continuous basis is paramount as health care moves forward.

To keep up with the momentum of change in health care, faculty members must provide valuable input on committees. Involvement gives faculty members a voice on important career development aspects related to tenure and promotion as well as policies and procedures for governing the everyday work for nurse educators. Standards for policies and procedures must be evidence based. Research in nursing education must provide evidence to produce positive outcomes for students (see the chapter titled *Competency and Certification*). Nursing faculty members are required to be knowledgeable of both clinical and educational research to keep up with the fast pace of health care and education in today's environment. The changes are related to the skills provided by students and the competencies required to practice nursing in a variety of settings.

SUMMARY POINTS

1. For the first time in history, the workplace is engaged with four distinctive generational cohorts: Traditionalists/Veterans, Baby Boomers, Gen Xers, and Millennials.
2. As with any grouping of individuals, the group members may display many of the same characteristics, but individuals will also have unique characteristics.
3. The Gen X and Millennial generations are considered to be technologically literate.
4. Faculty members should conscientiously consider the need to restructure course delivery to embrace the openness, civic focus, and self-reliant aspects presented by the Gen X and Millennial cohorts.

5. Faculty members must remember that the Millennial generation perceives education as being extremely expensive and thus must ensure that the majority of the educational process is viewed as realistic and meaningful.
6. Gen Xers look at the time to be committed to an experience, whereas the Millennials desire the uniqueness of the experience.
7. Both Gen Xers and Millennials expect to test authority repeatedly.
8. Gen Xers and Millennials seek to find individuals who have the experience and knowledge about how to get a message across.
9. Millennials treasure the ability to work with bright and energetic individuals.
10. Gen Xers appreciate freedom to approach problems and challenges in unique ways.
11. Communication and feedback are critical aspects of the learning process.
12. Gen Xers, overall, do not want public acknowledgement since they tend to be very private individuals.
13. Millennials want frequent feedback that is tied to goals and expectations.
14. As when working with any generation and culture, a sound knowledge of the group helps in understanding when and how group members can come to the table to work and/or learn.
15. Many different definitions can be found for the term *curriculum*.
16. Six types of learning have been identified: item, directive, rational, syntactical, contextual, and inquiry.
17. Once a program has determined the institutional philosophy, goals, and aims, specific instructional objectives and outcomes can be determined that will provide the underpinning for task analysis, content selection, and learning activities within a curriculum.
18. Curriculum development is a vigorous course of action and necessitates constant evaluation.
19. Within schools of nursing, curriculum is viewed as the responsibility of the faculty cohort.
20. The responsibility for learning does not fall to one group of individuals.
21. Each faculty member must develop skills and commitment to embrace a student-centered curriculum that will challenge individuals to take an active part in the learning process.
22. Faculty members from each generation provide a rich diversity necessary to achieve committee work.
23. The committee leadership (chair) must draw on the characteristics of each faculty generation to fulfill the committee tasks.

24. Tenure is the achievement of school-determined criteria for a designated period of time and is highly regarded and respected.
25. Not all faculty members will pursue tenure.
26. Promotion brings recognition and financial gains for faculty members.
27. Policies and procedures are a daily occurrence for nurse educators and must be based on solid evidence.

TIPS FOR NURSE EDUCATORS

1. Faculty members are dealing with the challenge of embracing and respecting the different generational needs within the faculty, student, and patient cohorts.
2. Faculty members must develop a sound foundational knowledge about generational strengths and challenges to ensure the success of the educational process while decreasing the frustrations that emerge when conflict and stress are present.
3. Faculty members must conscientiously consider the need to restructure course delivery to embrace the openness, civic focus, and self-reliant aspects within the Gen X and Millennial groups.
4. Material presented must be practical and realistic.
5. Clear delineation as to the rationale for each experience needs to be addressed, thus providing value for the encounter.
6. Gen Xers expect freedom to investigate innovative ways to address challenges and/or problems.
7. Gen Xers do not like teams and groups because singularity is a main principle in their value system.
8. Millennials desire teams and groups to be used to address the challenges presented in the classroom and clinical sites.
9. Email and voicemail are the primary means for communication used by the Gen X and Millennial groups.
10. Messages should be directed toward outcomes and goals/aspirations to gain support for the management of the interaction.
11. The Millennial generation strives to learn by questioning.
12. Faculty members would benefit by having a time at the beginning of courses for clarifying and validating the goals and expectations.
13. Developing generationally sensitive styles to effectively coach and motivate all members of the healthcare team is desired.
14. Active listing is imperative.
15. The learning types of item, directive, and rational are seen as fact-oriented learning.

16. The learning types of syntactical, contextual, and inquiry encourage critical thinking and a sense of investigation and analysis.
17. Each member of the faculty has to appreciate and comprehend the nuances within the curriculum to effectively provide the guidance required within the learning environment.
18. Students need to be actively involved and central to the learning process.
19. Utilize the strengths of your generational characteristics to plan your career development for tenure and/or promotion.
20. Become familiar with the policies and procedures of your educational institution, school, and clinical facilities where your students are assigned.
21. Provide feedback by taking an active role on committees at all levels of your institution, using the unique perspectives from your generational cohort.

Multiple Choice Questions

1. The four generation cohorts currently present in the workplace are:
   A. Traditionalists/Veterans, Baby Boomers, Gen Sers, Millennials.
   B. Traditionalists/Veterans, Baby Busters, Gen Xers, Millennials.
   C. Victorians, Baby Boomers, Gen Xers, Millennials.
   D. **Traditionalists/Veterans, Baby Boomers, Gen Xers, Millennials.**

   Rationale:
   The four cohorts currently present in the workplace are the Traditionalists/Veterans, the Baby Boomers, Gen X, and Millennials (Hahn, 2009; Wieck, 2008).

2. The different generations can have an influence on:
   A. **development of teams.**
   B. discouragement.
   C. decreasing efficiency.
   D. management of stress.

   Rationale:
   Hammill (2005) states that generational dissimilarities can influence everything from recruiting and fostering teams to managing change and encouraging, overseeing, and developing efficiency and output.

3. In regard to managing issues, the Baby Boomers tend to rely on:

A. an open-slate approach.
B. group activities.
C. **tested ways.**
D. mentors.

Rationale:

The tested ways are embraced by the Baby Boomers, whereas an open slate for managing the issues is celebrated by the Gen X group. Baby Boomer faculty members must allow the Gen X group to try out new approaches while respecting the teamwork orientation found with the Millennials.

4. Gen X individuals tend to prefer:
   A. **individual work.**
   B. group work.
   C. a mixture of both individual and group work.
   D. neither individual nor group work.

Rationale:

Gen Xers do not like teams and groups since singularity is a main principle in their value system. According to Wieck (2008), "The team orientation of the Millennials is in stark contrast to the more independent-minded Gen X" (p. 27). Millennial individuals desire teams and groups to be used to address the challenges presented in the classroom and clinical sites.

5. The Millennial cohort tends to communicate:
   A. with diplomacy and directness.
   B. **with politeness and active involvement.**
   C. with bluntness and directness.
   D. in a discreet and logical manner.

Rationale:

The Baby Boomers communicate with diplomacy and directness. Millennials desire communication that is polite and active in nature. Gen Xers, in contrast, did not develop as many of the networking skills, thus they expect blunt, immediate messages. See Table 2-4.

6. Gen Xers want messages to be tied to:
   A. goals and aspirations.
   B. consensus statements.
   C. **outcomes.**
   D. interactions.

Rationale:

Another interesting communication aspect is that Gen Xers want the messages tied to the outcomes, whereas Millennials value messages that are connected to goals and aspirations. This focus for the messages could be very valuable as faculty members strive to communicate with the different members within a class. Messages should be directed toward outcomes and goals/aspirations to gain support for the management of the interaction. See Table 2–4.

7. Feedback for Millennials should be:
   A. **tied to goals and provided often.**
   B. tied to freedom from public recognition.
   C. public in nature.
   D. subtle and private in nature.

Rationale:
Gen Xers overall do not want public acknowledgement since they tend to be very private individuals. Feedback to this group should be regular and constructive and should allow for freedom. Millennials want frequent feedback that is tied to their focus on goals and expectations. Communication, feedback, and interactions should concentrate on management and attainment of the goals and expectations established. See Table 2–4.

8. Curricula are viewed as:
   A. conceptual frameworks that are not useful in everyday life.
   B. documents that reflect the students' values and aims.
   C. **written documents used to direct the learning process.**
   D. written documents used to direct the accreditation process.

Rationale:
Each of these definitions implies written documents that are used to direct the learning process. Ironside (2007) takes a slightly different approach to the idea: "The most common agreement seems to be that curriculum is what actually occurs between and among persons in the educational enterprise and not some 'plan' for learning that is reflected in written materials" (p. 78). Curriculum moves from a document into a working process whereby learning can occur.

9. The learning types of item, directive, and rational serve to provide support for:
   A. **technical levels of learning.**
   B. the development of critical thinking.
   C. all types of learning.
   D. everyday learning.

Rationale:
The initial three types of learning (item, directive, and rational) provide a "black-and-white" involvement with materials to be used.

These three levels are considered to be at the technical level of learning. See Table 2-5.

10. Committees composed of members of each generation provide:
    A. dissention and chaos.
    B. **diversity and realism.**
    C. an environment of disagreement.
    D. unrealistic decisions.

    Rationale:
    A mix of the generations for faculty membership on committees allows for creativity and innovation that is realistic and necessary for committee decisions and/or recommendations.

11. Tenure is a process that:
    A. occurs only in university settings.
    B. all faculty members seek.
    C. can be obtained only by the Traditionalist/Veteran generation.
    D. **is based on specific criteria.**

    Rationale:
    Tenure occurs in all educational settings but is not sought by every faculty member. Some generations have characteristics that enhance their ability to achieve the specific criteria established by each school.

12. Promotion provides faculty members a method to:
    A. **gain recognition and a significant increase in salary.**
    B. give only one generation an opportunity to move up a career ladder.
    C. improve their community image.
    D. plan to decrease their stress.

    Rationale:
    Promotion can be viewed as a career ladder used to gain recognition and a higher salary. Promotion is possible for all generations but will require strict adherence to criteria established by individual schools, which may cause stress for some faculty members but motivate others.

13. Policies and procedures are:
    A. a necessary nuisance in all settings.
    B. a method to control faculty input.
    C. **a part of every aspect of the role of faculty members in academia.**
    D. based on "what's always been done" and do not require evidence.

Rationale:
Policies and procedures are a part of every aspect of the role of faculty in academia. Faculty members play an important role in the development, recommendation, and implementation of policies and procedures that must be evidence based.

14. Evidence required for policies and procedures must:
    A. be necessary in only the clinical settings.
    B. not be influenced by changes in the healthcare arena.
    C. **include accurate legal and ethical considerations.**
    D. address only matters that concern students' competence.

Rationale:
Currently, the emphasis is on evidence-based policies and procedures that allow for accurate legal and ethical considerations that are constantly changing as new information, new laws, and ethical situations emerge.

15. Faculty knowledge regarding clinical and educational research is:
    A. required only for faculty members involved in research.
    B. too much for faculty members to handle in today's fast-paced environment.
    C. nice to have but not necessary in the classroom, only in the clinical setting.
    D. **a requirement to provide students with the competencies to practice nursing in a variety of settings.**

Rationale:
All nursing faculty members are required to be cognizant of both clinical and educational research to keep up with the fast pace of health care and education in today's environment while still providing students with the competencies needed to practice nursing in a variety of settings.

DISCUSSION QUESTIONS

1. From the materials provided within the chapter and tables, select at least five to six characteristics that you think must be included in a plan to effectively address the needs and expectations for the different generational groups within a classroom experience.

    Considerations:
    Select several characteristics from each of the columns in Tables 2–1 through 2–4 to help determine a plan for meeting the educational needs related to the different generational groups.

2. From the materials provided within the chapter and tables, select at least five to six characteristics that you think must be included in a plan to effectively address the needs and expectations for the different generational groups within a clinical setting experience.
   Considerations:
   Select several characteristics from each of the columns in Tables 2–1 through 2-4 to help determine a plan for meeting the educational needs related to the different generational groups.
3. From the materials provided within the chapter and tables, select at least five to six characteristics that you think must be included in a plan to effectively address the needs and expectations for the different generational groups within a faculty committee.
   Considerations:
   Drawing from Tables 2–1 and 2–2, develop a plan that you as a chairperson would use to get all of the generational members to participate on the committee in a positive, functional manner.
4. Obtain examples of institutional policies and procedures for tenure and/or promotion. Establish criteria for your school that consider these policies and procedures while providing opportunities for growth of nursing faculty members.
   Considerations:
   Carefully consider the current policies and procedures in place within institutions of higher learning. Investigate which statements within the documents are based upon evidence. Consider what level of evidence would be appropriate for this type of document.
5. You are a faculty member lecturing to a group of junior nursing students in a traditional undergraduate program. A student stands up and loudly curses at a classmate with whom he has been texting. As a Baby Boomer, how would you handle the situation?
   Considerations:
   Consider generational characteristics of yourself as a faculty member, of the student cursing, and of the other students in the room. Also consider civility/incivility issues.

References

Conway, J., & Little, P. (n.d.). *From practice to theory: Reconceptualising curriculum development for PBL*. Australia: University of Newcastle.

Gaylor, D. (2002). Generational differences. Retrieved June 10, 2014, from http://www.chialpha.com/other-resources/127-generations/file.html

Giddens, J. (2010). The concept-based curriculum for nursing education. In L. Caputi (Ed.), *Teaching nursing and the art and science* (Chapter 24, Vol. 1). Glen Ellyn, Illinois: College of DuPage Press.

Hahn, J. (2009). Effectively manage a multigenerational staff. *Nursing Management,* *40*(9), 8–10.

Hammill, G. (2005). Mixing and managing four generations of employees. *FDU Magazine Online.* Retrieved June 10, 2014, from http://www.fdu.edu /newspubs/magazine/05ws/generations.htm

Ironside, P. M. (Ed.). (2007). *On revolutions and revolutionaries: 25 years of reform and innovation in nursing education.* New York, NY: National League for Nursing.

Madeus, G. F., & Stufflebeam, D. L. (1989). *Educational evaluation: The work of Ralph Tyler.* Boston, MA: Kluwer Academic Press.

O'Connor, M. (2009). Social networking and the role of technology in nursing education. *Voice of Nursing Leadership, 7*(6), 8–9.

Ohman, K. (2010). Revitalizing for success with active learning approaches. In L. Caputi (Ed.). *Teaching nursing and the art and science* (Chapter 36, Vol. 1). Glen Ellyn, Illinois: College of DuPage Press.

Oliva, P. F. (1988). *Developing the curriculum* (2nd ed.). Glenview, IL: Scott, Foresman and Company.

Penn, B. K. (2008). *Mastering the teaching role: A guide for nurse educators.* Philadelphia, PA: F.A. Davis Company.

Putre, L. (2013). Generations in the workplace. *Hospitals and Health Networks,* January, 26–31.

Roughton, S. E. (2013). Nursing faculty characteristics and perceptions predicting intent to leave. *Nursing Education Perspectives, 34*(4), 217–231.

Scanlan, C. (2013). Execuitve dialogue: Strategies for managing a generationally diverse workforce. *Hospitals and Health Networks,* October, 47–54.

Sherman, R. O. (2006). Leading a multigenerational nursing workforce: Issues, challenges, and strategies. *OJIN: The Online Journal of Issues in Nursing, 11*(2): Manuscript 2. Available online at http://www.nursingworld.org/Main MenuCategories/ANAMarketplace/ANAPeriodicals/OJIN/TableofContents /Volume112006/No2May06/tpc30_216074.aspx

Speakman, E. (2009). Student-centered, interactive, innovative programs and curricula: Needed to achieve excellence in nursing education. In M. H. Adams & R. M. Valiga (Eds.), *Achieving excellence in nursing education* (Chapter 5). New York, NY: National League for Nursing.

Tolbize, A. (2008). Generational differences in the workplace. In *Research and Training Center on Community Living.* Minneapolis, MN: University of Minnesota Press.

Wieck, K. L. (2008). Managing the millennials. *Nurse Leader, 6*(6), 26–29.

Wieck, K. L., Dols, J., & Northam, S. (2009). What nurses want: The nurse incentives project. *Nursing Economics, 27*(3), 169–177, 201.

Chapter 3

The Teaching Experience in Nursing

Theresa M. "Terry" Valiga and Beth C. Phillips

CHAPTER OBJECTIVES

At the conclusion of this chapter, the learner will be able to:

1. Describe the major tenets of at least three learning theories.
2. Explain how knowledge of the concept and utilization of *learning style/preference* can enhance teacher effectiveness.
3. Trace the evolution of the role of teacher from provider of information/facts (i.e., "sage on the stage") to facilitator of learning (i.e., "guide on the side").
4. Discuss ways in which external factors influence the role of the nurse educator.
5. Articulate one's own philosophy of an approach to teaching and the values influencing that philosophy.
6. Propose strategies to develop one's knowledge and skills related to implementation of the nurse educator role.

KEY TERMS

- Adult learning principles
- Andragogy
- Behavioral learning theory
- Brain-based learning
- Cognitive learning theory
- Collaborative and cooperative learning
- Concept-based thinking
- Constructivist theory of learning
- Educator
- Humanistic
- Interprofessional education
- Learning style/preference
- Pedagogy

- Problem-based learning
- Teacher
- Social learning theory

INTRODUCTION

As noted in the chapter titled *The Role of the Academician*, educators practice in colleges and universities and are expected to be "good citizens of the academy." Such "good citizenship" requires that educators be effective teachers and advisors. They also are responsible for participating in and contributing to the work of committees at the discipline (i.e., nursing) level and at the broader (i.e., department/college or university) level. Educators also are expected to design, implement, and evaluate the curricula in their discipline, taking into account the institution's mission, goals, and degree requirements. In addition, they are responsible for developing, implementing, evaluating, and revising (as needed) policies and procedures related to a number of areas, such as student admission, progression, and graduation; peer review; and tenure and promotion.

Indeed, the responsibilities of an academician are complex and broad. More importantly, they are ever-evolving. This chapter provides an overview of how the role of the academic educator has changed over time, some of the issues that faculty currently face, factors that influence the educator's role, and the uniqueness of the nurse educator role. It is intended to provide a broad context for discussions that follow—discussions related to classroom, online, and clinical teaching; program evaluation; competency assessment; and future directions for nursing education. Finally, it is intended to challenge the reader to "do philosophy" (Greene, 1973) and reflect on her or his values as a teacher and educator.

HISTORICAL BACKGROUND

There have always been **teachers** in our world. Parents teach their children values, skills, and ways of interacting with others. Religious leaders teach us about religious practices and beliefs. Community leaders teach us how we can contribute to the health and viability of our communities. "School marms" teach students about the world in which they live.

Educators, however, are something else. They are the individuals whose professional responsibility and major contribution to society relate to enhancing the total development of learners—their minds, their values, their skills—and to advancing knowledge and understanding in their field. These are individuals who have prepared for the role, who engage in a continual study of how to be most effective in that role, and who provide leadership within the educational community.

From the days of Socrates, educators have lived among us. Socrates, for example, spent his time talking with the youth of ancient Greek society using methods that stimulated them to think in new ways, to consider new possibilities, to contemplate deep issues, and to ponder the future and how they might influence it. There were no structured classrooms, there were no course syllabi, there were no rank or tenure systems, and there were few books from which to seek facts. Instead, knowledge and understanding were gained from deep thinking, and the role of the educator was to stimulate, guide, and challenge such thinking.

As societies evolved and there came to be a growing recognition of the need to educate more individuals who could lead those societies, educational systems became more structured. Tutors were employed to teach the children of aristocrats, and "public" schools were created to teach the children of less noble families. The responsibilities of such tutors or public school teachers were to help students learn to read, write, calculate, and understand the history of their world, which was being documented more carefully through textbooks, research reports, and presentations by experts. In some instances, individuals were prepared—often in an apprentice-type system, where they learned a specific role (e.g., physician, lawyer, clergyman) "at the elbow" of a master in the craft.

The focus of education was on the youth of society, assuming, perhaps, that adults were established in life and had no desire or need to learn. Because the number of children continued to grow, more efficient systems of education were needed. There seemed to be an assumption that all children needed to learn the same thing and in the same way, and that all should progress through this newly formed educational system at the same pace. No attention was paid to individualized learning, self-paced learning, or mastery learning; and those who could not "keep up" because of physical or mental disability, lack of commitment or interest, lack of aptitude to do the work, or inability or unwillingness to follow the rules of the system were "let go."

Those involved in such practices who were true educators, however, began to question the systems that were in place. They reflected on the nature of learning, the conditions that encouraged or got in the way of learning, and the role of the teacher. Theories of learning began to emerge, the role of the teacher/educator began to be more carefully defined, and the larger purposes of schooling began to be articulated.

LEARNING THEORIES AND APPROACHES

Theories of learning can be categorized, generally, into several areas—behavioral, cognitive, constructivist, social, humanistic, and brain-based. Each of these will be explained briefly, and the ways in which our thinking about learning has evolved will be noted.

Behavioral learning theories, espoused by scientists such as Skinner (1974), explained that learning was little more than a response to a stimulus. Learning was thought to be a form of operant conditioning (as articulated by Pavlov), and the role of the teacher was to manipulate the environment and be a "reinforcement machine" by providing rewards for "good" behavior or punishment for "bad" behavior. The basic premise was that a behavior would continue or be extinguished, depending on what was rewarded or punished.

In contrast to this perspective that placed emphasis on external factors, **cognitive learning theories** posited that learning had to do with what went on inside the learner's head. They argued that rewards and punishments were not necessary to facilitate learning, but one would stimulate learning through an environment that presented the learner with disequilibrium, imbalance, and tension. Indeed, scientists such as Gagne (1965) noted that past experiences, perceptions, and ways of incorporating and thinking about information created tension in the learner and affected learning.

Many of us are familiar with the work of Piaget (Atherton, 2009), who focused on cognitive processes and rational approaches to solving problems and how those processes and approaches evolved. Piaget studied children and outlined four stages of cognitive development, the highest of which was achieved by the mid-teen years. He noted that a child acquires knowledge by interacting with his or her physical and psychological environments.

The work of Piaget was challenged, in part, by Perry (1970), who asserted that cognitive/intellectual development is not achieved by the mid-teen years but continues into adulthood and, in fact, happens over and over again when individuals are placed in new situations that require knowledge and understanding they do not possess. Perry outlined a nine-stage model in which an individual moves from a dualistic, right/wrong perspective—where the world and problems in it are thought to have a single right answer known to some authority figure—to a more relativistic perspective, where one can appreciate and accept that different situations or circumstances lead one to hold views and make decisions that may be more varied, realizing that there may be more than one "right answer." One moves along this continuum, Perry said, by being challenged with thinking that is one stage higher than one's current position, while being supported through the cognitive struggles such challenges create.

Perhaps one of the best-known authorities on learning was John Dewey (1916), who proposed that knowledge is acquired through discovery and experimentation and whose work provided the basis for **constructivist theories of learning**. He asserted that if given enough time and guidance, almost anyone could learn anything. According to Dewey, then, the goal of education and educators was/is to actively involve learners in discovering processes and relationships, and giving them enough time and "freedom" to experiment, make mistakes, reflect on those mistakes, and eventually understand and comprehend the material under investigation.

Constructivism is based on experiential learning; that is, knowledge is constructed through real-life experience. It is problem-based, adaptive learning that challenges learners to integrate new knowledge with existing knowledge and allows for creation of original work or innovative procedures. Teachers guided by constructivist theory expect and help learners to be self-directed, creative, and innovative, and to draw upon *all* of the "intelligence" described by Gardner (1999) and explained later in this chapter. Such a theoretical base encourages discovery, hands-on, experiential, collaborative, project-based, and task-based learning, all of which are aligned with experiential learning as described by Kolb (1984).

The idea of active involvement and discovery was expanded by educational theorists such as Bandura (1977), who proposed that individuals learn from observing others and paying attention to what happens to them. Role modeling is important in **social learning theory**, and there is acknowledgement that individuals other than the assigned teacher could be the role models and the sources of learning. The environment for learning and all those in that environment were now identified as significant to learning.

Learning with and through others, as noted by Bandura, is congruent with the need to be more **humanistic**, rather than behavioristic, in our approaches to teaching and learning. As noted by Carl Rogers (1969), teachers need to attend to learners' feelings, draw on their life experiences, and strive to help them grow personally and be fulfilled as individuals. With this perspective in mind, educators construct learning environments in which learners participate completely and have control over what, how, when, and even where they learn. In essence, the educator transitions from being a "sage on the stage" to a "guide on the side," trusting the learner to confront problems in thoughtful ways, be open to changing his or her way of thinking, and engage in critical reflection and self-evaluation. In essence, the learning process is thought to be more significant than the specifics of what is learned.

A focus on the learning process is evident in current research that examines ways in which our brains work and how that influences how we learn, the environments that enhance our learning, the extent to which we retain or lose bits of information, and the ways in which we are able to make connections among what we know. Such **brain-based learning** theories (Jensen, 2008) build on the notions posited in the 1970s regarding left- and right-brain thinking:

> Left-brain thinking was described as analytic, logical, linear, and rulebound. It calls upon mathematical and verbal skills, focuses on parts more so than wholes, and allows us to discriminate and be explicit. This is the paradigm that has dominated our culture in general and our educational systems in particular.
>
> Right-brain thinking was described as artistic, holistic, and integrative. It involves feelings, intuition, and insight, and does not necessarily require verbal or math skills. The right brain allows us to integrate ideas into wholes, which are seen as more important than individual parts, and to look for tacit understanding of situations. This paradigm is culturally suppressed and not particularly evident in our educational systems.

Later, scientists proposed that the brain evolved in three parts: the lower brain, where survival learning occurs; the mid-brain, where emotions reside; and the upper brain, where higher-order thinking takes place. Current brain-based education embraces a more holistic view of the brain—one that is more systems-based and *gestalt* in nature—where the whole is greater than the sum of its parts.

Neuroscientists have done autopsies, experiments, and various types of scans (e.g., MRIs) to conduct research that has implications for improved teaching practices. We are coming to better understand how human learning actually occurs—how the brain processes and retains information. This research has led to the identification of the following core principles to guide brain-based education (Jensen, 2008):

- The brain is a parallel processor that can perform several activities at once.
- The brain perceives wholes and parts simultaneously.
- Information is stored in multiple areas of the brain and can be retrieved through multiple memory and neural pathways.
- Learning engages the whole body; thus, all learning is mind–body in nature.
- Humans' search for meaning is innate.

- The search for meaning comes through patterning.
- Emotions are critical to patterning, and they drive our attention, meaning, and memory.
- Meaning is more important than just information.
- Learning involves focused attention and peripheral perception.
- We have two types of memory: rote and spatial (i.e., knowing things in relation to other things).
- We understand best when facts are embedded in natural spatial memory.
- The brain is social and develops better in concert with other brains.
- Complex learning is enhanced by challenge and inhibited by stress.
- Every brain is uniquely organized.
- Learning is developmental.

A review of this list of core principles would seem to suggest that the theorists discussed earlier were all correct—to some extent. Meaning is important. We learn through focused attention as well as through exploration. Education must attend to the whole student, where learning with others is effective and each learner is unique. Indeed, findings from brain-based research and educational literature in general now embrace much of the work of the pioneers in educational theory.

Such insights from the field of brain-based learning are helping teachers understand the unique approaches to learning exhibited by digital natives (those who have grown up using digital technology) and how to effectively incorporate technology into the learning environments for these individuals (Prensky, 2010). In essence, in the 21st century, learning and technology must be considered together. Wise integration of our evolving and powerful technology demands that we rethink our curricula and our approaches to teaching.

Today, we hear increasing calls for **collaborative and cooperative learning**, and in professional fields like nursing, there are increasing expectations for **interprofessional education** where students in various health disciplines learn with and from one another. We are tasked with providing learners with problems that challenge them to construct new ideas or concepts—based on what they know and what they seek to find out—that allow them to manage those problems. And, among other things, we hear calls for more humanism in education, where learners' feelings and experiences are valued as important and acknowledged to lead to personal growth. The role of the educator who is guided by such perspectives, therefore, is to facilitate learning, rather than be the all-knowing authority who conveys information. So how do we do that as nurse educators?

CURRENT EDUCATIONAL PRACTICES AND CHALLENGES

Humanistic learning perspectives (Rogers, 1969) and brain-based learning theorists (Jensen, 2008) have led educators to see their central purpose as fostering curiosity, enthusiasm, initiative, and responsibility for one's own learning, rather than forcing the mastery of isolated facts. Knowles (1978), the "father" of adult learning, expanded these basic principles to identify characteristics of adult learners that must be attended to if learning is to be successful. Among those **adult learning principles** are the following:

- Allow adult learners to exercise autonomy and self-direction in the learning process.
- Help adult learners achieve the personal learning goals they have identified.
- Ensure that all learning experiences designed for adults are relevant.
- Encourage adult learners to solve practical problems.
- Develop learning experiences that build on the life experiences of adult learners.
- Help adult learners fulfill their potential.

As a result of his work with adult learners, Knowles introduced the concept of **andragogy**, which he defined as the education of adults. He asserted that the andragogical approach is learner-directed, focused on "the tasks of life," immediately applicable, and focused on learning how to learn. This, he proposed, is in direct contrast with the concept of **pedagogy**, which he defined as the education of children. A pedagogical approach calls for the learner to be passive, the subject matter to be central, motivation to come from external rewards, and learning to be focused on the future (i.e., "You'll need to know this someday").

In recent years, the line between andragogy and pedagogy has become blurred, and the term *pedagogy* is now receiving increased attention and being used widely. Educators are realizing that the principles initially outlined for adult learners have significance for any learner, regardless of age. Additionally, the term *pedagogy* has come to refer more to the art and science of teaching than it does to the learners engaged in the teaching/learning process (i.e., children or adults). We also hear talk of *critical pedagogy*, which focuses on helping learners question and challenge the dominant ways of thinking in our society—the beliefs and practices that dominate and the "sacred cows" that are embedded in our educational systems. We acknowledge publicly that learning is not an automatic consequence of teaching, but results from sound pedagogy that has been deliberately designed to promote learning and inspire critical inquisitiveness. Indeed, part of that deliberate design is to base one's educational approaches on research findings, thereby engaging in evidence-based teaching practices.

Today's students are increasingly diverse regarding culture, ethnic background, language ability, and past educational and life experiences. They are technologically savvy and want to be fully engaged with and see relevance in the material being studied. In other words, they want all learning experiences to have meaning for them. Additionally, the students of today have a wide variety of learning styles or preferences.

LEARNING STYLES/PREFERENCES

Learning styles/preferences can be thought of as the unique ways in which individuals perceive, interact with, process, and respond to information and learning situations. They involve cognitive, affective, and physiological factors, and they are thought to be relatively stable over time. All individuals learn through all modalities, but each of us prefers one or several modalities over the others. Therefore, they can be considered "preferences" as well "styles," and the literature often uses these terms interchangeably.

Gardner (1999) labelled these approaches to learning as "intelligences." He originally outlined seven such intelligences:

- Verbal/linguistic: Individuals with this preference prefer to read, write, talk, and share, and they "think in words."
- Mathematical/logical: These learners prefer to work with numbers, solve problems, experiment, ask questions, and think "logically" about solutions to problems or answers to questions.
- Visual/spatial: Learners who have strength in this area of intelligence "think in pictures." They prefer to draw, view pictures, create designs or models, think through mazes, and read.
- Bodily/kinesthetic: Individuals who have strength here prefer to move around, feel or manipulate things, use tools, dance, and use many senses.
- Musical: Learners who have strength in this area of intelligence "think in rhythms," preferring to pick out patterns, make up songs to help them remember, and listen to music.
- Interpersonal: These learners have many friends and like to talk to people, join and work in groups, share material and knowledge, collaborate with others, and resolve conflicts.

- Intrapersonal: Individuals who have strength in this area of intelligence prefer to work alone. They think deeply, are reflective, are comfortable with independent or self-paced activities, are aware of their own values, recognize their own strengths and weaknesses, and work diligently to pursue their personal interests and goals.

Recently, Gardner also noted that some learners are naturalistic (i.e., preferring to engage with nature to enhance learning), and some are existential (i.e., learning best from explorations of the lived experiences of human beings).

Many others have described learning styles. Gregorc (1984) described four types of learners:

- *Concrete/sequential learners* prefer structure and quiet environments.
- *Abstract/sequential learners* are global thinkers and need many facts.
- *Abstract/random learners* anchor their thinking processes in feelings and ask questions randomly, preferring a busy environment.
- *Concrete/random learners* are inquisitive, make intuitive leaps, and are more concerned with "why" than with "how."

Perhaps the most widely used framework is that outlined by Kolb (1984), who identified four learning styles that combine with one another to create a "gestalt" for each individual:

- *Convergent learners* prefer problem solving and practical application; they are the thinkers and doers.
- *Divergent learners* prefer to organize specific relationships into a meaningful whole and generate alternative ideas; they are the feelers and watchers.
- *Assimilative learners* prefer to reason, create models, and "play" with ideas; they are the watchers and thinkers.
- *Accommodative learners* prefer to do things, take risks, and rely on others for specific information; they are the doers and feelers.

Kolb noted that learning is a continuous process that is grounded in experience and is, by its very nature, full of tension.

Despite all of this work related to defining and measuring learning styles, questions and misconceptions remain. First of all, research does not support many of the claims and assumptions underlying learning style constructs. Second, attempting to match teaching strategies with specific learning styles or preferences is very difficult and does not often result in improved learning. Third, most learners are multimodal and learn in a variety of ways. Finally, as education moves toward more cooperative and collaborative learning environments, it may be more important to think about group dynamics and group interaction than the learning styles of individuals within those groups.

As educators, it may be valuable to help learners identify their own preferences for learning so that they can use that information most effectively. However, both we and they must be careful not to "pigeonhole" individuals into a single style and fail to challenge learners through a variety of experiences. We must realize as teachers that we, too, have our own preferences for how we learn. Those preferences influence how we teach. Therefore, it is essential that educators be attuned to designing learning experiences and evaluation methods that "tap into" many senses, are varied and do not result in an advantage or disadvantage for any particular group of students, and reflect the insights gained from pedagogical research efforts.

One thing that does evolve from all of these theories and all of the research on learning is a set of guiding principles that was formulated more than 25 years ago, but still has relevance today. In 1987—in response to criticisms of higher education (e.g., apathetic students, illiterate graduates, incompetent teaching, impersonal campuses)—Chickering and Gamson led a group of educators on a journey to define how students and faculty members could improve undergraduate education. They reviewed 50 years of research on "the way teachers teach and students learn, how students work and play with one another, and how students and faculty talk to each other" (Chickering & Gamson, 1987, p. 1).

The result of this careful and thorough analysis was the formulation of seven principles for good practice in undergraduate education. Though the focus of this work was on the undergraduate experience, the principles also apply to graduate education. In addition, the principles have been supported through research that has been done since the 1987 publication, which attests to their timelessness and significance. Those seven principles for good practice in education are as follows:

- Encourage student–faculty contact: Interaction between teachers and students is the most important factor in engaging students with the material to be studied and facilitating their learning.
- Encourage cooperation among students: Learning is enhanced when it feels like a team effort rather than a solo race. Good learning is collaborative and social, not competitive and isolated.
- Encourage active learning: Learning is not a spectator sport! Students must make what they learn part of themselves, and they do so by being actively engaged.

- Give prompt feedback: Knowing what you know and do not know focuses learning. Learning is dependent on frequent feedback if it is to be sustained, practice if it is to be nourished, and opportunities to use what has been learned if it is to have meaning.
- Emphasize time on task: Learning to use one's time well is critical to effective learning, and students may need help in learning effective time management skills.
- Communicate high expectations: Expecting students to perform well becomes a self-fulfilling prophecy, so teachers must "set the bar high" and then work with students to help them achieve that goal.
- Respect students' diverse talents and ways of learning: Students bring different talents and styles of learning to the learning experience. They need opportunities to show their talents and their intelligences (Gardner, 1999), and to learn in ways that work best for them.

The individual who routinely and thoughtfully employs these principles of good education in combination with insights gained from a study of various learning theories is well positioned to evolve as an effective educator.

COMPETENCIES OF NURSE EDUCATORS

Educators, particularly in nursing, are influenced by many factors, and those factors, in turn, influence curriculum design and our approaches to teaching and learning. Among other factors, accreditation standards and Board of Nursing regulations specify expectations of nursing programs, technological innovations challenge educators to "think outside the box," the power of social media offers new ways to "connect" with students, and policy changes like the Affordable Care Act direct reconceptualization of the role and expectations of nurses. As a result, educators must consider curricula and teaching/learning strategies that provide for interprofessional experiences, **concept-based thinking**, **problem-based learning**, team-based learning, "flipped classrooms," and other emerging phenomena.

Ultimately, educators need to strive to create learning systems that are learner-centered (Weimer, 2013), focus on inquiry, attend to the total development of the learner, actively involve learners, call upon many senses, and challenge learners to think about their thinking. Learning together, educators and learners need to allow for individualized learning, encourage expression and exploration of personal feelings and values, provide opportunities to work and learn in teams, and constantly raise questions about the world around us.

The role of the educator is to facilitate learning, encourage collaboration, help students learn how to learn, empower learners, challenge students to take responsibility for their own learning, and encourage and support a spirit of inquiry. Of course, the educator also gives information, helps learners know where and how to find information on their own, and helps them develop skills to critique and judge the information they find. Educators assess learning needs, create positive and empowering learning environments, provide feedback, coach, inspire, challenge, and genuinely care about the learners and their success. The way in which each of us implements the many dimensions of this role is influenced in large part by our philosophy; thus, it is important for educators to "do philosophy" so that we can be most effective in the role.

What does it mean to "do philosophy," and why is it important? Greene (1973), an educational philosopher, challenged educators to "do philosophy" by taking the risk of thinking about what we do when we teach, and what we mean when we talk of enabling others to learn. She also challenged educators to look, if we can, at our presuppositions and to examine critically the principles underlying what we think and what we say as educators. Although Green laid out these challenges more than 40 years ago, they are still relevant today. In fact, they have been presented over and over again—though with different words or changing emphases—by educational scholars, including Palmer (2007).

In his personal account of his journey as a teacher, Palmer (2007) concluded that "good teachers must live examined lives and try to understand what animates their actions for better and for worse" (p. ix). He talked about the importance of knowing those whom we teach and being connected to them, knowing ourselves because "we teach who we are" (p. xi), and trusting ourselves and all those engaged in the educational enterprise. Palmer's basic premise is that "good teaching cannot be reduced to technique; good teaching comes from the identity and integrity of the teacher" (p. 10). Thus, one's personal philosophy and self-understanding are critical to effective teaching.

Although we often have to ask and answer painful questions to "do philosophy," we must think about what we are doing in order to be most effective at what we are doing. Do we not ask our students to reflect on their values, what drives them, and how the assumptions they make about themselves and others affect the care they provide? We can do no less. Such a "heightened self-consciousness and greater clarity" (Greene, 1973, p. 11) about our philosophy of education and our conceptualizations about teaching and learning will enhance the teaching experience in nursing and help us achieve and continually improve our competence in the role.

The educator competencies we need to develop and continually refine were articulated by the National League for Nursing (2005) and further explicated by Halstead (2007). They include the following:

- *Facilitate learning.* Nurse educators are responsible for creating an environment in classroom, laboratory, and clinical settings that facilitates student learning and the achievement of desired cognitive, affective, and psychomotor outcomes.
- *Facilitate learner development and socialization.* Nurse educators recognize their responsibility for helping students develop a nursing identity and integrate the values and behaviors expected of those who fulfill that role.
- *Use assessment and evaluation strategies.* Nurse educators use a variety of strategies to assess and evaluate student learning in classroom, laboratory, and clinical settings, as well as in all domains of learning.
- *Participate in curriculum design and evaluation of program outcomes.* Nurse educators are responsible for formulating program outcomes, designing curricula that reflect contemporary healthcare trends and prepare graduates to function effectively in the healthcare environment, and designing relevant methods to assess student achievement of program outcomes.
- *Function as a change agent and leader.* Nurse educators function as change agents and leaders to create a preferred future for nursing education and nursing practice.
- *Pursue continuous quality improvement in the nurse educator role.* Nurse educators recognize that their role is multidimensional and that an ongoing commitment to develop and maintain competence in the role is essential.
- *Engage in scholarship.* Nurse educators acknowledge that scholarship is an integral component of the faculty role and that teaching itself is a scholarly activity.
- *Function within the educational environment.* Nurse educators are knowledgeable about the educational environment within which they practice and recognize how political, institutional, social, and economic forces impact their role.

As educators, we must have a sound knowledge base about teaching and learning so that we can most effectively help our increasingly diverse students learn the complexities of what it means to be a nurse and to engage in the practice of nursing. We must continually refine our teaching skills so that we can develop effective case studies, games, simulations, discussions, online resources, lectures, visuals, group projects, and values clarification exercises, as well as lab and clinical learning experiences. We must also continually reflect on how the practice of nursing is changing and ensure that our curricula and learning activities prepare students for those ever-changing roles. For example, with increasing expectations of team practice in clinical settings, educators would do well to integrate more interprofessional learning activities and possibly develop courses in which students from a variety of disciplines learn and grow together.

It also is critical—in this age of "where's the evidence?"—to emphasize the increasing need for all nursing educators to engage in scholarly teaching through the design of evidence-based curricula and the implementation of evidence-based teaching practices. We teach our students the value of evidence-based practice and expect them to integrate that perspective into what they do as nurses. Can we expect less of ourselves? Additionally, more of us need to engage in the scholarship of teaching (Boyer, 1990), which involves studying the effect of our curricula and the learning experiences we create with students and then sharing with the broader nursing education community what we have learned from such study.

Such ongoing development and improvement as educators will occur through deliberate efforts. Just as clinicians continually keep current and advance their knowledge and skills related to practice and the care of the patients for whom they provide care, so, too, must educators keep current and advance their knowledge and skills related to the practice of teaching and the ways they interact with and guide the total development of their students. How can such ongoing development occur?

One route to continued growth as an educator is to enroll in academic courses that are relevant. Courses in innovative teaching practices, the integration of technology into nursing education, building the science of nursing education, new advances in clinical education, the history of and current issues facing higher education, or other relevant topics are all areas that need to be considered.

Additionally, there are many professional conferences offered for educators. Examples of educational activities that can be used to support and prepare the educator include conferences and webinars offered by the National League for Nursing (NLN) and the American Association of Colleges of Nursing (AACN), as well as those offered by the Association for Research in Higher Education, American Association of Higher Education, other national organizations, and individual colleges/universities. At such conferences, educators are introduced to the latest innovative practices and research efforts, and they have opportunities to engage in dialogue with others in that same role.

The number of books about education, teaching strategies, evaluation of learning, brain-based research, and so on is ever-increasing. Nurse educators would do well to engage with this literature outside our own field. In medicine, for example, there is a fair amount of research being done about new curriculum designs, the use of simulation, and collaborative learning. In addition, we can learn a great deal from educators in businesses that have extensive experience with problem-based education, where students work in groups to complete projects that have real-world relevance and use. And literature related to broad education goals—such as those often associated with the arts and humanities—keep educators "grounded" in the fact that our purpose is more than to prepare students for a job or a specific career.

In addition to books, educators can continue to learn and grow in that role through reading a wide variety of journals and/or staying connected with listservs, blogs, websites, or social networking pages that specifically address education issues. **Table 3–1** presents a list of such resources that is by no means all-encompassing, but does point out the variety of resources available to us as educators to learn more about our "craft."

Teachers can further challenge themselves to develop expertise in the educator role by seeking certification in that specialty through the NLN's program (www.nln.org/certification/index.htm). Sitting for the nurse educator certification exam requires reading education-focused literature,

Table 3–1   Selected Education-Focused Journals and Other Resources

Academic Leader	*International Journal of Nursing*
Action Learning: Research and Practice	*Journal of Curriculum Studies*
American Educational Research Journal	*Journal of Further and Higher Education*
Biomedical Education	*Journal of Multicultural Education*
British Educational Research Journal	*Journal of Nursing Education*
Change (publication of the Carnegie Foundation for the Advancement of Teaching)	*National Forum of Applied Educational Research Journal*
Chronicle of Higher Education	*Nurse Educator*
Community College Journal of Research and Practice	*Nursing Education Perspectives* (National League for Nursing journal)
Comparative and International Education	*Phi Delta Kappan* (journal of Phi Delta Kappa)
Education Media, Technology and Science	*Studies in Higher Education*
Education Policy	*Teacher Education*
Education Scholarship (online)	*Teachers & Teaching*
Educational Action Research	*Teaching in Higher Education*
Educational Researcher	*The Internet and Higher Education*

engaging in dialogue with colleagues about teaching and learning, and thinking deeply about our role as educators. Receiving such certification attests to one's evolving expertise as an educator. With certification comes the expectation that the educator be a change agent, seeking out ways to improve programs, curricula, and teaching methodologies. This is a dynamic certification; it is not one that is accomplished and set aside, but one that inspires further seeking of best practices, challenging the status quo in the profession for the betterment of nursing education and ultimately patient care.

Certainly, another way to continue to develop one's mastery as a teacher is to seek out a mentor or seek help from and dialogue with colleagues who have expertise in education. Think about contacting one of the Fellows in the Academy of Nursing Education, or one of the individuals who participated in the NLN/Johnson & Johnson Faculty Leadership and Mentoring Program, or someone who has been inducted into the American Academy of Nursing because of her or his sustained and significant contributions to nursing education. You might also consider contacting an author whose ideas truly "resonate" with your own passions about a mentor relationship or collaboration. You might consider applying to participate in programs sponsored by the NLN's Leadership Institute (www.nln.org/facultyprograms/leadershipinstitute.htm), Sigma Theta Tau International's Nurse Faculty Leadership Academy (www.nursingsociety.org/LeadershipInstitute/nursefaculty/Pages/default.aspx), or any number of other such initiatives, to receive personalized and individualized guidance on your journey toward excellence in nursing education. Finally, you will want to continue to challenge yourself, always remain open to change, and be enthusiastic about the opportunities before you as an educator.

As educators, we must continually pursue excellence as teachers, facilitators of learning, pedagogical scholars, educational leaders, and citizens of the academy. This lifelong journey will take us to new places, and we will continue to be energized and grow. After all, we are adult learners ourselves!

SUMMARY THOUGHTS

In this chapter, we have explored various theories of learning and examined how an understanding of the concept of "learning style or preference" can enhance our effectiveness as teachers. We have followed the evolution of the educator role from that of a "sage on the stage" (who provides a great deal of information, focuses on the content more so than on the student, and assumes that if something was taught, it also was learned) to that of a "guide on the side." The guide challenges students to think deeply, engenders in them a spirit of inquiry, helps them understand who they are as human beings and evolving nurses, and allows them to have more control over the educational experience.

We hope you have been challenged to "do philosophy" and reflect deeply on the insights to which such self-exploration leads. Knowing who we are as human beings and what we value will strengthen our ability to guide students on their journey to reach personal and professional goals. It serves to ensure that we do not attempt to "create students in our own image."

Finally, this discussion has outlined the complexity of the educator role and the multiple competencies associated with that role. It is hoped that you have been stimulated to outline a plan for the ongoing development of the knowledge and skills you need as an educator, as well as to consider a scholarly path you might pursue that will enable you to contribute to the evolving science of nursing education.

The nurse educator role and the teaching experience in nursing are both challenging and incredibly rewarding. Do not hesitate to allow your passion for teaching to be evident to students, and do not hesitate to continually question how we can improve the nursing education experience for students and faculty.

SUMMARY POINTS

1. "Good citizenship" requires that educators be effective teachers and advisors.
2. Educators are expected to design, implement and evaluate the curricula in their discipline, taking into account the institution's mission, goals, and degree requirements.
3. Faculty members are responsible for developing, implementing, evaluating, and revising (as needed) policies and procedures related to a number of areas, such as student admission, progression, and graduation; peer review; and tenure and promotion.
4. Educators are different from teachers. They are the individuals whose professional responsibility and major contribution to society relate to enhancing the total development of learners—their minds, their values, their skills—and to advancing knowledge and understanding in their field.
5. Faculty members must provide learners with problems that challenge them to construct new ideas or concepts—based on what they know and what they seek to find out—that allow them to manage those problems.

6. Learning styles/preferences can be thought of as unique ways in which individuals perceive, interact with, process, and respond to information and learning situations.

7. Educators need to strive to create learner-centered systems that focus on inquiry, attend to the total development of the learner, actively involve learners, call upon many senses, and challenge learners to think about their thinking.

8. The role of the educator is to facilitate learning, encourage collaboration, help students learn how to learn, empower learners, challenge students to take responsibility for their own learning, and encourage and support a spirit of inquiry.

TIPS FOR NURSE EDUCATORS

1. Use a variety of teaching strategies in order to "connect" with the diversity of students and the array of learning styles/preferences and intelligences they present.

2. Question the assumptions you make about students and teachers that influence what you do as a teacher.

3. Read extensively about teaching/learning and incorporate new ideas into what you do as a teacher.

4. Ensure that your teaching practices are based on evidence, rather than solely on tradition and past practice.

5. Use a variety of evaluation methods that attend to affective-domain learning, as well as the cognitive and psychomotor domains.

6. Reflect carefully and often on what you do as a teacher and how it can be improved to best serve students.

7. Seek out colleagues or mentors with whom you can engage in serious dialogue about teaching, learning, curriculum development, implementing the educator role, and issues in higher education.

8. Allow your passion for teaching to shine for students and faculty colleagues.

MULTIPLE CHOICE QUESTIONS

1. Which of the following learning activities would most likely appeal to a student whose strength is Gardner's visual/spatial intelligence?
   A. Study groups, discussion boards, and group projects.
   B. Independent work and self-paced activities.
   C. **Drawing, working with colors, pictures, and puzzles.**
   D. Reading, writing, and debating.

Rationale:

Visual/spatial intelligence refers to an individual's strength in using visual materials to learn (e.g., maps, charts, pictures).

2. Which of the following principles related to learning styles is a correct statement?

A. Learning styles cannot be determined through any form of measurement.

B. **We teach how we learn.**

C. Knowing one's own learning style interferes with effective learning.

D. Teachers should use strategies that best match the learning style that is preferred by most students in the class.

Rationale:

Learning styles can be measured, and when learners know their own learning style, they can use their strengths to enhance learning. Teachers should use a variety of strategies in order to meet the needs of all learners and to ensure that the strategies used are not overly influenced by our own preferences, because we do tend to teach how we learn.

3. Which of the following sets of characteristics best describes left-brain thinking?

A. **Sequential, rule-bound, logical.**

B. Analytic, tacit, linear.

C. Nonverbal, integrative, emotional.

D. Artistic, parts more important than the whole, synthesis.

Rationale:

Characteristics such as artistic, emotional, tacit, and synthesis are characteristics of right-brain thinking.

4. The concrete/random learner described by Gregorc prefers a trial-and-error approach, with breakthroughs through intuitive insights. Which of the following learning activities would be *least* likely to be preferred by this kind of learner?

A. Independent study.

B. Computer games and simulations.

C. Model development.

D. **Lecture.**

Rationale:

The concrete/random learner likes a stimulus-rich environment and thrives on competition. A lecture would not engage this learner to the extent the other activities would.

5. Which of the following is the most significant "driving force" when deciding what learning activities to design to facilitate student learning?
   A. Students' learning styles.
   B. Teacher's learning style.
   C. **Learning objectives.**
   D. Experience with using a particular activity.

   Rationale:
   The goals or objectives of a learning experience are the most important factors that guide the development or selection of teaching strategies. Many other factors (such as those noted in the options above) can and should be taken into consideration, but the goals of learning must take priority.

6. Which of the following statements is most closely aligned with the perspectives on teaching and learning expressed by John Dewey?
   A. **Learners are motivated by intrinsic goals and the opportunity to learn through discovery.**
   B. Learners are motivated by rewards, reinforcement, and punishment.
   C. Advancement in one's cognitive development occurs through being challenged with thinking that is one stage higher than one's current position.
   D. Individuals learn through observing others and what they do.

   Rationale:
   Rewards and punishment reflect Skinner's perspectives, one-plus stage challenging reflects Perry's model, and social learning is congruent with Bandura's theory. Dewey's perspective promotes intrinsic goal motivation and discovery.

7. Currently, the term *pedagogy* is most closely aligned with which of the following statements?
   A. Teaching should be learner-directed and focus on "the tasks of life."
   B. Learners are passive and subject matter is central.
   C. **Teaching is both an art and a science.**
   D. Teachers should encourage cooperation among students.

   Rationale:
   Pedagogy no longer refers to the teaching of children, but to the art and science of teaching.

8. Which of the following *Principles of Good Practice in Undergraduate Education* (Chickering & Gamson, 1987) is identified as the most

important factor in engaging students with the material to be studied and facilitate their learning?

A. Give prompt feedback.
B. Communicate high expectations.
C. Encourage cooperation among students.
D. **Encourage student–faculty contact.**

Rationale:

Though the first three responses are among the *Principles*, the
authors note that research indicates that student–faculty contact is
the most significant factor in engaging students.

9. When an educator "does philosophy" (Greene, 1973), he or she takes
the risk of doing which of the following?

A. Receiving less-than-positive feedback from peers.
B. **Discovering that what we say we value as teachers is not
always congruent with what we do in that role.**
C. Failing when a new teaching approach is used.
D. Preparing students who are unable to pass the licensing
examination.

Rationale:

"Doing philosophy" is an introspective process that leads us to
think carefully about who we are, what "drives" us, and whether our
actions/behaviors match our words or expressed values.

10. Which of the following is *not* a nurse educator competency articulated by the National League for Nursing (2005)?

A. Function as a change agent and leader.
B. **Maintain certification in a clinical specialization.**
C. Engage in scholarship.
D. Use assessment and evaluation strategies.

Rationale:

The NLN's list of nurse educator competencies notes that the individual pursues continuous quality improvement in the nurse educator role, which may include maintaining some level of expertise
and/or certification in a clinical specialty area, but the NLN does
not specify that such certification is essential for all nurse educators.

DISCUSSION QUESTIONS

1. Who is the "adult learner"? How do approaches to teaching need to
be modified when dealing with an adult learner population?

Considerations:
Adult learners are self-directed, goal oriented, and problem oriented, and they want learning to be relevant. Learning experiences designed by the teacher should encourage students to draw on their past experiences to solve new problems, and the problems presented should be "real-life" challenges so they have relevance.

2. Which theories of learning are most congruent with your own philosophy of education? Which are most incongruent? Which of those theories do you think have (or would have) the greatest influence on you as a teacher?

   Considerations:
   Highlight major themes of various learning theories. Thoughtfully reflect on their meaning and which are most closely aligned with your own philosophy. Discuss how a learning theory influences the role of the learner, the role of the teacher, the teaching strategies used, learner/teacher relationships, the nature of the learning environment, and the evaluation methods used.

3. Given that a teacher may know individual students' learning styles/preferences, is it possible to accommodate those individual preferences when that teacher is involved with many students during the course of a semester or program? If so, how can you avoid teacher "burnout"? If not, what's all the "fuss" about learning styles/preferences, and why bother to find out what they are?

   Considerations:
   Summarize the major learning styles. Discuss identification of learning styles/preferences through self-assessment, completion of tools/instruments, or dialogue and reflection with others (e.g., the teacher). Discuss the usefulness of knowing one's style to "play to one's strengths." Consider the need to match teaching strategies and learning experiences with learning goals, more so than with learning styles.

4. Some assert that nursing faculty want students to be humanistic with patients, yet they themselves are behavioristic with students. What do the two perspectives mean in the context of education, and why might this phenomenon occur in nursing?

   Considerations:
   Reflect on the meaning of humanism and behaviorism in the context of education. Develop insights regarding the realities of nursing education (e.g., licensure examination, accreditation standards).

TEACHING SCENARIO

Judy Mack is a new faculty member who has been assigned to teach a lower-division (i.e., freshman or sophomore) course on health assessment at a nearby baccalaureate nursing program. She must teach the theory/lab course within the framework of the approved course objectives, but otherwise she has the freedom to develop the course in any way she sees fit. Judy is excited about the possibilities this course presents and wants to implement all of what she learned in graduate school about teaching and learning.

The sophomore students who will be enrolling in the course have completed a one-credit "Introduction to Nursing as Profession" course as freshmen as well as foundational courses in the biological and social sciences. Judy realizes that each of the 30 students in her class has developed her or his own approach to learning, and she is hopeful that she can satisfy everyone's needs, including her own.

- How can Judy identify each student's learning style/preference without using large amounts of class time?
- What learning styles/preferences should Judy expect to find among this student group that ranges in age from 19 to 52 years and includes males and females, several students whose basic education was completed outside the United States, and students who have transferred to this school from another nursing program?

Judy decides to structure the course as follows: lecture on one aspect of assessment on Monday, demonstrate it in lab on Wednesday, remind students of the hours the lab will be open for them to practice the assessment, and test them on that aspect of assessment the following Wednesday in lab. She is careful to correlate the class session with the "Anatomy and Physiology" content the students are learning simultaneously and is patient in answering individual students' questions about how this assessment knowledge will help their nursing practice.

- What learning principles has Judy applied appropriately?
- What learning principles has Judy violated?
- How could Judy better structure this course to fulfill more principles of learning and meet a wider array of learning styles/preferences?

Judy has now been asked to teach a similar course for registered nurses through the school's continuing education department.

- What modifications should Judy make in the course, given this particular learner population?
- What principles of adult learning are evidenced by these modifications?

BIBLIOGRAPHY

Amerson, R. (2006). Energizing the nursing lecture: Application of the theory of multiple intelligence learning. *Nursing Education Perspectives, 27*(4), 194–203.

Ard, N. (2009). Essentials of learning. In C. M. Shultz (Ed.), *Building a science of nursing education: Foundations for evidence-based teaching/learning* (pp. 25–131). New York, NY: National League for Nursing.

Ashley, J. A., & LaBelle, B. M. (1976). Education for freeing minds. In J. A. Williamson (Ed.), *Current perspectives in nursing education—The changing scene* (Vol. I, pp. 50–65). St. Louis, MO: Mosby.

Carter, S. L. (1978). The nurse educator: Humanist or behaviorist? *Nursing Outlook, 26*(9), 554–557.

Coffield, F., Moseley, D., Hall, E., & Ecclestone, K. (2004). Learning styles and pedagogy in post-16 learning: A systematic and critical review. Retrieved March 1, 2014, from http://www.voced.edu.au/print/content/ngv13692

Glenn, D. (2009, December 16). Matching teaching style to learning style may not help students. *The Chronicle of Higher Education*. Retrieved August 6, 2014, from http://chronicle.com/article/Matching-Teaching-Style-to/49497/

Greer, A. G., Pokorny, M., Clay, M. C., Brown, S., & Steele, L. L. (2010). Learner-centered characteristics of nurse educators. *International Journal of Nursing Education Scholarship, 7*(1), Article 6.

Hartley, M. P. (2010). Experiential learning using Kolb's cycle of learning [Syllabus Selection]. *Journal of Nursing Education, 49*(2), 120.

Honigsfeld, A., & Dunn, R. (2006, Winter). Learning-style characteristics of adult learners. *The Delta Kappa Gamma Bulletin*, 14–17, 31.

Jewell, M. L. (1994). Partnership in learning: Education as liberation. *Nursing & Health Care, 15*(7), 360–364.

Kohlberg, L., & Mayer, R. (1972). Development as the aim of education. *Harvard Educational Review, 42*(4), 449–496.

Kostovich, C., Poradzisz, M., Wood, K., & O'Brien, K. L. (2007). Learning style preference and student aptitude for concept maps. *Journal of Nursing Education, 46*(5), 225–231.

McDaniels, O. B. (1983). Existentialism and pragmatism: The effect of philosophy on methodology of teaching. *Journal of Nursing Education, 22*(2), 62–66.

Philosophy of teaching statements: Examples and tips on how to write a teaching philosophy statement. (2009). *Faculty Focus*, Special Report, May 2009. Madison, WI: Magna Publications.

Robinson, F. P. (2009). Servant teaching: The power and promise for nursing education. *International Journal of Nursing Education Scholarship, 6*(1), Article 5.

Smoyak, S. A. (1978). Teaching as coaching. *Nursing Education, 26*(6), 361–363.

Tabak, N., Adi, L., & Eherenfeld, M. (2003). A philosophy underlying excellence in teaching. *Nursing Philosophy, 4*, 249–254.

Thompson, C., & Crutchlow, E. (1993). Learning style research: A critical review of the literature and implications for nursing education. *Journal of Professional Nursing, 9*(1), 34–40.

References

Atherton, J. S. (2009). Learning and teaching: Piaget's developmental theory. Retrieved March 1, 2014, from http://www.learningandteaching.info/learning/piaget.htm

Bandura, A. (1977). *Social learning theory.* Englewood Cliffs, NJ: Prentice Hall.

Boyer, E. L. (1990). *Scholarship reconsidered: Priorities of the professoriate.* Princeton, NJ: The Carnegie Foundation for the Advancement of Teaching.

Chickering, A. W., & Gamson, Z. F. (1987). Seven principles for good practice in undergraduate education. *The Wingspread Journal, 9*(2), 1–5. Retrieved March 1, 2014, from http://files.eric.ed.gov/fulltext/ED282491.pdf

Dewey, J. (1916). *Democracy and education: An introduction to the philosophy of education.* New York, NY: The Free Press.

Gagne, R. M. (1965). *The conditions of learning.* New York, NY: Holt, Reinhart & Winston.

Gardner, H. (1999). *Intelligence reframed: Multiple intelligences for the 21st century.* New York, NY: Basic Books.

Greene, M. (1973). *Teacher as stranger: Educational philosophy in the modern age.* Belmont, CA: Wadsworth.

Gregorc, A. F. (1984). *Gregorc Style Delineator: Development, technical, and administration manual.* Columbia, CT: Gregorc Associates.

Halstead, J. A. (2007). *Nurse educator competencies: Creating an evidence-based practice for nurse educators.* New York, NY: National League for Nursing.

Jensen, E. P. (2008). *Brain-based learning: The new paradigm of teaching* (2nd ed.). Thousand Oaks, CA: Sage Publications.

Knowles, M. S. (1978). *The adult learner: A neglected species* (2nd ed.). Houston, TX: Gulf.

Kolb, D. A. (1984). *Experiential learning: Experience as the source of learning and development.* London: Prentice Hall.

National League for Nursing. (2005). *Nurse educator core competencies.* New York, NY: Author. Retrieved March 1, 2014, from http://www.nln.org/facultyprograms/competencies/educator_core_competencies.htm

Palmer, P. (2007). *The courage to teach: Exploring the inner landscape of a teacher's life* (10th anniversary edition). San Francisco, CA: Jossey-Bass.

Perry, W. (1970). *Forms of intellectual and ethical development in the college years: A scheme.* New York, NY: Holt, Reinhart & Winston.

Prensky, M. (2010). *Teaching digital natives: Partnering for real learning.* Newbury Park, CA: Corwin.

Rogers, C. R. (1969). *Freedom to learn.* Columbus, OH: Charles E. Merrill.

Skinner, B. F. (1974). *About behaviorism.* New York, NY: Vintage Books.

Tosteson, D. C. (1979). Learning in medicine. *New England Journal of Medicine, 301*(13), 690–694.

Weimer, M. (2013). *Learner-centered teaching: Five key changes to practice* (2nd ed.). San Francisco, CA: Jossey-Bass.

Chapter 4

Ethics in Teaching

Carol Boswell and Sharon Cannon

CHAPTER OBJECTIVES

At the conclusion of this chapter, the learner will be able to:

1. Discuss policies impacted by legislative and regulatory agencies.
2. Distinguish the differences in HIPAA and FERPA in relation to ethics in nursing education.
3. Discuss ethics.
4. Discuss ethical issues in teaching in higher education.

KEY TERMS

- Accreditation Commission for Education in Nursing
- Care ethics
- Commission on Collegiate Nursing Education
- Commission for Nursing Education Accreditation
- Deontology
- Ethics
- FERPA
- HIPAA
- The Joint Commission
- Legislative policy
- Regulatory policy
- Rights ethical theory
- Utilitarianism
- Virtue ethical theory

INTRODUCTION

Nurses and nurse educators are challenged daily by legal and ethical considerations in their practice. Nurse educators are in a unique position of having to balance legal/ethical issues from two perspectives: as a nurse and as a nurse educator. The two are intertwined and yet, at times, are separate.

There are legal/ethical issues unique, yet similar, to each, such as laws that govern the release of students' grades to parents and the restriction of patient information to families. The only similarity in this example is release of information, but the actual laws and ethics for each are different in the enactment, audience, and setting. The nurse at the bedside does not need to know the information disclosure law for students, but the nurse educator must be cognizant of both.

To fully understand the relationship of ethics to legal aspects of nursing and nursing education, a definition of each is in order. Sumner (2011) indicated that the term **ethics** comes from the Greek word *ethos* and reflects societal standards. The term *legal* pertains to laws that are established by society. Keep in mind that though primitive societies such as remote tribes in South America can differ greatly from a populations, say, in the United States, each has norms for standards of behavior. Violations in either society bring repercussions for unacceptable behaviors. Aiken (2004) states that "ethics are declarations of what is right or wrong and what ought to be" (p. 100). Regardless of societal sophistication, there are governing bodies and guidelines relating to acceptable behavior. In nursing and nursing education, legal and ethical standards guide nursing practice and education.

LEGISLATIVE AND REGULATORY POLICY

Many nurses, regardless of their practice setting, equate legislation with politics, and thus ignore the huge impact that legislation has upon their practice. Sad to say, but the fact that few nurses are informed voters (if they vote at all) is common knowledge. Boswell, Cannon, and Miller (2005) suggested political involvement is a responsibility, not a privilege. Laws (**legislative policy**) and regulations (**regulatory policy**) are embedded in nursing practice and nursing education. Laws come from city, county, state, and national policy. Rules and regulations follow the same path by establishing guidelines based upon laws. Both have governing bodies to carry out the required standard. In addition, professions such as medicine, nursing, pharmacy, and so forth have codes of ethics and governing bodies to regulate the profession. For example, many national nursing organizations have a code of ethics that involves doing no harm to patients under nursing care. State Boards of Nursing, whose sole purpose is to protect patients, are present to regulate nursing practice and nursing education. To further comprehend legislative/regulatory policies and their interactions in nursing education, an examination of two legislative acts is necessary.

HIPAA AND FERPA

The Health Insurance Portability and Accountability Act (**HIPAA**) was enacted in 1996 to protect health information through a "privacy rule" to establish standards about the use and disclosure of health information (Department of Health and Human Services, n.d.). The final form of the Privacy Rule was published in 2002. HIPAA determines:

1. who is covered,
2. what information is protected,
3. principles for use and disclosure,
4. permitted use and disclosure,
5. authorized uses and disclosure,
6. limiting uses and disclosures to the minimum necessary,
7. notice and other individual rights,
8. administrative requirements,
9. organizational options,
10. personal representative and minors,
11. state laws,
12. enforcement and penalties for noncompliance, and
13. compliance dates.

Obviously, HIPAA has huge implications for nurses and has become more complex with the advent of new methods of communication, especially computer technology such as emails, iPods, texting, and blogs. Communication is no longer limited to what is faxed or talked about in the hallways and elevators, but has expanded through technology to include multiple new modalities. This affects the nurse educator in the areas of developing case studies, conducting pre- and postclinical conferences, creating care plans, reviewing student logs/journals and student papers, conducting simulation lab scenarios, and giving lectures, to name just a few. Care must be taken that patient identification is not apparent regardless of the instructional methodology employed in the classroom, clinical setting, or online courses by faculty or students.

The Family Educational Rights and Privacy Act (**FERPA**) was enacted in 1974 and is commonly known as the Buckley Amendment. This law protects the privacy of student education records and applies to all schools receiving federal funds. Prior to the age of 18, a student's parents have the right to their child's education records. After the age of 18, the rights transfer to the student (Department of Education, n.d.). FERPA spells out:

1. who is eligible to receive information,

2. how to correct inaccurate or misleading information,
3. how student information can be released,
4. the type of information that may be disclosed without consent,
5. notification about directory information with allowances for a non-disclosure request, and
6. annual notification of rights under FERPA.

FERPA appears simple but is extremely complex and far reaching. The use of the Internet, external regulations, and accrediting bodies all play a major role in how FERPA affects students. Guidelines state where and how grades can be posted. For instance, posting grades on a bulletin board outside a faculty member's office isn't allowed. In addition, use of a student's identification number or social security number is a violation.

Faculty actions must be based on legally sanctioned facts. Faculty are being compared to national standards rather than the prior "locality rules" (Gumby, 2008). In other words, faculty members cannot act on whether or not they like a student, or claim that the local norm allows faculty members to act in contradiction to standards set by national organizations/agencies.

Faculty, as well as students, can be held accountable for clinical negligence. "Do no harm" to patients can also be extended to faculty to protect students from harm related to exposure to violence and needlesticks. Another consideration that has changed over the years is that students do not practice under their faculty's nursing licensure, and faculty may need to intervene to protect the patients.

In addition, FERPA has implications for students with disabilities. In this instance, the student must provide evidence and documentation of the disability with proposed accommodations. Caution is advised here depending on the disability and requirements necessary to complete assignments in the clinical setting. Faculty and school administrators must work to effectively manage those disabilities that are documented. Some examples of the different means that have been used are (1) longer time periods to complete examinations, (2) readers for those individuals who are hearing or sight impaired, and (3) computers provided for those with physical disabilities.

As in all education systems, policies and procedures must exist to allow students due process for academic dishonesty and failing grades and to protect them in unsafe clinical settings. HIPAA and FERPA apply to both students and patients. A school's policies and procedures must incorporate all rights for both students and their patients.

REGULATORY AGENCIES

Accreditation is addressed in the chapter titled *Program Evaluation*, but its influence on the education of nurses and the faculty role must be mentioned at this point. **The Joint Commission** accredits healthcare organizations and sets standards required for consumers of health care, especially hospitals and clinics where nurses are employed. Thus, faculty members are required to maintain competence in nursing practice to be able to teach students in these settings. Without accreditation, hospitals are ineligible for federal funds and are often not financially viable, thus lacking high standards of care. There are several educational organizations that set standards for higher education institutions. They are organized by region and are designated as a commission, such as the Southern Association of Colleges and Schools Commission on Colleges or the Northwest Commission on Colleges and Universities. These commissions accredit colleges and universities that have schools of nursing. Colleges and universities without accreditation are also ineligible for federal funds, especially for Pell Grants, traineeships, and so forth, which can result in students being unable to afford an education in nursing.

Schools of nursing are also accredited by two national nursing organizations. The National League for Nursing (NLN) accredits all levels of nursing programs through the **Accreditation Commission for Education in Nursing** (ACEN), which was formally called the National League for Nursing Accrediting Commission (NLNAC). The NLN is currently developing an innovative accreditation commission called the **Commission for Nursing Education Accreditation** (CNEA). The American Association of Colleges of Nursing (AACN) provides accreditation for baccalaureate and graduate nursing programs through the **Commission on Collegiate Nursing Education** (CCNE).

The two most important regulatory agencies for nursing are the National Council of State Boards of Nursing (NCSBN) and the Board of Nursing (BON) of each state, commonwealth, and/or territory. The NCSBN states its purpose as follows: "To ensure public protection, each jurisdiction requires candidates for licensure to meet set requirements that include passing an examination that measures the competencies needed to perform safely and effectively as a newly licensed, entry-level practical/vocational nurse (LPN/VN)" (NCSBN, 2014, p. 3).

The second regulatory agency is each state's BON. State BONs protect and promote the welfare of their citizens. Unfortunately, many nurses think that their BON is for nurses, but it is not; BONs regulate the practice of nursing and the approval of nursing education programs. Each state has laws with rules and regulations for the practice of nursing, often derived from the Nursing Practice Act of the state. The services of BONs range from licensing school approval to enforcement of laws to provision of information. Faculty members must have a current, valid license to practice nursing and the appropriate education credentials to teach nursing.

As can be seen, legislative/regulatory agencies, HIPAA, and FERPA, along with accrediting bodies, are integral to the role of faculty. Each of these affects ethical issues in higher education regarding the practice of nursing and the teaching of nursing.

ETHICS

According to Rainbow (2002), "Ethical theories and principles are the foundation of ethical analysis because they are the viewpoints from which guidance can be obtained along the pathway to a decision" (para. 1). When ethics are used effectively, decisions are based upon specific guidelines and information. The different ethical theories and principles provide the societal standards on which decisions can be made. O'Connor (2010) states that "learning to acknowledge personal moral views, to analyze and evaluate moral opinions, to reflect on moral situations, to defend moral choices, and to work with other healthcare team members on resolutions of ethical/moral situations and dilemmas is critical to the development of the ethical nurse" (p. 621). Nurses and nurse educators must accept the responsibility for incorporating personal moral views, opinions, situations, and choices into the day-to-day experiences of peers and students. All aspects within the delivery of health care are transformed by an understanding and acknowledgement of the moral/ethical obligations that the nursing profession embraces.

Nelson (2003) further supports these ideas because the ethical principles that provide the foundation for ethical decision making are founded upon moral values. These subtle moral ideals are not enforceable by any laws. The principles subsumed within ethical decisions are not laws in and of themselves, but are the foundational components that guide the behaviors used when confronted by situations outside the control of laws. The six major ethical principles are autonomy, veracity, nonmalfeasance, confidentiality, beneficence, and justice. Each of these tenets is used to maneuver toward an outcome when a situation is not covered by legal precedents.

As one begins to investigate the different principles foundational for ethical decisions, the first one to be considered is autonomy. According to Nelson (2003), autonomy is related to the idea that each of us has the right to self-determine the aspects within our lives. Laws have been established to protect the ability for individuals to choose independently concerning situations encountered. All persons are understood to have the right and responsibly to make free choices about the decisions that are key to their private lives. The independent control over individual existence is held as a critical principle for the uniqueness of each person. Rainbow (2002) states that "each man deserves respect, because only he has had those exact life experiences and understands his emotions, motivations, and body in such an intimate manner" (para. 5). These emotions, motivations, and life experiences shape how an individual comes to the unique decisions encountered in the ethical dimension. Within the principles of autonomy, each individual is allowed to pull from his or her culture and environment when making those decisions not addressed by legal rules.

A second principle of ethical decision making is the concept of veracity. Veracity is understood to represent truth telling. The confines of ethical decisions are closely linked with informed decision making and informed consent (Nelson, 2003). For each decision with which a person is confronted, the expectation is that truthful information will be provided by all involved parties, so the affected individual can use the entirety of the information to make the appropriate decision. All decisions rest upon the idea that the individuals involved in the determination have all of the necessary information to make a full and complete decision about the situation encountered. Without factual and complete information, the effectiveness of the decision-making process is compromised.

Another tenet in ethical decision making is the concept of nonmalfeasance. This is a busy term that basically means "do no harm." Within health care particularly, the idea of doing no harm to individuals is paramount. This principle of not harming someone is foundational in ethical aspects and is vital to the fabric of legal determination. Nonmalfeasance is one of the key aspects when negligence and/or malpractice issues are raised. According to Rainbow (2002), individuals could "reasonably argue that people have a greater responsibility to 'do no harm' than to take steps to benefit others" (para. 4). Someone who chooses to harm a person tends to be directly in opposition to the fabric of societal standards. In all situations, the expectation is that individuals will endeavor to not harm others. Though this aspect is not always possible, the thought is that in all situations the imperative is to not do any harm, or at least as little harm as possible.

A fourth principle used for ethical decision making is the idea of confi-dentiality. Confidentiality is viewed as the securing of all privileged infor-mation that is obtained as a result of functioning in a professional capacity with a patient or client. In each and every situation, the maintaining of private information in a secure and protected manner is viewed as the stan-dard. Materials and/or information gained as a consequence of providing care to an individual is considered to be privileged communication. For all information controlled due to the manner or setting in which it was collected, the protection and privacy of the information must be closely guarded. Within the arena of ethical decision making, the materials gained from this type of discussion remain the sole property of the patient and/ or client.

Another aspect of ethical decision making is the concept of beneficence. Frequently, this component is viewed as "doing good." Rainbow (2002) states that "this principle stipulates that ethical theories should strive to achieve the greatest amount of good because people benefit from the most good" (para. 2). For each situation, the focus is expected to be on the actions that will bring about the greatest good or most beneficial outcome for those involved.

The final principle subsumed under ethical decision making is the idea of justice. Justice is viewed as the fairness of the situation. This concept entails striving to ensure equality for all individuals in regard to goods, ser-vices, and protection. Consistency within the determination of decisions for each and every individual is the mind-set when considering a decision to be founded on justice. When resolving ethical situations, basing deci-sions on a consistent logical foundation is imperative and essential.

After carefully considering the foundational principles utilized within ethical theories, a discussion of the different ethical theories can be under-taken. Books have been written on the different ethical theories; thus, an in-depth dialogue concerning these theories is outside the scope of this chapter. An overview of the different theories will be provided: deontology, utilitarianism, virtue ethics, care ethics, and rights ethics. Each of these theories considers the ethical situation from a different approach, result-ing in discrete management of the state of affairs.

Deontology for ethical considerations is founded on rules. Deontologi-cal theory obliges the addressing of any ethical situation based on the idea that correctness originates from rules and duty (O'Connor, 2010; Rainbow, 2002). The upholding of a person's obligation is the foundation on which this theory is based. The rules, regulations, standards, and/or policies are the underpinning for all decisions related to ethical situations. Rain-bow (2002) states that a person utilizing this theory "will produce very consistent decisions since they will be based on the individual's set duties" (para. 10). Though the strength of this theory is the steadiness and reliability of the resulting management of ethical situations, the challenge relates to the requirement of implementing the rules without consideration for the welfare of those involved. The entire focus for this theory is the use of those selected rules in a consistent manner. Within the use of this theory, the rules, regulations, standards, and/or policies are expected to be established on what is best for the individuals involved. Thus, when the foundation of rules is based upon this concept, the application of the rules should benefit those involved.

The second theory used within ethical decision making is **utilitarianism**. It is also called the consequentialist, teleology, or situation theory (Aiken, 2004). This theory is based upon outcomes. The decisions made using this theory would endeavor to envision the consequences of each action possible. As a result of considering all of the possible outcomes, the best decision for the most individuals can be selected. This theory works to provide the solution that prompts the maximum advantage for the majority of the people involved in the situation. Within this theory, the focus can be directed in two different directions. One is the act of utilitarianism that omits personal feelings or societal constraints when making the decision. This type of outcome is based on benefitting the most individuals without considering any other aspect. The other focus is called rule utilitarianism. For this focus, laws and fairness are utilized when the decision is being made. Fairness and justice are viewed as foundational in this focus, and these concepts are used to help determine the solution that will benefit the majority of the individuals involved. The primary concern when using utilitarianism as a method for decision making is the aspect of effectively predicting outcomes. This predicting of outcomes requires that the decisions be made based on knowledge of the future. The need to foresee into the future is a flaw of this theory.

The **virtue ethical theory** has grown in support and functionality over the last few years. According to O'Connor (2010), "Virtue ethics focuses on the traits of good character that individuals develop over years, influenced by family, faith communities, education, and society" (p. 627). The foundation for this theory is character rather than actions or rules. The character of a person in normal behavior is used as the groundwork for determining the plan for managing an ethical situation. One of the primary concerns ensuing from this theory relates to the changing views of "normal" behavior. As individuals encounter different situations and learning opportunities, their behaviors frequently reflect the evolving knowledge and culture. With every change in behavior, prior ethical decisions are then called into question, as they were based on "normal" behavior at that time. Normal behavior can be significantly modified as societal aspects change. Another concern with the use of this theory is the problem encountered when an individual is labeled by society as not engaging in "normal" accepted behavior. The labeling of individuals becomes the problem, not necessarily the behavior being used within the decision-making process. A person can demonstrate both normal and abnormal behaviors reflective of a specific setting. For this theory, the behavior used at the time of the decision-making process is the criterion for the decision.

A fourth ethical theory that can be used in the decision-making process is the **rights ethical theory**. In this theory, rights as established by society and endorsed by the larger, ruling population are used as the foundation for the decisions made. As long as the rights set forth by this population are ethically correct, the resulting decisions will be ethical in nature. The determination of the societal rights becomes a key aspect when utilizing this theory.

The final ethical theory for consideration is **care ethics**. According to O'Connor (2010), this theory centers on the interaction of the specific nurse and the individual patient or family. As an individual uses this process, the participants are expected to contemplate the milieu of the circumstances, preserve the interactions involving the individuals, and ensure that everyone is supported and strengthened. Within the care theory of ethics, the persons involved in the decision are key to the determination of the action plan to be enforced. Only when everyone is in agreement with the direction to be taken is the situation effectively managed. One grave problem with this theory is the realization that getting everyone to agree to a plan of action is sometimes very difficult, if not impossible.

Ethical situations provide everyone with the opportunities to grow and develop. At times, it is difficult and frustrating. Since ethical standards are based upon a moral foundation, the stressors involved frequently become personal in nature. Each participant in the decision-making process comes to the table with different moral backgrounds. Individuals can move on several different paths toward a goal or outcome based upon those principles and theories used within the decision-making process.

ETHICS OF TEACHING IN HIGHER EDUCATION

As we move from general consideration of ethical aspects to their application to teaching, several different thoughts and challenges become evident. Nurses at the bedside deal with ethical situations that tend to relate to the physical side of their professional practice. Life, death, quality of life, quantity of life, informed consent, privacy/confidentiality, and other aspects tend to be the focus for ethical situations that impact the physical care of the client. Ethics within the teaching realm moves toward the management of individuals. Usually in the teaching realm, faculty members do not worry about whether their students are going to live or die. It is more about the moral development of the individual instead of the physical management of the individual. Thus, the application moves to the determination and application of the moral behaviors resulting in the clarification of a decision.

Each of the six principles within ethics is critical when considering both the HIPAA and FERPA aspects within the educational process. Since both of these laws tend to deal more with information, the principles of veracity, confidentiality, and justice are highly important within the finalization of a decision. Having acknowledged the importance of these three does not negate the contributions of autonomy, nonmalfeasance, and beneficence. Faculty members and school administrators must constantly remember that each student is unique. Though the rules and regulations can be used to ensure nonmalfeasance and beneficence in the management of the educational environment, each student comes with a unique history that must be carefully considered when addressing the different aspects controlled by HIPAA and FERPA regulations.

According to O'Connor (2010), "Teaching ethics is an important area that can be used as an area of content to emphasize the importance of attitude and fair thinking" (p. 620). The teaching and utilization of ethical principles within the classroom/clinical experience serves to serendipitously reinforce the students' capacity to distinguish individual values, to critically cogitate, to act as a team, and to evade any violation of academic integrity, such as plagiarism. Faculty members can provide these opportunities in many ways. As stated by Condon (2008), "One's ethics provides the grounds for every action taken or not taken in relation to students and faculty colleagues" (p. 402). Some examples of ethical behavior are (1) acting as an ethical role model as decisions are made, (2) using student discussion groups to struggle with ethical dilemmas, (3) facilitating values-clarification activities to allow students to safely investigate their values, and (4) using case studies that incorporate ethical principles in the management of the scenario. Providing safe environments where the students can dissect the ethical situations and arrive at alternative decisions allows the students to test out conduits for use when they are confronted with similar situations in less structured settings. The American Nurses Association (ANA) in 2001 revised and updated the *Code of Ethics for Nurses with Interpretive Statements.* This document provides a universal foundation used by American nurses as they work within an ethical framework. The ANA code is regularly revised and is due for revision in 2013–2014 (Badzek, 2013). Though we do not at this time have a unique code for nurse educators, the ethical principles maintained within the ANA code provide an underpinning that is acceptable in practice and educational settings. The International Council of Nurses (ICN) also has a Code of Ethics for Nursing (approved in 2000). Within this code, the expectations of ethical behavior are presented with an international focus. A code of ethics is a "written list of a profession's values and standards of conduct" (Aiken, 2004, p. 100). Such codes form the pedestal on which a profession practices. The aspects noted within a code of ethics do not provide specific examples but do provide the values and expectations by which the professionals are expected to function.

Tippitt, Ard, Kline, Tilghman, Chamberlain, and Meagher (2009) presented several interesting thoughts related to ethics and academic integrity. Within their article, academic integrity was defined as "a commitment, even in the face of adversity, to five fundamental values: honesty, trust, fairness, respect, and responsibility" (Tippitt et al., 2009, para. 2). Since academic integrity is a key aspect of ethical behavior within higher education, it becomes very important that faculty members provide effective role modeling of the practices that reflect integrity. This article suggests some questions to focus a faculty member's thoughts toward academic integrity, including (Tippitt et al., 2009, paras. 10–12):

- Does the academic institution itself demonstrate a culture of academic integrity?
- Are rules/policies created for the sake of having them, or do faculty and administrators explain the rationale for policies to students and faculty?
- Does the curriculum lend itself to integrity?
- Are the objectives for assignments clear?
- Are assignments being given as busywork, or do they facilitate significant learning?
- Are specific program outcomes in place related to the affective domain, such as honesty, integrity, and values?
- How do faculty model and mentor students in acquiring and living within these values?

As faculty members strive to apply the ideas of ethical decision making and academic integrity to the educational setting, several strategies can be employed to diminish or avert academic misconduct, such as assigning seats for students, jumbling up the order of the test questions, restricting the things students are allowed to have available during an exam, having all examinations proctored, and having clear policies regarding the use of social media. Though these strategies are effective in reducing the potential for academic misconduct, they are frequently viewed as negative in nature. These strategies seek to prevent students from engaging in problematic behavior, which implies that faculty members expect students to engage in academic misconduct. Using strategies that showcase the expectation that students should not participate in academic misconduct sets up a positive and supportive environment for learning. Hutchinson, Shedlin, Gallo, Krainovich-Miller, and Fulmer (2014) recommend providing students with opportunities to examine ethical challenges and ways to resolve them. They propose an "ethics-in-the-round" approach to obtain knowledge for ethical skill acquisition.

One particular current evolution regarding ethics in nursing and nursing education is that of the use of social media. Specific information on the use of social media is discussed in the chapter titled *Social Media and Incivility*, but the subject cannot be omitted when discussing ethics and nursing. As Beard (2013) indicates:

> Over 193,000 text messages are sent every second.... Even more telling is the fact that 48% of all adults use social networking sites such as Facebook or Twitter and that such use accounts for a quarter of the time spent on the Internet. (p. 38)

Priority and confidentiality of student and patient information become ethical issues if/when that information is shared on the Internet. As a nurse educator and leader, faculty must ensure that technology is used professionally and appropriately.

SUMMARY THOUGHTS

Ethical issues are all around us within the academic arena and the health arena. As faculty members, it becomes vital and essential for each of us to carefully consider the message we are providing in regard to ethics. Each faculty member must develop a firm foundation related to key legislative and regulatory policies such as HIPAA and FERPA. In addition to this underpinning, nursing faculty members must also be very aware of the different codes of ethics of the nursing and education professions. O'Connor (2010) states that "faculty members must be prepared to facilitate thinking about ethics in their students by acting as ethical persons of integrity both personally and professionally" (p. 621). As faculty members, it is our responsibility to present an effective role model for ethical behavior based upon a firm understanding of legislative and regulatory policies. To demonstrate any less is to provide the example that ethics is not an integral part of effective health and educational practices.

SUMMARY POINTS

1. The term *ethics* comes from the Greek word *ethos* and reflects societal standards.
2. When using ethics effectively, decisions are based upon specific guidelines and information. The different ethical theories and principles provide the societal standards on which decisions can be made.
3. All aspects within the delivery of health care are transformed by an understanding and acknowledgement of the moral/ethical obligations which the nursing profession embraces.
4. The independent control over individual existence is held as a critical principle for the uniqueness of each person.
5. Deontological theory obliges the addressing of any situation based on the idea that correctness originates from rules and duty.
6. Utilitarianism theory endeavors to envision the consequences of each action possible.
7. The virtue ethical theory focuses on the aspects of good character.
8. Rights ethical theory uses rights established by society and endorsed by the larger, ruling population.
9. Care ethical theory centers on the interaction of the specific nurse and the individual patient or family.
10. Legislative and regulatory policies are embedded in nursing practice.
11. The Health Insurance Portability and Accountability Act (HIPAA) was enacted in 1996 to protect health information.
12. The Family Educational Rights and Privacy Act (FERPA) was enacted in 1974 to protect the privacy of students.
13. Both HIPAA and FERPA have implications for teaching nursing.
14. Educational accrediting commissions and The Joint Commission have standards governing nursing educational programs and the practice of nursing.
15. The National League of Nursing (NLN) and the American Association of Colleges of Nursing (AACN) accredit programs of nursing.

16. The National Council of State Boards of Nursing (NCSBN) and state Boards of Nursing (BONs) have as their mission to protect the welfare of the public.
17. The NCSBN developed a test to measure competence needed to perform safely and effectively as a newly licensed, entry-level registered nurse, regardless of state, commonwealth, or territory of the United States.
18. State BONs regulate the practice of nursing and approval of nursing education programs.
19. Ethics within the teaching realm moves toward the management of individuals.
20. The teaching and utilization of ethical principles within the classroom/clinical experience serves to serendipitously reinforce the students' capacity to distinguish individual values, to critically cogitate, to act as a team, and to evade any violation of academic integrity, such as plagiarism.
21. Using strategies that showcase the expectation that students should not participate in academic misconduct sets up a positive and supportive environment for learning.
22. Emerging technology may involve issues of confidentiality and primary ethical considerations, especially with the evolution of social media.

TIPS FOR NURSE EDUCATORS

1. The nurse educator must be politically active to be an advocate for students, patients, and the nursing profession.
2. Having a solid foundation of HIPAA and FERPA policies enhances the effectiveness of nursing faculty.
3. Legislative/regulatory agencies mandate standards by which nurse educators must abide.
4. The NCSBN and the state BONs are concerned with the competence of entry-level registered nurses and the safety of the public.
5. Accrediting agencies for health care and higher education promote quality outcomes for patients and students.
6. Ethical and moral development involve the determination and application of moral behaviors within the clarification of a decision.
7. Some examples of ethical behavior are (1) acting as an ethical role model as decisions are made, (2) using student discussion groups to

struggle with ethical dilemmas, (3) facilitating values-clarification activities to allow students to safely investigate their values, and (4) providing case studies that incorporate ethical principles in the management of the scenario.

8. Several strategies can be employed to diminish or avert academic misconduct, such as assigning seats for students, jumbling up the order of the test questions, restricting the things students are allowed to have available during an exam, having all examinations proctored, and having clear policies regarding the use of social media.

MULTIPLE CHOICE QUESTIONS

1. The role of nursing faculty includes:
   A. **ethical and legal implications in teaching nursing as well as the practice of nursing.**
   B. ethical and legal implications only in nursing practice.
   C. ethical and legal implications only in teaching nursing.
   D. None of the above

   Rationale:
   Ethical and legal implications for teaching nursing require a balance of two perspectives—that of a practicing nurse and that of a nurse educator.

2. Ethics and laws are based on:
   A. individual behaviors.
   B. opinions of the public.
   C. **the norms for societal behavior.**
   D. the values of family and friends.

   Rationale:
   The term *ethics* stems from the Greek word *ethos* and reflects standards. Laws are the norms for standards of societal behavior.

3. State Boards of Nursing protect:
   A. students.
   B. faculty.
   C. administration.
   D. **the public.**

   Rationale:
   The purpose of state Boards of Nursing is to protect the welfare of the public and approve schools of nursing programs.

4. The Health Insurance Portability and Accountability Act (HIPAA) established standards about the use and disclosure of:
   A. student information.
   B. faculty information.
   C. financial information.
   D. **health information.**

   Rationale:
   The Health Insurance Portability and Accountability Act (HIPAA) was enacted in 1996 to protect health information through a Privacy Rule to establish standards about the use and disclosure of health information.

5. For faculty members, HIPAA has:
   A. no impact on their teaching role.
   B. **major impact on their teaching role.**
   C. implications for only hospitals/clinic staff.
   D. no implications for either the teaching or practice role.

   Rationale:
   HIPAA has a major impact on the role of nursing faculty members to ensure confidentiality of patient information on student clinical assignments, case study presentations, pre-/postclinical conferences, student papers, and simulation lab scenarios.

6. The Family Educational Rights and Privacy Act (FERPA) protects:
   A. parents.
   B. faculty.
   C. **students.**
   D. patients.

   Rationale:
   B. FERPA protects the privacy of student education records. After the age of 18, the right of access to the records transfers from the parents to the student.

7. FERPA applies to:
   A. **students, students with disabilities, and patients.**
   B. parents, patients, and faculty.
   C. hospitals, clinics, and health departments.
   D. kindergarten, elementary, and high school students.

   Rationale:
   FERPA applies to students at all levels, students with disabilities, and students in clinical practice.

8. Regulatory agencies for health care, nursing, and nursing education set standards that apply to:
    A. the entertainment industry, television, and newspapers.
    B. **higher education, hospitals/clinics, and consumers of health care.**
    C. all people in all countries for protection of endangered species.
    D. engineers, social workers, respiratory therapies, and nutritionists.

Rationale:
Regulatory agencies for health care, nursing, and nursing education set standards for higher education, hospitals/clinics, and consumers of health care. The legislative/regulatory agencies' standards are integral to the role of the nursing faculty.

9. When ethics and ethical principles are used effectively, decisions are based upon:
    A. **specific guidelines and information.**
    B. general protocols and data.
    C. specific guidelines and general data collected.
    D. general protocols and information.

Rationale:
When ethics are used effectively, decisions are based upon specific guidelines and information. The different ethical theories and principles provide the societal standards on which decisions can be made. O'Connor (2010) states that "learning to acknowledge personal moral views, to analyze and evaluate moral opinions, to reflect on moral situations, to defend moral choices, and to work with other healthcare team members on resolutions of ethical/moral situations and dilemmas is critical to the development of the ethical nurse" (p. 621).

10. The six major ethical principles are:
    A. trust, caring, autonomy, confidentiality, holism, and veracity.
    B. nonmalfeasance, caring, autonomy, confidentiality, veracity, and beneficence.
    C. **autonomy, veracity, nonmalfeasance, confidentiality, beneficence, and justice.**
    D. autonomy, trust, holism, nonmalfeasance, beneficence, and justice.

Rationale:
The principles subsumed within ethical decisions are not laws in and of themselves but are the foundational components that guide the behaviors used when confronted by situations outside the control of laws. The six major ethical principles are autonomy, veracity,

nonmalfeasance, confidentiality, beneficence, and justice. Each of these tenets is used to maneuver toward an outcome when a situation is not covered by legal precedents.

11. The areas that help to shape an individual's unique decisions within the ethical dimension are:
    A. stress, justice, and emotions.
    B. motivation, work experiences, and emotions.
    C. **motivation, emotions, and life experiences.**
    D. life experiences, work experiences, and emotions.

Rationale:
Rainbow (2002) states that "each man deserves respect because only he has had those exact life experiences and understands his emotions, motivations, and body in such an intimate manner" (para. 5). These emotions, motivations, and life experiences shape how an individual comes to the unique decisions encountered in the ethical dimension. Within the principle of autonomy, each individual is allowed to pull from his or her culture and environment when making those decisions that are not addressed by legal rules.

12. Several different ethical theories are available to be used for the determination of an ethical decision. The theories are:
    A. deontology, utilitarianism, telepathy, and consequentialism.
    B. virtue, care, and justifications.
    C. deontology, virtue, individualism, care, and rights.
    D. **deontology, consequentialism, virtue, care, and rights.**

Rationale:
Several different theories are currently embraced—deontology, utilitarianism (consequentialist or teleological), virtue ethics, care ethics, and rights ethics. Each of these theories considers the ethical situation from a different approach, thus resulting in discrete management of the state of affairs.

13. Within the teaching realm, ethical decision making frequently addresses:
    A. **the management of individuals instead of their physical care.**
    B. the physical care of individuals instead of their management.
    C. both the physical and the individual component.
    D. neither the physical nor the individual component.

Rationale:
The nurse at the bedside deals with ethical situations that tend to relate to the physical side of professional practice. Life, death, quality of life, quantity of life, informed consent, privacy/confidentiality,

and other aspects tend to be the focus for ethical situations that impact the physical care of the client. Ethics within the teaching realm moves toward the management of individuals. Usually within the teaching realm, faculty members do not worry about whether their students are going to live or die. It is more about the moral development of the individual instead of the physical management of the individual.

14. An example of demonstrating ethical behavior by a faculty member would be:
    A. assigning seats for the students within the classroom setting.
    B. restricting the objects a student can bring into a testing area.
    C. **using student discussion groups to struggle with an ethical dilemma.**
    D. telling students that they do not need to be concerned with values clarification.

Rationale:

Some examples of ethical behavior are (1) acting as an ethical role model as decisions are made, (2) using student discussion groups to struggle with ethical dilemmas, (3) facilitating values-clarification activities to allow students to safely investigate their values, and (4) providing case studies that incorporate ethical principles in the management of the scenario.

15. What documents can be used as an underpinning for ethical discussions?
    A. Medical journals, articles, and lawyer briefs.
    B. Nursing research articles.
    C. HIPAA and FERPA documents.
    D. **ANA Code of Ethics and ICN Code of Ethics.**

Rationale:

The ANA in 2001 revised and updated the *Code of Ethics for Nurses with Interpretive Statements*. This document provides a universal foundation used by American nurses as they work within an ethical framework. Though we do not at this time have a unique code for nurse educators, the ethical principles maintained within the ANA code provide an underpinning that is acceptable in practice and educational settings. The ICN Code of Ethics is an international code provided for the global provision of nursing care.

16. When considering strategies related to ethical academic integrity, faculty members should:

A. **identify positive methods for ensuring that students maintain academic integrity.**
B. institute any measure that will prevent students from employing unethical behaviors.
C. expect students to use whatever means that they can to be successful.
D. set students up for problems early in the course to demonstrate that academic misconduct will not be tolerated.

Rationale:
As faculty members strive to apply the ideas of ethical decision making and academic integrity to the educational setting, several strategies can be employed to diminish or avert academic misconduct, such as assigning seats for students, jumbling up the order of the test questions, restricting the things students are allowed to have available during an exam, having all examinations proctored, and having clear policies regarding the use of social media. Though these strategies are effective in reducing the potential for academic misconduct, they are frequently viewed as negative in nature. These strategies seek to prevent students from doing the problematic behavior, which implies that faculty members expect students to engage in academic misconduct. Using strategies that showcase the expectation that students should not participate in academic misconduct sets up a positive and supportive environment for learning.

DISCUSSION QUESTIONS

1. How does your school of nursing address HIPAA and FERPA guidelines and standards?
   Considerations:
   Examine the two federal acts. Review your school's policies and procedures for confidentiality of students and patients. Ask questions of yourself about how you use both HIPAA and FERPA in your role as a nurse educator.
2. Apply the ethical principles of autonomy, veracity, nonmalfeasance, confidentiality, beneficence, and justice to the following scenario:
   You are a novice nursing educator who is confronted by a group of students who have worked together to complete an assignment that was expected to be done as individual work. The syllabus does not clearly state that the assignment was to be individual work. From

the instructions provided within the syllabus, it could be inter-preted to allow for working as a group. The students did not clarify the assignment but just assumed that group work was allowed.

Considerations:

- The six major ethical principles are autonomy, veracity, nonmal-feasance, confidentiality, beneficence, and justice. Each of these tenets is used to maneuver toward an outcome when a situation is not covered by legal precedents.
- According to Nelson (2003), autonomy is related to the idea that each of us has the right to self-determine the aspects within our lives. Laws have been established to protect the ability of individuals to make decisions independently about situations encountered. Each person is understood to have the right and responsibly to make free choices about the decisions that are key to their private lives.
- Veracity is understood to represent truth telling. In each decision that a person confronts, the expectation is that truthful informa-tion will be provided by all involved parties so that the affected individual can use the entirety of the information to make the appropriate decision.
- The concept of nonmalfeasance basically means "do no harm." Within health care particularly, the idea of doing no harm to indi-viduals is paramount. This principle of not harming someone is foundational within ethical aspects and is vital in the foundation of legal determination.
- Confidentiality is viewed as the securing of all privileged informa-tion that is obtained as a result of functioning in a professional capacity with a patient or client. In each and every situation, the maintaining of private information in a secure and protected manner is viewed as the standard.
- The concept of beneficence means "doing good." For each situa-tion, the focus is on making a decision that will lead to the best outcome for the greatest number of individuals involved.
- Justice is viewed as the fairness of the situation. This concept strives to ensure equality for all individuals in regard to goods, services, and protection.

3. What educational activities do you provide so that students can examine ethical issues and potential resolutions?

Considerations:

Provide the codes of ethics of professional organizations to stu-dents and allow a forum for a debate or roundtable discussion of an identified ethical issue such as end-of-life management or the problem of students posting pictures of patients on Facebook.

REFERENCES

Aiken, T. D. (2004). *Legal, ethical, and political issues in nursing* (2nd ed.). Philadelphia, PA: F.A. Davis Company.

Badzek, L. (2013). Issues up close: Enduring and evolving: Code of ethics for nurses. *American Nurse Today, 8*(9), 30–32.

Beard, E. (2013). Nurse leaders and the use of social media: Becoming literate to lead. *Nurse Leader, 11*(6), 38–40.

Boswell, C., Cannon, S., & Miller, J. (2005). Nurses' political involvement: Responsibility versus privilege. *Journal of Professional Nursing, 21*(1), 5–8.

Condon, E. H. (2008). Ethical issues in teaching nursing. In B. K. Penn (Ed.), *Mastering the teaching role: A guide for nurse educators* (Chapter 30). Philadelphia, PA: F.A. Davis Company.

Department of Education. (n.d.). Family Educational Rights and Privacy Act. Retrieved June 13, 2014, from http://www2.ed.gov/policy/gen/guid/fpco/ferpa/index.html

Department of Health and Human Services. (n.d.). Health information privacy. Retrieved June 13, 2014, from http://www.hhs.gov/ocr/hipaa

Gumby, S. S. (2008). Legal issues in teaching nursing. In B. K. Penn (Ed.), *Mastering the teaching role: A guide for nurse educators* (Chapter 3). Philadelphia, PA: F.A. Davis Company.

Hutchinson, M. K., Shedlin, M. D., Gallo, B., Krainovich-Miller, B., & Fulmer, T. (2014). Ethics-in-the-round: A guided peer approach for addressing ethical issues confronting nursing students. *Nursing Education Perspectives, 35*(1), 58–60.

National Council of State Boards of Nursing. (2014). NCLEX-PN test plan. Retrieved June 13, 2014, from https://www.ncsbn.org/2014_PN_TestPlan.pdf

Nelson, M. J. (2003). Ethical, legal, and economic foundations of the educational process. In S. B. Bastable (Ed.), *Nurse as educator: Principles of teaching and learning for nursing practice* (2nd ed.). Sudbury, MA: Jones and Bartlett Publishers.

O'Connor, K. F. (2010). Teaching nursing ethics. In L. Caputi (Ed.), *Teaching nursing: The art and science* (2nd ed., Vol. I). Glen Ellyn, IL: College of DuPage Press.

Rainbow, C. (2002). Descriptions of ethical theories and principles. Retrieved June 13, 2014, from http://www.bio.davidson.edu/people/kabernd/indep/carainbow/Theories.htm

Sumner, J. (2011). Ethics and nursing research. In C. Boswell & S. Cannon (Eds.), *Introduction to nursing research: Incorporating evidence-based practice* (2nd ed., pp. 55–91). Sudbury, MA: Jones and Bartlett Publishers.

Tippitt, M. P., Ard, N., Kline, J. R., Tilghman, J., Chamberlain, B., & Meagher, G. P. (2009). Creating environments that foster academic integrity. *Nursing Education Perspectives, 30*(4), 239–244.

Chapter 5

Social Media and Incivility

Sharon Cannon and Darlene Del Prato

CHAPTER OBJECTIVES

At the conclusion of this chapter, the learner will be able to:

1. Discuss the impact of social media on the nursing profession.
2. Compare legal/ethical issues regarding the use of social media in nursing education and nursing practice.
3. Discuss the evidence-based teaching approach as it relates to advanced Internet technology.
4. Define academic incivility.
5. Identify uncivil student and faculty behaviors.
6. Explain factors that contribute to student incivility.
7. Summarize ways that faculty can create a supportive learning environment that fosters professional formation and discourages incivility.
8. Apply strategies for preventing/managing uncivil student behavior.

KEY TERMS

- Blog
- Facebook
- Faculty incivility
- Incivility
- Professional formation
- Social media
- Socialization
- Stress
- Student incivility
- Twitter

INTRODUCTION

Advanced technology has changed the way the world communicates. The exchange of information has exploded following the birth of the Internet, giving rise to a new age of **social media** that allows family, friends, colleagues, and even strangers to connect with one another more conveniently than ever before (Huston, 2014). The ability to reach a wide audience is exciting and can provide opportunities and challenges inconceivable even 5 years ago. This connectivity is of particular importance to nurse educators responsible for teaching students the role of the professional nurse in preparation for joining the healthcare team to provide safe, effective care to patients. To fully convey the scope of the impact of social media on nursing education and nursing practice, this chapter will focus on defining social media, the types of social media, myths regarding social media, and benefits and consequences related to social media. In addition, **incivility** related to social media and uncivil communication within nursing education and nursing will be explored.

OVERVIEW OF SOCIAL MEDIA

Definition and Types of Social Media

Social media has been described as any type of public forum that has a web-based social medical platform. The National Student Nurses' Association (NSNA, 2014) lists the following types of social media:

- **Blogging** (e.g., Blogger, LiveJournal, Xanga)
- Microblogging (e.g., Foursquare, Google Buzz, Posterous, Tumblr, **Twitter**)
- Postcasting (e.g., Blubrry)
- Social networking (e.g., Beto, **Facebook**, Google+, LinkedIn, Myspace, Orkut)
- Social news sharing (e.g., Digg, Reddit)
- Social bookmarking/social tagging (e.g., Delicious, Diigo, StumbleUpon)
- Video hosting (e.g., Vimeo, YouTube)

Obviously with advances in technology and the need for social connections, this list is not all inclusive.

MYTHS ABOUT SOCIAL MEDIA

Multiple myths surround the use of social media. The National Council of State Boards of Nursing (NCSBN) published *White Paper: A Nurse's Guide to the Use of Social Media* (NCSBN, 2011) due to growing concerns about the issues regarding confidentiality and privacy in health care. The American Nurses Association (ANA) *Code of Ethics for Nurses* offers guidelines (Barry, 2013). Student nurses and nurses may not intend to use social media in a negative way, but they are not aware that multiple myths about social media exist. Some myths that abound include the following:

- *Content can be deleted so that no one can access it.* Unfortunately, even though content may be deleted, it has been sent to multiple users who may in turn have sent it to others.
- *Content is private to only the individuals receiving it.* See preceding comment.
- *Content is harmless if clarifiers (name, age, sex, etc.) are not used.* Sharing information about patients and work-related information, regardless of efforts to exclude identifying information, constitutes a potential violation of confidentiality.
- *As long as consent has been given, it is okay to share medical information.* Distributing information to a patient, family, or friend, even when consent has been obtained, can be a violation when there is no need to give the information.

BENEFITS OF SOCIAL MEDIA

Before making any judgement about the use of social media, a thoughtful examination of some benefits of using social media is necessary. In many ways, the world has become a small place thanks to connections between students and/or nurses who are separated geographically. Professional networks, research results, innovative approaches to patient care, and increased communications are possible for educational purposes. Opportunities for networking regarding evidence for patient care abound. Nurse educators can also connect regarding curriculum, innovative teaching strategies, and effective classroom management. For example, the American Association of Colleges of Nursing has a listserve that allows deans, associate deans, assistant deans, and directors to query others regarding unusual student issues, politics, and curriculum design.

Consequences of Misusing Social Media

Any instance of a nurse using social media inappropriately, even if inadvertently, is a reportable event to a Board of Nursing (BON) (Cronquist & Spector, 2011). The NCSBN (2011) indicates that any BON can take disciplinary action that may include a "reprimand or sanction, assessment of a monetary fine, or temporary or permanent loss of licensure" (p. 2). In addition, state or federal laws may be violated and result in civil or criminal penalties such as fines and incarceration. Personal liability is another consequence to be considered. Individual nurses and nurse educators can be sued for violation of confidentiality. This concern about legal actions can impact their personal finances and obviously be very expensive. Finally, employers may decide to terminate an employee—and not just because of patient privacy and confidentiality. Inappropriate statements on a social media platform about coworkers or the organization are considered grounds for termination.

Student nurses are also not exempt from consequences even though they are in a learning environment. Schools of nursing, the NCSBN, and the NSNA are working diligently to develop policies and guidelines to assist students in understanding the distinction between a social life and a professional life. Students can be counseled, receive a failing grade, or be expelled from their program as a result of using social media inappropriately.

Misuse of social media impacts the healthcare team, whether the act is committed by a student or a practicing nurse. This misuse is often considered bullying or lateral violence as a form of incivility and can occur student to student, student to faculty, faculty to student, faculty to faculty, faculty to staff, and staff to faculty. Incivility is a major concern.

INCIVILITY

Creating learning environments that facilitate student learning and **socialization** to the nursing role is an important responsibility of nurse educators (Halstead, 2007). Increasingly, faculty report uncivil student behaviors that hinder their ability to create effective learning environments. In fact, Forni (2008) noted that civility, the foundation of respect that once distinguished the academe, has eroded over the last several decades in response to waning cultural norms and digital technologies.

Uncivil student behavior causes distress for college faculty across disciplines. However, incivility raises particularly grave concerns in nursing education, where the risk is that uncivil behavior may persist after graduation as students enter clinical practice and assume professional responsibilities for patient care (Suplee, Lachman, Siebert, & Anselmi, 2008). This section of the chapter examines the phenomenon of academic incivility, focuses on factors that contribute to **student incivility**, and describes strategies nurse educators can use to create supportive learning environments that prevent or address uncivil behavior that is inconsistent with becoming a professional.

Socialization and Professional Formation

Socialization is the process whereby students acquire nursing knowledge, skills, and attitudes. Students are formally socialized to professional behaviors and norms in the classroom and clinical practice setting. However, socialization to professional values such as caring and civility also occurs in the informal (hidden) curriculum that is communicated in how faculty teach and relate to students (Bevis & Watson, 1989). In nursing, socialization is a process of **professional formation** that indicates "a way of being and acting in practice and in the world" (Benner, Sutphen, Leonard, & Day, 2010, p. 166).

Uncivil Student Behaviors

Uncivil student behavior presents a major challenge to nurse educators charged with forming students into compassionate, civil, and ethical practitioners. Researchers have identified uncivil behaviors that range from mild forms of disrespect to highly aggressive and threatening behavior (Clark & Springer, 2007a; Lashley & de Meneses, 2001). A national survey conducted by Lashley and de Meneses identified uncivil student behaviors such as lack of attendance, inattentiveness in class, arriving late or leaving early, yelling, and physical contact. Other uncivil student behaviors include cheating, using cell phones during class, conversing with friends, making sarcastic remarks or gestures, sleeping, using a computer for purposes not related to class, demanding makeup exams or other favors, making disapproving groans, and dominating class discussions (Clark & Springer, 2007a).

Contributing Factors

Experts speculate that uncivil behavior is largely a learned behavior associated with less formal societal norms, inadequate parenting, and repeated exposure to crude popular culture portrayed in movies, on television, and on the Internet (Forni, 2008; Thomas, 2003). At the same time, the widespread reliance on social media, email, and text messaging has led to major changes in the way people communicate with one another. A recent survey of 2,698 individuals conducted by VitalSmarts found that hostility is increasing on social media and negatively impacting people's lives. Furthermore, younger people were four times more likely than Baby Boomers to require instruction in how to communicate effectively online (Glenn, 2013). Thus, some students may lack basic skills and knowledge about how to communicate appropriately.

High levels of **stress** may provoke uncivil behavior, especially in less motivated and less prepared students (Luparell, 2004). There is substantial evidence that the journey of becoming a nurse is a major source of nursing students' anxiety and stress (Del Prato, 2010; Oermann, 1996). The stressful nature of nursing education, faculty arrogance, and student entitlement are key contributors to academic incivility (Clark, 2008a).

Lashley and de Meneses (2001) examined problematic student behavior in 409 undergraduate nursing programs. Over 50% of the program directors who responded reported that students at their institution were less prepared than previous students had been 5 years earlier. Almost 50% of respondents felt that the quality of student work had declined.

Luparell (2004) studied faculty experiences with uncivil nursing students and found that student incivility often revolved around receiving criticism, failing a course, or disagreeing with grading protocols. Of the 36 encounters identified, 23 ensued following criticism of a student's unsatisfactory performance, and 8 involved testing or grading protocols.

Complicating matters further, some students view themselves as consumers with certain rights. For these students, paying for their education entitles them to make certain demands such as makeup exams or other special treatment (Robertson, 2012). Other students may feel justified in resorting to cheating or plagiarism.

Finally, the impersonal atmosphere of large universities and lack of connected relationships may contribute to academic incivility. In one study, students felt a lack of connection with impersonal teachers who focused on evaluation, offered exclusively negative feedback, and "watched them like a hawk" (p. 7). In contrast, connected teacher–student relationships include both personal and professional dimensions characterized by caring, knowing, trust, respect, and mutuality (Gillespie, 2002).

Respondents in Lashley and de Meneses's (2001) study of problematic student behavior described student absence, tardiness, and inattention in the clinical setting. Yelling or verbal abuse of classroom instructors and cheating on exams was reported more often in programs with 200 nursing students or more. The researchers speculated that problematic student behavior might have occurred more often in larger nursing programs due to a less personal learning environment and less connected faculty–student relationships.

Faculty Incivility

There is growing evidence that some faculty contribute to academic incivility. **Faculty incivility** occurs when faculty create a stressful, hostile learning environment by demeaning and belittling students, setting unrealistic expectations for performance, being overly critical, evaluating subjectively and showing favoritism, and targeting students for failure (Clark, 2008a; Del Prato, 2013). Within this context, uncivil student behavior can be understood as a form of protest to a high-stakes learning environment perceived as hostile and unjust (Clark, 2008b; Del Prato, 2010).

Altmiller (2012) examined 24 baccalaureate nursing students' perspectives about incivility. Participants expressed empathy for faculty who were confronted with uncivil student behavior that seemed unwarranted. However, participants also identified faculty behaviors that "fueled student incivility" (Altmiller, p. 16) and believed that student incivility was justified in the context of faculty incivility. Faculty incivility included unprofessional behavior, disrespectful communication, a power gradient in clinical evaluations perceived as subjective, gender and racial bias, a stressful clinical environment, authority failure, and difficult peer behavior.

Strategies to Prevent Student Incivility

Academic incivility prevents the creation of supportive learning environments that foster positive socialization and professional formation. While research focused on interventions for incivility is lacking, the following best practices may prevent or discourage student incivility.

Create a Supportive Learning Environment

Preventing incivility begins with the faculty and the nature of the learning environment created. Faculty create a supportive learning environment that mitigates students' stress and discourages incivility when they listen, demonstrate a willingness to hear the students' point of view, maintain an attitude of respect, and communicate empathy for the challenges students experience (Del Prato, 2010; Thomas, 2003). This is not to say that faculty must agree with everything a student says or does; rather, it is meant as a reminder that students observe *everything* faculty say and do. Just as faculty teach students to use therapeutic communication with patients who are angry or afraid, faculty should role model therapeutic communication with students (Del Prato, 2010). Listening to students when they are anxious or upset demonstrates caring and a desire to understand the students' view, an approach that can deescalate conflict and incivility (Thomas, 2003).

Establish Connected Relationships

Establishing connected relationships with students is an effective strategy for promoting positive behavior. Learning students' names, being approachable and available, and creating a learning environment of mutual respect and trust can foster connected relationships with students that contribute to feeling supported (Del Prato, 2010). For students at risk of failing, connected faculty–student relationships may prevent incivility by deemphasizing the teacher's traditional role as impersonal evaluator, maintaining students' dignity and self-worth, and preserving the prospect of student success (Del Prato, 2010; Gillespie, 2005).

Establish Policies

It is important to establish college policies that prevent incivility or decrease its occurrence. Policies should establish clear guidelines for student behavior with a description of unacceptable behaviors, the consequences of enacting those behaviors, and the ramifications of repeated offenses (Suplee et al., 2008).

Identify and Communicate Course Requirements and Norms for Behavior

The syllabus serves as a written contract between faculty and students (Suplee et al., 2008). The course learning outcomes, assignments, grading criteria, and expectations regarding student and faculty engagement and behavior should be clearly described in the syllabus. An ambiguous or poorly written syllabus can lead to misunderstandings and contribute to student anger and incivility (Morrissette, 2001). Conversely, a well-written syllabus can establish a positive tone for the course by establishing clear guidelines and creating a sense of community.

Reviewing key aspects of the syllabus during the first class session enhances communication and prevents misunderstandings. Faculty should review expected behaviors, inappropriate behaviors, and sanctions for inappropriate behavior as delineated in college policies. Faculty enhance communication and prevent misunderstandings by allowing time for students to ask questions and discuss or clarify norms for faculty and student behavior.

Be Explicit in Promoting Professional Formation

Facilitating the development of students' professional values is an important faculty responsibility that begins with educating students about the ideals, ethical norms, and behaviors expected of them as future members of the profession. According to the ANA *Code of Ethics for Nurses* (2001), "Individuals who become nurses are expected to adhere to the ideals and moral norms of the profession but also to embrace them as part of what it means to become a nurse." To stimulate dialogue about unethical and uncivil behaviors and expectations for professional behaviors, faculty can highlight the ANA *Code of Ethics for Nurses* (2001) provision that the nurse must practice with compassion and respect in all professional relationships.

Hold Students Accountable

As future professionals, nursing students must be held accountable for their behavior. The course syllabus is a contract that should include clearly written behavioral outcomes that students must demonstrate to be successful. For example, an instructor might include the following sentence in the outcomes section: "Student will demonstrate professional behaviors that reflect the standards, values, and ethical behaviors of the nursing profession." When well written, course outcomes foster students' understanding of expected behavior and allow faculty to hold students accountable for uncivil behavior.

Providing Constructive Feedback

Faculty must assess whether students have met identified clinical competencies and provide formative feedback that supports student learning and development. However, impersonal evaluation of a student's unsatisfactory performance that instills fear may leave students feeling vulnerable and angry (Del Prato, 2010; Reutter, Field, Campbell, & Day, 1997), a context that can set the stage for uncivil behavior (Luparell, 2004).

Within this context, the way feedback is delivered is critical. In one study, students felt supported by faculty who provided constructive feedback about knowledge, skills, or attitudes that needed improvement but also provided feedback about something they had done well (Del Prato, 2010). Participants felt invalidated and threatened by exclusively negative criticism that, while important to hear, was "hard to take" because it made them question whether they were capable of becoming a nurse. In contrast, participants shared that criticism was "easier to swallow" when it was accompanied by feedback that acknowledged their strengths. Students who had received this type of balanced feedback reported feeling motivated to persist and work on areas of needed improvement.

Responding to Student Incivility

Students expect faculty to maintain classroom decorum and demonstrate a positive example (Atmiller, 2012). The following teaching and learning strategies, gleaned from the education and nursing education literature, can be implemented to respond to student incivility.

Engage Inattentive or Unprepared Students

Students are more likely to prepare for class and remain engaged when they know they will be held accountable for understanding information in assigned readings. Strategies that can be used to engage students' preparation and attention include quizzing techniques that provide instant feedback to students, small group work, and learning activities such as think-pair-share that allow faculty to respectfully ask students to report for their group (Wingert & Molitor, 2009).

Faculty can discourage uncivil behavior by moving around the classroom to engage students' attention. A remote control allows faculty to move from behind the podium and control the computer or advance a slideshow from anywhere in the classroom. Pausing respectfully near any inattentive or disruptive students and making brief eye contact, as if talking with them, can also be effective (Wingert & Molitor, 2009).

Reframe Uncivil Behavior to Prevent Power Struggles

Despite every effort to create a supportive learning environment, faculty are likely to encounter incivility and should plan ahead for how they will address uncivil student behavior. Keeping in mind that students learn a great deal in the informal curriculum, the importance of modeling professional behavior when responding to an uncivil student's comment or behavior by remaining nondefensive and respectful cannot be overemphasized. To avoid conflicts and power struggles with students, experts recommend that faculty reframe uncivil behavior by acknowledging the student's concerns and communicating empathy (Morrissette, 2001). As discussed earlier in this chapter, faculty create a supportive learning environment that discourages incivility when they respectfully listen to and understand the student's point of view and communicate empathy (Del Prato, 2010; Thomas, 2003). As Morrissette (2001) points out, faculty should never underestimate "the value in having other students observe one's concern and regard for a student who may be struggling to articulate an idea or response" (p. 6).

SUMMARY THOUGHTS

Social media and incivility are two issues gaining prominence in the field of nursing education. Knowledge regarding the proper use of social media and communicating effectively is essential in today's healthcare arena. Nurse educators must become cognizant of the proper use of social media and civil communication to provide students with the knowledge and boundaries of ethical behavior. Creating learning environments that facilitate student learning and socialization to the nursing role is a responsibility of nurse educators (Halstead, 2007).

Student incivility is a significant problem because it hinders the faculty's ability to create an effective learning environment. Furthermore, and of most concern, uncivil behavior may persist after graduation when students enter practice and assume professional responsibilities for patient care (Suplee et al., 2008).

Faculty create a supportive learning environment that discourages incivility when they demonstrate a willingness to listen, maintain an attitude of respect, and communicate empathy for the challenges students experience (Del Prato, 2010; Thomas, 2003). Faculty promote students' professional formation by teaching and role modeling professional behavior, addressing student incivility, and holding students accountable for uncivil behavior.

SUMMARY POINTS

1. Use of social media is on the rise due to the availability of advanced technology.
2. Myths, benefits, and consequences of inappropriate use of social media are impacting the education of and practice of the professional nurse.

3. Schools of nursing and the NCSBN, NSNA, ANA, and other professional nursing organizations are recommending and developing guidelines, policies, and codes of ethics regarding the use of social media in nursing.
4. Uncivil behaviors range from mild forms of disrespect to highly aggressive behavior.
5. Stress, negative faculty attitudes, and student entitlement contribute to academic incivility.
6. Preventing incivility begins with the faculty and learning environment created.
7. Faculty create a hostile learning environment by demeaning students, setting unrealistic expectations for performance, being overly critical, showing favoritism, and targeting students for failure.
8. Uncivil student behavior may be associated with receiving criticism, failing a course, or disagreeing with grading protocols.
9. Faculty create a supportive learning environment that discourages incivility when they take time to listen, maintain an attitude of respect, and demonstrate caring.
10. Faculty promote students' professional formation by teaching and role modeling professional behavior, addressing student incivility, and holding students accountable for uncivil behavior.

TIPS FOR NURSE EDUCATORS

1. Study and review the NCSBN and NSNA guidelines for use of social media in nursing.
2. Incorporate appropriate social media in the educational arena, especially with examples to guide students.
3. Be sure your school has clear policies regarding the use of social media by students.
4. Role model civility and professionalism.
5. Create a supportive learning environment by listening, acknowledging students' concerns, and communicating empathy.
6. To stimulate class discussion about unethical and uncivil behaviors and expectations for professional behavior, use the ANA *Code of Ethics for Nurses* (2001) provision that the nurse must practice with compassion and respect in all professional relationships.
7. Review the syllabus during the first class session to ensure students understand course requirements as well as expectations for professional behavior.

8. Maintain classroom decorum by implementing strategies that encourage student engagement during class.
9. Use a supportive approach to deliver feedback to students by telling them what they need to work on to improve as well as what they are doing well.
10. Ensure that your school has clear policies for student behavior that include a description of unacceptable behaviors, the consequences of enacting those behaviors, and the ramifications of repeated offenses.
11. Strive to role model professional values and behavior.

MULTIPLE CHOICE QUESTIONS

1. Social media is limited to:
   A. **no one; it is available to the world at large.**
   B. only friends.
   C. colleagues.
   D. school and work.

   Rationale:
   The rapid expansion of electronic media connects any person with the world at large.

2. Social media is defined as:
   A. only professional platforms.
   B. only personal platforms.
   C. **a public forum.**
   D. a private forum.

   Rationale:
   Social media is defined as a public forum.

3. Social media contains information that cannot be:
   A. public information.
   B. **deleted and restricted.**
   C. harmful or hostile.
   D. a violation if distributed.

   Rationale:
   One myth is that content can be deleted and restricted.

4. Benefits of social media include:
   A. confidential information sharing.
   B. privacy of patient rights.
   C. **geographic connections.**
   D. patient identifiers.

Rationale:

Social media allows individuals to connect with others when geographically separated.

5. Consequences of inappropriate use of social media:
    A. do not apply to students in nursing programs.
    B. do not apply to faculty in nursing programs.
    C. result in free speech for students and faculty.
    D. **may result in monetary fines, jail time, and lawsuits.**

Rationale:

Consequences of inappropriate use of social media may result in civil or criminal penalties to students and faculty members alike.

6. Creating learning environments that facilitate student learning and socialization to the nursing role is an important responsibility of:
    A. nursing students.
    B. students' parents.
    C. **nurse educators.**
    D. nurse administrators.

Rationale:

Creating learning environments that facilitate student learning and socialization to the nursing role is an important responsibility of nurse educators (Halstead, 2007).

7. An example of uncivil student behavior is:
    A. arriving late or leaving class early.
    B. logging onto Facebook during class.
    C. cheating on exams.
    D. **all of the above.**

Rationale:

Uncivil student behaviors include lack of attendance, inattentiveness, arriving late or leaving early, yelling, making physical contact, using cell phones, conversing with friends, making sarcastic remarks or gestures, sleeping, using a computer for purposes not related to class, demanding makeup exams or other favors, making disapproving groans, and dominating class discussions (Clark & Springer, 2007a; Lashley & de Meneses, 2001).

8. Which of the following factors contributes to student incivility?
    A. The stress of nursing education.
    B. Faculty arrogance.
    C. Student sense of entitlement.
    D. **All of the above.**

Rationale:
The stressful nature of nursing education, together with faculty arrogance and student entitlement, are key contributors to academic incivility (Clark, 2008a).

9. Faculty create a stressful learning environment that may contribute to student incivility by:
   A. belittling students.
   B. expecting perfect performance.
   C. criticizing students.
   D. **all of the above.**

Rationale:
Faculty create a stressful, hostile learning environment by demeaning and belittling students, setting unrealistic expectations for performance, being overly critical, evaluating subjectively and showing favoritism, and targeting students for failure (Clark, 2008a; Del Prato, 2013).

10. Faculty create a supportive learning environment that mitigates students' stress and discourages incivility when they:
    A. display an attitude of superiority.
    B. **listen to and understand students' perspectives.**
    C. agree with everything a student says or does.
    D. establish friendships with students.

Rationale:
Faculty create a supportive learning environment that mitigates students' stress and discourages incivility when they listen, demonstrate a willingness to hear the students' point of view, maintain an attitude of respect, and communicate empathy for the challenges students experience (Del Prato, 2010; Thomas, 2003).

11. By responding to uncivil student behavior in a respectful way that acknowledges the student's concerns and communicating empathy, faculty:
    A. role model professional values of caring and respect.
    B. teach what it means to be a professional.
    C. prevent power struggles with students.
    D. **all of the above.**

Rationale:
Reframing uncivil behavior by acknowledging the student's concerns and communicating empathy can help faculty avoid conflicts and power struggles with students (Morrissette, 2001).

Discussion Questions

1. What types of social media issues have you encountered when teaching students? Consider whether use of social media has been appropriate or inappropriate. How would you resolve an issue of inappropriate use?

   Considerations:

   Carefully review and examine the NCSBN white paper on the use of social media. All too frequently we consider the use of social media to be private and harmless, without realizing the gray area of communicating our thoughts and feelings about our patients, students, colleagues, or organization. Social media has its place in the educational arena, but nursing faculty must be cautious and provide examples of appropriate use of social media. The potential for blurring our professional and social lives has led professional nursing organizations to establish guidelines and codes of ethics.

2. What types of incivility have you encountered when teaching students? Think about an experience you had with uncivil behavior and how you responded. In what ways might you modify your approach next time to prevent and/or respond to uncivil behavior in a way that minimizes incivility while also modeling the values of the profession?

   Considerations:

   Carefully review the ANA *Code of Ethics for Nurses*. Faculty often focus on teaching students nursing knowledge and clinical skills. While teaching knowledge and skills is important, faculty are also charged with socializing students to the values, ethical norms, and behaviors of the profession and forming students as professionals. The potential for uncivil behavior to continue after students graduate and enter clinical practice has prompted nursing programs to establish policies for addressing incivility.

References

Altmiller, G. (2012). Students' perceptions of incivility in nursing education: Implications for educators. *Nursing Education Perspectives, 33*(1), 15–20.

American Nurses Association. (2001). *Code of ethics for nurses.* Silver Springs, MD: Author.

Barry, M. E. (2013). Social media: Proceed with caution. *The American Nurse.* November/December, 9.

Benner, P., Sutphen, M., Leonard, V., Day, L. (2010). Educating nurses: A call for radical transformation. Stanford, CA: The Carnegie Foundation for the Advancement of Teaching.

Bevis, E., & Watson, J. (1989). Toward a caring curriculum: A new pedagogy for nursing. New York, NY: National League for Nursing.

Clark, C. M. (2008a). Student voices on faculty incivility in nursing education: A conceptual model. *Nursing Education Perspectives, 29*(5), 284–289.

Clark, C. M. (2008b). Student perspectives on the faculty incivility in nursing education: An application of the concept of rankism. *Nursing Outlook, 56*, 4–8.

Clark, C. M., & Springer, P. J. (2007a). Incivility in nursing education: A descriptive study of definitions and prevalence. *Journal of Nursing Education, 46*(1), 7–11.

Clark, C. M., & Springer, P. J. (2007b). Thoughts on incivility: Student and faculty perceptions of uncivil behavior in nursing education. *Nursing Education Perspectives, 28*(2), 93–97.

Cronquist, R., & Spector, N. (2011). Nurses and social media: Regulatory concerns and guidelines. *Journal of Nursing Regulation, 2*(3), 37–40.

Del Prato, D. 2010. The lived experience of associate degree nursing education: Conditions and barriers in the learning environment that shaped students' learning, identity development, and success. Unpublished dissertation. Syracuse, NY: Syracuse University.

Del Prato, D. (2013). Students' voices: The lived experience of faculty incivility as a barrier to professional formation in associate degree nursing education. *Nurse Education Today, 33*(3), 286–290.

Forni, P. M. (2008). The civil classroom in the age of the net. *Thought & Action: The NEA Higher Education Journal,* 15–22.

Gillespie, M. (2002). Student–teacher connection in clinical nursing education. *Journal of Advanced Nursing, 37*(6), 566–578.

Gillespie, M. (2005). Student–teacher connection: A place of possibility. *Journal of Advanced Nursing, 52*(2), 211–219.

Glenn, D. (2013). Survey: Is social media making us hostile? Retrieved June 14, 2014, from http://socialtimes.com/survey-is-social-media-making-us-hostile_b123830

Halstead, J. A. (Ed.). (2007). Nurse educator competencies: Creating an evidence-based practice for nurse educators. New York, NY: National League for Nursing.

Huston, C. (2014). The impact of emerging technology on nursing care: Warp speed ahead. *The Online Journal of Issues in Nursing, 18*(2). Manuscript 1.

Lashley, F. R., & de Meneses, M. (2001). Student civility in nursing programs: A national survey. *Journal of Professional Nursing, 17*(2), 81–86.

Luparell, S. (2004). Faculty encounters with uncivil nursing students: An overview. *Journal of Professional Nursing, 20*(1), 59–67.

Morrissette, P. J. (2001). Reducing incivility in the university/college classroom. *International Electronic Journal for Leadership in Learning, 5*(4). Retrieved June 14, 2014, from http://iejll.journalhosting.ucalgary.ca/iejll/index.php/ijll/article/view/497

National Council of State Boards of Nursing. (2011). White paper: A nurse's guide to the use of social media. Retrieved June 14, 2014, from https://www.ncsbn.org/Social_Media.pdf

National Student Nurses' Association. (2014). Recommendations for social media usage and maintaining primary confidentiality and professionalism. Retrieved January, 2014, from http://www.nsna.org/Portals/0/Skins/NSNA/pdf/NSNA_Social_Media_Recommendations.pdf

Oermann, M. (1996). Differences in clinical experiences of ADN and BSN students. *Journal of Nursing Education, 37*(5), 197–201.

Reutter, L., Field, P. A., Campbell, I. E., & Day, R. (1997). Socialization into nursing: Nursing students as learners. *Journal of Nursing Education, 36,* 149–155.

Robertson, J. E. (2012). Can't we all just get along? A primer on student incivility in nursing education. *Nursing Education Perspectives, 33*(1), 21–26.

Suplee, P. D., Lachman, V. D., Siebert, B., & Anselmi, K. K. (2008). Managing nursing student incivility in the classroom, clinical setting, and on-line. *Journal of Nursing Law, 12*(2), 68–77.

Thomas, S. P. (2003). Handling anger in the teacher–student relationship. *Nursing Education Perspectives, 24*(1), 17–24.

Wingert, D., & Molitor, T. (2009). Best practices: Preventing and managing challenging classroom situations. *Currents in Teaching and Learning, 1*(2), 4–18.

Chapter 6

Connection Between Evidence-Based Practice and Nursing Education

Carol Boswell and Sharon Cannon

CHAPTER OBJECTIVES

At the conclusion of this chapter, the learner will be able to:

1. Recognize the key definitions and elements related to evidence-based practice and evidence-based teaching.

2. Analyze the different evidence-based practice theories/models to see how they apply to evidence-based teaching.

3. Discuss motivation of learners in nursing education.

4. Identify steps to foster motivation in students.

5. Compare compliance in nursing education to patient education.

KEY TERMS

- ACESTAR model
- ARCC model
- Benner's model
- The Cochrane Collaboration
- Compliance
- Iowa model
- Joanna Briggs Institute
- Johns Hopkins model
- Model
- Motivation
- Quality improvement
- Rosswurm-Larrabee model
- Stetler/Marran model
- Theory

INTRODUCTION

At this point, the literature does not provide any theory or model for nursing evidence-based teaching (EBT). Since no theory/model for EBT exists, the models and theories related to evidence-based practice (EBP) must be used to contribute key aspects. From these EBP theories and models, key elements can be combined to address the process of EBT. The application of the elements and concepts requires manipulation to address the academic and educational aspects of EBT. Most of the different pieces can be readily applied with a change in focus from a clinical to an educational concentration.

Melnyk (2013) states, "Faculty in academic institutions cannot teach what they themselves do not know" (p. 185). Melnyk was quoting what she and Fineout-Overholt, Feinstein, Sadler, and Green-Hernandez state in 2008 regarding faculty who continue to teach research and EBP without really comprehending the relationship of EBP and research. Each nursing professional must carefully look at how to integrate evidence in the practice that they are involved in completing, whether that is clinical or academia. Benner, Sutphen, Leonard, and Day (2009) have advocated for a radical transformation within the education of nurses. Benner et al. (2009) argue that despite the substantial external challenges facing health care, nursing practice, and nursing education, changes within nursing education are imperative and essential. Within this text, the authors demand that nursing education deliberate and undertake a drastic and revolutionary change in the manner of delivery for nursing education. Some of the changes demanded by this call reflect the necessity of embracing EBT. The recommendations for nursing programs include changing:

- from a focus on covering decontextualized knowledge to an emphasis on teaching for a sense of salience, situated cognition, and action in particular situations,
- from a sharp separation of clinical and classroom teaching to an integration of the two,
- from an emphasis on critical thinking to an emphasis on clinical reasoning and multiple ways of thinking, and
- from an emphasis on socialization and role taking to an emphasis on formation (Benner et al., 2009, p. 4).

Each of these recommendations strongly supports the idea that the educational process used within the classroom and clinical settings must assimilate the process of confirming the appropriateness and effectiveness of the different teaching strategies utilized. To simply teach as we have always taught or been taught does not demonstrate the commitment to excellence that is mandated by this call for an uncompromising transformation in the educating of nursing professionals. Parse (2013) presented ideas voiced during an international nursing conference related to evidence-based practice within the academic venue. The article states that "frequently faculty in these programs (higher degree nursing programs) were mandated to add to all course outlines the words *evidence-based practice*, because accrediting agencies had added these words to the criteria for evaluation of nursing programs" (Parse, 2013, p. 109). The consensus of the faculty at the meeting was the lack of any additions or changes within the actual course materials. The words were added, but content and management of the process were not modified or included within the delivery of the course.

DEFINITIONS AND ELEMENTS

As thoughts turn toward EBT, many different words come to mind that play a part in understanding the facets involved. Terms such as *theory*, *model*, *philosophy*, *nursing process*, *critical thinking*, *evidence-based practice*, *research*, *practice-based evidence*, and *research utilization* will be discussed. Though these terms are sometimes used interchangeably, each term provides a different dimension in the management of evidence. *Encarta World English Dictionary* (2009) defines *philosophy* as an investigation into the foundational concepts, a discipline of thought, the foundational or fundamental principles, and/or a compilation of beliefs and goals. The philosophical aspects are those items that come together to form the foundation on which the other building blocks can be laid. As one moves from the philosophy, theories are developed. *Encarta World English Dictionary* (2009) characterizes a **theory** as (1) a set of rules and/or techniques that can be applied to a subject and/or abstract thoughts and (2) the ideas that form the underpinning that is used to move a distinct practice into reality. Theories come in multiple levels and formations. Theories can be very structured and clearly delineated, or they can be the initial work toward understanding the abstract thoughts and ideas about a particular subject.

According to *Encarta World English Dictionary* (2009), a **model** is a simplified version of the complex analysis and problem solving related to a topic and/or an explanation of a theory and/or the concepts related to that theory. The model is usually an illustration of the complex facts, beliefs, rules, and thoughts that are subsumed within a theory. The model provides an attempt to visually represent the diverse interconnections of the concepts within a theory. Complexity theory is an example that demonstrates diversity through informal networking that involves interlocking relationships. The model for complexity theory includes patient care beyond the hospital setting and provides a microsystem approach to the level of care for populations of individuals, families, and population groups (Roussel, Godfrey, & Williams, 2010). According to Holistic Health and Healing (2012), "Nursing could be viewed as a dissipative system, a self-organizing system that gains energy from the environment, is responsive to feedback, and evolves over time" (para. 5). These characteristics reflect the complexity of the nursing profession as it functions within this type of theory. Complexity theory strives to identify and react to the interrelationships of multiple components as they intertwine collectively to establish the complex form of structure on which an idea is built. Models provide the foundation for the manner in which relationships are formed and managed.

Within EBP, many different terms come into play. As is true with any involvement with evidence, thought and analysis are key. Terms such as *nursing process, critical thinking, research*, and *research utilization* all depict some form of thinking and scrutinizing. The nursing process includes assessment, diagnosis, planning, implementation, and evaluation. Each of these different steps comes together to move a patient treatment plan forward toward success. These same five steps are critical for the provision of appropriate and effective nursing education. The nursing process provides a foundation for the effective management of EBT; that is, EBT is best initiated using these same five steps. A second term that is directly involved in analysis is *critical thinking*. According to The Critical Thinking Co. (2005), "Critical thinking is the identification and evaluation of evidence to guide decision making. A critical thinker uses broad in-depth analysis of evidence to make decisions and communicate his/her beliefs clearly and accurately" (para. 1). The concepts included in thinking critically require that each problem and/or topic be considered from all sides. Each and every potential aspect housed within critical thinking compels the participants to seek innovative ways to address the various components in an evaluation of the evidence. Paul and Elder (2009) stipulate that critical thinking should be timely and self-directed while requiring individualized management and monitoring for success. In addition, critical thinking showcases a process of self-correcting any errors and challenges encountered. Critical thinking, though imperative for nursing care, is also vital to the process of educating the student. It is important that faculty members model the process of critical thinking in the classroom and clinical setting, use it when making decisions about management of the classroom, and employ it with every discussion during the educational process.

Other terms frequently included during a discussion of EBP are *research* and *research utilization*. Research is defined as the systematic examination of a topic to ascertain facts, to determine or modify a theory/model, or to cultivate a plan of action established on the evidence revealed (*Encarta World English Dictionary*, 2009). Research utilization builds on the idea of research. Research utilization considers the evidence presented as a result of one study. When multiple research projects are summarized, the outcome includes a systematic review.

The final terms to consider are *evidence-based practice, practice-based evidence, quality improvement,* and *evidence-based teaching.* These terms are carefully contemplated within the chapter titled *Overview of Evidence-Based Practice.* A comparison of the different definitions for EBP is provided in the first table of that chapter. In that chapter, six different definitions are contrasted. The characteristics within each of the definitions are provided to determine the consistency among the definitions. According to Boswell and Cannon (2014), the constant characteristics found within the multiple definitions relate to the decision-making scheme, clinical application, provider expertise, and client contribution. According to Drisko (2012b):

> EBP is a mix of (a) learning what treatments "work" based on the best available research (whether experiential or not), (b) discussing client views about the treatment to consider cultural and other differences, and to honor client self-determination and autonomy, (c) considering the professional's "clinical wisdom" based on work with similar and dissimilar cases that may provide a context for understanding the research evidence, and (d) considering what the professional can, and cannot, provide fully and ethically. (para. 2)

Each of these four components is essential to the provision of EBP. The evidence, client, setting, and provider are all crucial as effective and appropriate care is considered and determined. We would suggest that while research evidence is tested and analyzed, other evidence is also appropriate to consider when determining the best practices to be implemented. As we move EBP to practice-based evidence, the process takes on a convoluted appearance. Salmond (2013) sponsored the idea that an "evidence-based approach to practice calls for practitioners to question why they do things in a particular fashion, whether there may be a better approach, and what the evidence suggests may be best for a particular clinical context and patient population" (p. 16). Developing an inquisitive mind-set allows the nursing profession to seek and embrace optimum avenues for delivering professional services. Only when individuals appreciate the dynamics of EBP and the value of best practices will true support and engagement with EBP occur. EBP is viewed as the general level of identifying and validating the evidence presented and related to the different topics under investigation. Practice-based evidence takes the evidence as it moves from the "research to practice" level. Thus, practice-based evidence is the day-to-day engagement of the evidence into the practice arena for the betterment of the provision of care.

Most often, **quality improvement** (QI) in nursing is associated with the improvement of nursing care at the point of care. QI efforts have become a recognized form of EBP and are now considered to be essential in the provision of nursing care. QI also has implications for EBT, as demonstrated in the process of evaluation for programs, courses, faculty, and students. Evaluation is discussed in other chapters, but must be considered in the parallel between EBP and EBT. In EBP, QI is considered in relation to improvements needed specific to an organization providing patient care. In EBT, QI is also improvement specific to an educational institution providing nursing education.

One last term to consider for this discussion is *evidence-based teaching*. As stated in the *Overview of Evidence-Based Practice* chapter, EBT is a dynamic, holistic system using educational principles validated by evidence to support, maintain, and promote a new level of knowledge for a learner in a variety of settings. Drisko (2012a) suggested that "educational efforts. . . could be oriented to provide beginning professionals with effective tools and a model for the continuing improvement and renewal of their professional practices" (para. 1). EBT takes the ideas and concepts included within EBP to improve management of the educational process within the health disciplines. According to Mitchell (2013), "It is important for nurses to ask provocative questions about the use of evidence to sustain the status quo, for instance, or to extend colonization of dominant ideologies and agendas" (p. 149). As educators and professionals, the idea of becoming increasingly engaged in seeking the best answers to all types of practice—clinical and educational—is imperative. The *Overview of Evidence-Based Practice* chapter provides several figures and a discussion concerning the process of EBT for use within this text.

THEORY/MODELS

Many different types of EBP theories and models exist. According to Vratny and Shriver (2007), EBP models concentrate on the scientific nature, not the "art," of EBP. Nursing knowledge tends to primarily emerge from clinical experiences, human sources, opinion, folklore, rituals, and/or traditions, but not as much from research. It seems that up to this point in the nursing profession, the knowledge used by nurses has been based on subjective types of evidence instead of embracing the objective management of evidence. Burman, Robinson, and Hart (2013) noted the importance of "developing organizational cultures and resources that empower nurses to develop the knowledge, skills, and authority to implement all components of the EBP model" (pp. 236–237). EBP has been showcased for over 20 years, yet we continue to encounter nurses who do not know how to actively engage in EBP. They can perform simple tasks, but the process of EBP is not ingrained in the fiber of nursing practice. As a result of these types of knowledge sources, the boundaries between research, research utilization, and EBP have been clouded. Only in the last few years has the nursing profession embraced the concept of EBP. With this transition to evidence as the foundation for the care provided by nurses, nursing research has increased. In addition, discussions have multiplied and focused on areas concerning such questions as: What is evidence? Where can evidence be found? How much evidence is needed? What about the "art" of nursing care as a source for this evidence? While some progress toward the answers to these questions has been made, additional attention and thought are needed.

Since multiple models and theories about EBP have been developed, Gawlinski and Rutledge (2008) provided an evaluation tool for critiquing the different EBP models. This tool provides an initial method for selecting a model that could be utilized in the unique practices of nursing care. Each setting has to carefully consider the different models and theories to select one that works best within the unique environment. This tool is one method developed to facilitate the selection of a model that would address the concerns and problems distinctive to a given setting.

At this point, we need to look at several of the EBP models. Although these models are EBP models, they have aspects that can be related to EBT. Since only one EBT model related to higher education can be located at this time, the application of EBP models is the primary method for viewing the process. One evidence-based education model is provided by Evidence Based Practice and Curriculum (2011). This model utilizes professional wisdom and empirical evidence. Professional wisdom is viewed to include both individual experiences and expertise. Empirical evidence brings the scientific research along with the empirical information to the table for consideration. Foundational within this model is the expectation of rigorous research to be supported by successful utilization of the educational aspects. The validity of the process is based on the reliability and trustworthiness of the evidence as seen within the practice arena.

Two overarching groups—the Joanna Briggs Institute and The Cochrane Collaboration—will be discussed first. These two agencies do not directly have models but are strategic when looking at EBP. After discussing these two agencies, several EBP models will be presented: the Stetler/Marran, Rosswurm-Larrabee, ACESTAR, ARCC, Iowa, Benner, and Johns Hopkins. These models are not the only models but tend to be the ones that are frequently utilized.

The **Joanna Briggs Institute** (JBI) was established in 1996. Evidence-based health care is regarded as a cyclical opportunity by the members of this institution. The JBI strives to incorporate all levels of evidence from opinion up to the rigorous randomized controlled trials (RCTs) while endeavoring to focus on the effectiveness of interventions and activities. In order to ensure that the information and resources provided by the JBI are of global importance, they must:

- consider international evidence related to the feasibility, appropriateness, meaningfulness, and effectiveness of healthcare interventions (evidence generation),
- include these different forms of evidence in a formal assessment called a systematic review (evidence synthesis),
- globally disseminate information in appropriate, relevant formats to inform health systems, health professionals, and consumers (evidence transfer), and
- offer designated programs to enable the effective implementation of evidence and evaluation of its impact on healthcare practice (evidence utilization) (JBI, 2008).

The JBI uses as its primary crux feasibility, appropriateness, meaningfulness, and effectiveness (FAME) of health practices and delivery methods (JBI, 2008). These four principal designations make up the "FAME" scale of evidence. In addition to the JBI Levels of Evidence scale, the JBI utilizes a JBI Grades of Recommendation scale that also uses the four designations. These two scales mirror the Appraisal of Guidelines Research and Evaluation (AGREE) Collaboration. The AGREE tool is used by individuals to assess guidelines related to the depth of evidence used to develop the guideline.

The **Cochrane Collaboration** is an international, not-for-profit network established in 1993 to help healthcare providers and others to make well-informed healthcare decisions. This collaboration was named after Archie Cochrane, a British epidemiologist, who is viewed as the individual who conceptualized EBP (The Cochrane Collaboration, n.d.). This group pledges to keep up-to-date and accurate information about health care and its effects for the global community. One of the major contributions from this agency is the production and dissemination of systematic reviews concerning healthcare interventions. It also is dedicated to promoting the ongoing search for evidence in the form of clinical trials and other studies of intervention. Those who generate the reviews are primarily volunteer healthcare professionals who function in one of the many Cochrane Review Groups. These groups work with an editorial team to prepare and maintain the reviews while applying the rigorous quality standards for which Cochrane Reviews are known. The Cochrane Reviews are viewed as the gold standard in regard to the process and quality of the publications.

The **Stetler/Marran model** of research utilization was developed in 1976, making it one of the oldest of the models. It was revised in 1994 with the addition of conceptual underpinnings and a set of assumptions and is now referred to as the Stetler model. According to Gawlinski and Rutledge (2008), this model is one of the few that does not pivot on only formal changes accomplished by nurses within the organizational setting. This model assimilates the individual nurse while promoting the use of both internal and external data/evidence. According to Melnyk and Fineout-Overholt (2005), "The Stetler model outlines a prescriptive series of steps to assess and use research findings, thereby facilitating safe and effective EBP" (p. 188). The Stetler model is a practitioner-oriented model that focuses on critical thinking and the incorporation of the findings of knowledgeable individuals. The steps included within the model are (McClinton, 1997):

- Preparation (ascertaining the rationale and core of the review)
- Validation (confirming the research as to applicability and relevancy)
- Comparative evaluation (reviewing findings from comparable studies)
- Decision making (selecting from four choices—to use the findings, to consider using the findings, to delay using the findings, or to reject the findings in total)
- Translation/application (determining how to implement the findings into practice)
- Evaluation (validating the consequence on the practice, policy, and/or patient)

Overall, the changes to this model have been constructed to address the utilization of focused integrative review methodology, targeted evidence concepts, and ongoing encounters as the model has been used by clinical nurse specialists and nurse practitioners. Although this model is not a true EBP model, it serves as the forerunner to the models that have been developed as a result of moving from research utilization toward practice based on sound evidence.

The **Rosswurm-Larrabee model** was developed in 1999. This model was established for use in primary care settings with advanced practitioners. It strives to guide the individual through the entire process of EBP. The steps used within this model follow the steps of the nursing process. The six steps are assessing the needs of stakeholders, building bridges while making connections, synthesizing the evidence to determine its relevancy, planning the practice change, implementing the changes culminating in evaluating those changes, and integrating the practice changes for sustainability. This model aspired to move the existing medical EBP model to include a focus on nursing phenomena. The ultimate goal within this model is to change clinical practice as a result of the evidence. According to Gawlinski and Rutledge (2008), the preliminary need for change was ascertained by equating the internal data with data resulting from studies conducted outside of the organization. Thus, the internal data were supported by the external information that was collected and analyzed.

Another model was developed by the Academic Center for Evidence-Based Practice (ACE). The model is titled the ACE Star Model of Knowledge Transformation, or the **ACESTAR model**. According to the ACE (2012), the ACESTAR model is a representation for how to interpret the sequences, description, and features of knowledge that are used in different phases of evidence-based practice. The model is depicted as a star with the five points embracing: knowledge discovery, evidence summary, translation into practice recommendations, integration into practice, and evaluation. According to Gawlinski and Rutledge (2008), this model supports EBP by depicting knowledge as it evolves. This model does not discuss the use of non-research evidence. Knowledge gained from other venues outside of research is not integrated within the model. Although the model does not completely restrict the incorporation of knowledge gained in this manner, the assimilation of other knowledge is done by the individual, not within the explanation of the stages.

The Advancing Research and Clinical Practice Through Close Collaboration model, or **ARCC model**, has as its goals (1) the advancement of EBP among advanced practice nurses, (2) the establishment of a network of clinicians to act as EBP mentors, and (3) dissemination of the best evidence. Initially, this model focused on RCTs. As it has matured, other levels of evidence have been accepted, but the focus continues to be directed toward research findings. Gawlinski and Rutledge (2008) designate the key focus for this model to be at the departmental and/or unit level within the organization. The ARCC draws on the use of EBP mentors to champion the development of the advanced practice nurse. This model endeavors to consolidate the integration of practice and research in the form of EBP with a foundation of benchmarking.

The Iowa Model of Evidence-Based Practice to Promote Quality Care, or the **Iowa model**, was originally developed in 1994 with a goal of helping to guide bedside nursing staff members toward the use of research findings to improve the care provided. This model emphasizes the organization, primarily acute care settings. Melnyk and Fineout-Overholt (2005) state that the utilization of this model "gives a strong message to the organization about its role in the support of EBP" (p. 197). The Iowa model was cultivated to promote quality care in multiple academic and clinical settings. It works to mesh QI with research utilization. One item unique to this model is the use of "triggers" of EBP. The triggers are those items identified within the practice arena that raise a question as to the validity of the current practice. By identifying and acknowledging these triggers, EBP projects can be instituted to determine the optimum way to address the issue that will result in quality care for clients.

Benner's model of novice to expert (1982) for nursing practice initially provided a pathway for nurses to develop patient care skills and knowledge through education and experience. The emergence of evidence-based practice expanded the novice-to-expert model to include best evidence in decision making (Purvis & Gabb, 2013) in an online program. However, Benner's model can be used by all types of nursing programs to assist students in applying best practices regardless of the level of learner in an undergraduate program or graduate program.

The final EBP model to be discussed within this chapter is the **Johns Hopkins model**. According to Johns Hopkins Nursing and Evidence-Based Practice (n.d.), this model "is a powerful problem-solving approach to clinical decision-making and is accompanied by user-friendly tools to guide individual or group use" (para. 1). This model was developed for use by the nurses and nursing students at Johns Hopkins to answer clinical, administrative, and education practice questions.

While multiple EBP models and tools are available, their application to teaching has not occurred at this time. Each of these models has concepts that could be adapted to address the EBT viewpoint. In the *Overview of Evidence-Based Practice* chapter, the second figure reflects the multiple areas that must be considered when conceptualizing the aspects indicative of EBT. The facets and features encompassed by the teaching role are multiple and complex. Care must be given to ensure that while the academic teaching role is a huge component of the educational process, other educational venues such as staff development are also of paramount importance. As evidence is collected on the different facets and features included in the teaching role, the application of the evidence needs to embrace the multiplexity of the teaching role and environment.

MOTIVATION, COMPLIANCE, AND BEHAVIORS OF THE LEARNER

Along with examining EBP theories, models, definitions, and elements, understanding the **motivation** of students is essential. Reams of evidence regarding motivation abound in the literature, especially in the behavioral science and education areas. Theories of motivation are provided by Skinner, Piaget, Bandura, Maslow, and Knowles, to name just a few. However, few studies have been conducted in nursing education. An examination of motivational theories will be discussed first.

Ard (2009) suggests that motivation may look simple but is actually complex; Ard applies Wlodkowaki's 1978 definition of motivation as involving processes promoting and directing the purpose of behavior. Ard (2009) builds on that definition by indicating that "motivation is a complex interaction" (p. 41) that is both intrinsic (internal) and extrinsic (external). However, Biehler and Snowman suggest, "Motivation is only intrinsic but circumstances can be created to influence motivation" ("Motivation," 1997, p. 2).

We are all familiar with Skinner's model of operant conditioning that involved rats in a maze seeking a piece of cheese. Skinner indicates that positive or negative reinforcement determines motivation ("Motivation," 1997). Ever wonder what Skinner might have thought about "Who moved my cheese?" Within this text about managing change, the use of positive and/or negative reinforcement can help greatly as change is addressed. The use of reinforcements to drive the conditioning is a key strategy incorporated into Skinner's model.

Piaget took a more cognitive approach to motivation by explaining it as a balance between old and new experiences using organizing and balancing schemes. As a result, learners want to "master their environment" ("Motivation," 1997, p. 3). Piaget developed his cognitive theory around the ideas of schemas, equilibrium, assimilation, accommodation, and stages of development. McLeod (2009) affirms the expectation that the role of the teacher in the process of learning and motivation is as a facilitator. Within this approach, a teacher uses active methods to allow for discovery and construction of the end products of learning. Atherton (2011) supports these ideas and further develops the idea that each person must be allowed to grow into knowledge at her or his own rate of processing. Learning could be visually represented as stairs within this model. As an individual becomes comfortable at one level, she or he can then be motivated to move to the next level of complexity. This suggestion by Atherton fits well with Benner's model of novice to expert.

Sweetland (2010) defines motivation as "the force that drives a person to do something" (p. 1). He further emphasizes that motivation comes from within the individual, which Bandura identifies as goal setting and modification of prior behavior models that are successful. Hodson-Carlton (2009) also points out the importance of Bandura's theory related to self-efficacy, which "is the result of previous learning attempts" (p. 312).

According to Biehler and Snowman ("Motivation," 1997), Maslow's hierarchy of needs ranges from a deficiency of needs to a growth need (self-actualization) to achieve self-fulfillment. Cognitive needs for growth influence motivation. As individuals become increasingly secure with the different levels Maslow included within the hierarchy of needs model, the realization of seeking self-achievement and accomplishment can be grasped. One idea within this model reflects the desire to strive for the higher levels once the lower levels have been satisfied.

In higher education, Malcolm Knowles's theory of adult learning is considered essential to motivating students. Knowles proposes that adults are self-directed, need to be involved, rely on prior experiences, need relevance, and should center on problems rather than content (Knowles, 1980). In many ways, one could postulate that Knowles's theory incorporates all of the motivational theories previously discussed.

For the purpose of this text, motivation is considered to be both intrinsic and extrinsic. Motivation involves satisfaction derived from prior learning prompting the desire to learn more. As each individual carefully considers his or her professional goals, the intrinsic and extrinsic aspects resulting in individualized motivation can be determined. By understanding the different ideas related to motivation, leaders can formulate a plan to engage and support faculty members to be motivated toward excellence.

Now let's investigate evidence regarding motivation of students in nursing education. Ard (2009) suggests that a "literature review revealed only five studies on motivation in nursing" (p. 4) and all were conducted outside of the United States. Thompson (2009) supports Ard's suggestion that there is a lack of nursing education research and little evidence to validate learning theories. Most of the motivational literature in nursing education is descriptive applications or strategies that provide nurse educators information about motivation. Research about what motivates student nurses and how nurse educators influence motivation of students are two areas worthy of intense study.

Inherent to education, patient education, and nursing education is the notion of compliance. **Compliance** is discussed in almost every aspect of the management of health care, especially in relation to patient education. You can often hear comments such as, "I gave them the information but they don't use it," or "I taught it, so why don't they incorporate the knowledge?" Obviously, compliance is closely related to motivation (i.e., the impetus to move/change/act). Getting patients or nursing students to change behavior and act on information given is a phenomenal task and may overwhelm novice or even expert nurse educators. Though little research has been conducted in this area, it does not mean that there aren't strategies to increase compliance and motivation.

Based on the motivational theories discussed previously, tips proposed by the authors will be examined. One of the first tips to consider in motivation directed toward changing the behaviors of the learners is the differences among the generations of learners, as discussed in the chapter titled *The Role of the Academician*. Patient education has focused more heavily on adult learning and literacy, especially health literacy. However, nursing education has recognized the importance of generational differences. Use of these generational considerations is discussed throughout this text, as it is an important aspect to incorporate into motivating students to learn.

ARCS motivation theory (Keller, 2010) suggests that to motivate, the educator must address attention, relevance, confidence, and satisfaction (ARCS). Attention can be achieved through novel and uncertain events, through posing problems, and through variations of instructional elements. Relevance relates to using familiar language and examples, identifying goals to be accomplished, and matching teaching strategies with profiles of students. Confidence is gained when learners know how to perform at multiple achievement levels and are given supportive feedback. Satisfaction involves opportunities to use knowledge in real or simulated settings, provision of positive feedback and reinforcement, and use of consistent standards and consequences to accomplish tasks. To effectively incorporate this theory into the classroom, faculty members strive for active learning such as role play, case studies, simulation activities, or problem-solving exercises. Through these different activities, the ideas of ARCS can be incorporated into the different activities utilized within the learning setting to provide the required materials.

Knowles (1980) focuses heavily on relevance of task-orientation, discovery, experimentation, involvement in the instructions, and problem-oriented content. Process is emphasized more than content being taught, with faculty more in the role of facilitator than lecturer. As a faculty member attempts to use this method in the learning environment, care must be given to the idea of concept-based learning. To get at the processes that are used within health care, concepts would be the emphasis of the learning. This method of motivation works toward establishing the foundation for the transference of knowledge to other situations.

In discussing motivation theories, Sweetland (2010) offers 14 suggestions to increase motivation. The suggestions include discussion about variables (ability, luck, efforts, etc.), positive feedback on progress, opportunities to create knowledge, relearning concepts and correcting errors, listening and teaching how to listen, maintaining high expectations, and problem solving with critical thinking. Each instructor carefully and thoughtfully considers the different ways that motivation can occur. In addition, the faculty member must contemplate the cohort that is being taught. Each cohort of individuals has unique needs and expectations. Faculty members must reevaluate the types of motivational efforts used based upon the makeup of the cohort. Different generational groups lean toward certain motivational techniques while others gravitate toward a totally different stimulus for learning. Effective teachers will modify approaches and grow as educators to accommodate the current cohort of learners.

Biehler and Snowman ("Motivation," 1997) suggest the use of behavioral techniques, addressing what is required with the process and achievement, satisfying deficiency needs, emphasizing rewards and consequences, focusing on success, and having a sense of adventure. They incorporate both operant conditioning and social learning theory. Behavioral aspects can be used effectively with some groups to address their motivational needs. An effective manager will strive to understand which techniques work best with which groups of individuals. The same techniques do not work for every person.

Tips and strategies for addressing the behaviors of the learners will be given in additional chapters for online, clinical, and simulation settings. Motivational concepts should be carefully applied for the different educational environments. One method of motivating does not work in all settings. Faculty members must be willing to try new facets of the concepts for unique settings and groups of students.

As we strive to integrate generational components and motivational theories, care must be given to the use of generalizations. Generalizations must be considered with the awareness that each individual is unique. Utilizing the information provided in the chapter titled *The Role of the Academician* regarding generational characteristics, some assumptions related to motivation can be ascertained.

The Traditionalists/Veterans (born before 1946) tend to reflect the concepts found within the ARCS motivation theory. This generation strives to serve while working hard and respecting authority. To motivate students within this cohort, attention should be given to clearly (1) determine the goals or tasks expected; (2) embrace the attributes of discipline, order, structure, and logic; and (3) address the idea of duty.

Moving to the Baby Boomer cohort (born 1946–1964), the mechanisms to consider would center on this generation needing to be in the spotlight. While embracing the idea of "making a difference," they tend to be focused on themselves—the "Me" generation. Members of this generation, though team players, desire personal gratification. As faculty members attempt to challenge and motivate these individuals, thoughts should be directed toward providing recognition for activities completed. The Baby Boomer cohort embraces challenges and risks. They function well when allowed to discover answers, experiment with options, and problem solve, particularly within groups.

The next cohort for consideration is Generation X (born 1965–1976). When trying to motivate this group, it is wise to remember that they are self-starters and results-driven. Providing goals for them and then getting out of their way to allow them to creatively and individually complete the goals is beneficial. This cohort expects to influence the terms and conditions employed to research the goals and outcomes.

The final group currently at the higher education level is the Millennial generation (born 1977–1997). This cohort tends to be very competitive, civic-minded, and materialistic. When endeavoring to motivate this group, employing challenges based on "real-world" situations allows them the opportunity to compete with peers to solve an identifiable problem. Service learning is an effective strategy for this group. Students learn while contributing to an organization in their community. The Millennial cohort is goal-driven. Motivation is increased as the goals are set and confronted within a team orientation.

The Traditionalists/Veterans and Generation Xers want to work independently toward their goals. Baby Boomers and Millennial individuals value the benefits of teamwork to reach a goal/outcome. Another aspect to consider related to motivating the different generations concerns time orientation. Members of the Traditionalist/Veteran and Baby Boomer groups are more structured concerning time; they are therefore more linear. The other two cohorts (Generation X and Millennial) tend to be more "outside the box" due to their technology orientation. Technology allows these groups to work flexibly, any time and any place.

Although the generational characteristics are useful when considering motivation, care must be used to ensure that each individual is still considered in relation to personal needs and expectations. Faculty members need to contemplate the distinctive and idiosyncratic characteristics of each student and/or class cohort. Each class tends to take on a distinct group personality. The generational characteristics that are included in the class cohort can offer the faculty member a beginning place from which to seek to engage and motivate the class.

SUMMARY THOUGHTS

Evidence-based practice and evidence-based teaching share elements and concepts applicable to the advancement of nursing education. While research utilizing EBP elements and concepts is becoming more prolific, a dearth of research exists in nursing education. EBP models can and should be applied to nursing education. Benner et al. (2009) advocate for drastic change in the delivery of nursing education. Evidence for promoting best practices in the classroom and clinical setting must incorporate the motivation and compliance of students to critically think when providing nursing care, especially to patients from diverse settings and having complex healthcare needs.

The Institute of Medicine and Robert Wood Johnson recommendations for the future of nursing and the Affordable Care Act all require that evidence be apparent for educating nurses to provide care based on best practices. To assist with this initiative through EBP and EBT, Sigma Theta Tau International and the National League for Nursing collaborated in an effort to promote EBT through research in nursing education. In 2014, the two organizations arranged for a national conference on research in nursing education. This spotlight will result in podium and poster presentations promoting EBT.

SUMMARY POINTS

1. The literature has only recently begun to provide any type of theory or model for EBT.
2. The recommendations presented by the call for a radical change in nursing education strongly support the idea that the educational process used within classroom and clinical settings must assimilate the process of confirming the appropriateness and effectiveness of the different teaching strategies utilized.

3. EBT is a dynamic, holistic system using educational principles validated by evidence to support, maintain, and promote a new level of knowledge for a learner in a variety of settings.

4. Nursing knowledge tends to emerge from clinical experiences, human sources, opinion, folklore, rituals, and/or traditions, but not usually from research.

5. The Joanna Briggs Institute strives to incorporate all levels of evidence, from opinion up to rigorous randomized controlled trials, while endeavoring to focus on the effectiveness of interventions and activities.

6. The Joanna Briggs Institute uses as its primary crux feasibility, appropriateness, meaningfulness, and effectiveness (FAME) of health practices and delivery methods.

7. One of the major contributions from The Cochrane Collaboration is the production and dissemination of systematic reviews concerning healthcare interventions.

8. As evidence is collected on the different facets and features included in the teaching role, the application of the evidence needs to embrace the multiplexity of the teaching role and environment.

9. Motivation is intrinsic and extrinsic.

10. Motivation appears simple but is complex.

11. Few studies have been conducted in the United States that involve the learning motivation of nursing students.

12. Consideration of generational characteristics can be effective when determining how to motivate a cohort of students.

TIPS FOR NURSE EDUCATORS

1. Develop a clear definition of EBP and EBT.

2. Incorporate an evidence-based model approach to EBT.

3. Consider generational differences when seeking to motivate students.

4. Promote attention, relevance, confidence, and satisfaction (ARCS) to engage students in the learning process.

5. Utilize feedback, listening, and problem solving/critical thinking.

6. Emphasize rewards, consequences, and success while maintaining high expectations.

7. Incorporate operant conditioning and social learning theory.

MULTIPLE CHOICE QUESTIONS

1. The nursing process that provides a beginning organization for thinking includes:
   A. **assessment, diagnosis, planning, implementation, and evaluation.**
   B. assessment, data mining, implementation, and evaluation.
   C. planning, organizing, diagnosis, implementation, and evaluation.
   D. planning, diagnosis, data mining, implementation, and evaluation.

   Rationale:
   The nursing process includes the phases of assessment, diagnosis, planning, implementation, and evaluation. Each of these different steps comes together to move a patient treatment plan forward toward success.

2. The characteristics routinely found in the multiple evidence-based practice definitions are:
   A. decision making, educational application, and client contribution.
   B. clinical application, physician expertise, and client contribution.
   C. critical thinking, clinical application, and provider expertise.
   D. **decision making, provider expertise, and clinical application.**

   Rationale:
   According to Boswell and Cannon (2014), the constant characteristics found within the multiple definitions are the decision-making scheme, clinical application, provider expertise, and client contribution.

3. Evidence-based teaching is a:
   A. complex process using educational principles legalized by data to aid the learner to gain knowledge.
   B. **dynamic, holistic system using educational principles validated by evidence to support, maintain, and promote knowledge for a learner in a variety of settings.**
   C. energetic system employing principles of education to provide knowledge to a learner in a variety of settings to support and maintain the process.
   D. holistic system using educational principles validated by evidence to support, maintain, and promote a new level of knowledge for a learner in a classroom setting.

Rationale:

Evidence-based teaching is a dynamic, holistic system using educational principles validated by evidence to support, maintain, and promote a new level of knowledge for a learner in a variety of settings.

4. The Joanna Briggs Institute uses four principles and/or criteria when determining the scale of evidence, which are:

   A. assessment, planning, implementation, and evaluation.
   B. feasibility, assessment, meaningfulness, and effectiveness.
   C. **feasibility, appropriateness, meaningfulness, and effectiveness.**
   D. assessment, appropriateness, meaningfulness, and evaluation.

Rationale:

The Joanna Briggs Institute uses as its primary crux feasibility, appropriateness, meaningfulness, and effectiveness of health practices and delivery methods (JBI, 2008). These four principal designations make up the "FAME" scale of evidence.

5. The two scales used by the Joanna Briggs Institute for assessing evidence mirror what other guide?

   A. **Appraisal of Guidelines Research and Evaluation (AGREE) Collaboration**
   B. FAME scale of evidence
   C. The Cochrane Collaboration
   D. Appraisal Related to Competency and Completeness (ARCC)

Rationale:

In addition to the JBI Levels of Evidence scale, JBI also utilizes a JBI Grades of Recommendation scale that similarly uses the four designations. These two scales mirror the Appraisal of Guidelines Research and Evaluation (AGREE) Collaboration.

6. The gold standard in regard to the process and quality of systematic reviews is the:

   A. Joanna Briggs Institute.
   B. Academic Center for Evidence-Based Practice.
   C. Institute of Medicine.
   D. **Cochrane Reviews.**

Rationale:

One of the major contributions from The Cochrane Collaboration is the production and dissemination of systematic reviews concerning healthcare interventions. It also is dedicated to promoting the ongoing search for evidence in the form of clinical trials and other studies of intervention. Those who generate the reviews are primarily volunteer healthcare professionals who function in one of the many Cochrane Review Groups. These groups work with an editorial team to prepare and maintain the reviews while applying the rigorous quality standards for which Cochrane Reviews are known. The Cochrane Reviews are viewed as the gold standard in regard to the process and quality of the publications.

7. The model that serves as the forerunner for evidence-based practice models is the:
   A. Rosswurm-Larrabee model.
   B. ACESTAR model.
   C. **Stetler model.**
   D. ARCC model.

   Rationale:
   Overall, the changes to the Stetler model have been accomplished to address the utilization of focused integrative review methodology, targeted evidence concepts, and ongoing encounters as the model has been used by clinical nurse specialists and nurse practitioners. Although this model is not a true EBP model, it serves as the forerunner to the models that have been developed as a result of moving from research utilization toward practice based upon sound evidence.

8. The evidence-based practice model that focuses on knowledge is the:
   A. Rosswurm-Larrabee model.
   B. **ACESTAR model.**
   C. Stetler model.
   D. ARCC model.

   Rationale:
   The ACESTAR model, according to the Academic Center for Evidence-Based Practice (2012), "is a model for understanding the cycles, nature, and characteristics of knowledge that are utilized in various aspects of evidence-based practice" (p. 1).

9. Motivation is:
   A. intrinsic.
   B. extrinsic.
   C. **both intrinsic and extrinsic.**
   D. neither intrinsic nor extrinsic.

   Rationale:
   Motivational theories postulate that motivation is both intrinsic and extrinsic.

10. Motivation involves processes that:
    A. **look simple but are complex.**
    B. conflict with established research.
    C. have little relevance to teaching.
    D. apply only to the science of psychology.

    Rationale:
    Ard (2009) suggests that motivation may look simple but is actually complex.

11. Validation of learning is:
    A. found in empirical studies in nursing education.
    B. seldom discussed in descriptive applications.
    C. not necessary to be an effective nurse educator.
    D. **found in only five studies, all of which were conducted outside of the United States.**

    Rationale:
    Ard (2009) notes that a "literature review revealed only five studies on motivation in nursing" (p. 4), and all were conducted outside of the United States.

12. Changing behavior and acting on information given are two aspects to consider for:
    A. self-confidence.
    B. apathy.
    C. indifference.
    D. **motivation.**

    Rationale:
    Compliance is closely related to motivation (i.e., the impetus to move/act/change).

13. According to Keller, the ARCS motivation theory must address:
    A. **attention, relevance, confidence, and satisfaction.**
    B. activity, response, caring, and satisfaction.
    C. attention, response, commonalities, and satisfaction.
    D. activity, response, complexity, and sources.

    Rationale:
    Keller's (2010) ARCS motivation theory suggests that to motivate learners, the educator must address attention, relevance, confidence, and satisfaction.

14. To motivate learners, Biehler and Snowman suggest the use of:
    A. textbooks.
    B. **adventure.**

C. failure.

D. society.

Rationale:

Biehler and Snowman ("Motivation," 1997) suggest the use of behavioral techniques, addressing what is required with the process and achievement, satisfying deficiency needs, emphasizing rewards and consequences, focusing on success, and having a sense of adventure.

15. Clinical simulation activities require the formation of a group to manage the client scenario. Which generational groups would function better in this type of learning situation?

A. Traditionalist/Veteran and Baby Boomer

B. **Baby Boomer and Millennial**

C. Traditionalist/Veteran and Generation X

D. Generation X and Millennial

Rationale:

The Traditionalist/Veteran and Generation X cohorts want to work independently toward goals. Baby Boomers and Millennials value the benefits of teamwork to reach a goal/outcome.

16. To motivate Generation Xers, the faculty member should work to establish:

A. **goals, then let them do it their own way.**

B. goals and paths for them to use.

C. groups, then let them come up with their own goals.

D. goals and stay with them to direct the process.

Rationale:

When endeavoring to motivate the Generation X group, it is wise to remember that they are self-starters and results-driven. Providing goals for them then getting out of their way to allow them to creatively and individually complete the goals is beneficial.

DISCUSSION QUESTIONS

1. Design a model for evidence-based teaching in your setting.

Considerations:

· Future directions of nursing education

· Target audience characteristics

· Outcomes to achieve

· Evaluation of the model; how to test

2. What motivates the students in your program to learn?
   Considerations:
   - Identify generational characteristics.
   - Identify strategies that students indicate motivate them.
   - Explore strategies that are new/different from yours.
   - Select a motivational theory that is relevant to your setting.

TEACHING SCENARIO

1. You have been assigned to teach a nursing theory course. Students consider nursing theories to be abstract and to have no relevance to nursing practice. How would you motivate the students to incorporate a nursing theory in their approach to nursing care? What evidence would you use to demonstrate the need for a relationship of theory to practice?
2. As a new faculty member, you are assigned to teach an evidence-based beginning course within an accelerated BSN program. These students come to the course with a background of having already completed a degree within a different discipline. Many of them have worked within that discipline for a significant time. They have now elected to change professions to become nurses. What type of motivational ideas and other aspects do you need to consider when setting up the assignments and course flow? What aspects related to generational differences do you need to consider?

REFERENCES

Academic Center for Evidence-Based Practice. (2012). ACE: Learn about EBP. Retrieved August 20, 2013, from http://www.acestar.uthscsa.edu/acestar-model.asp

Ard, N. (2009). Essentials of learning. In C. M. Schultz (Ed.), *Building a science of nursing education: Foundation for evidence-based teaching–learning* (Chapter 3, pp. 125–131). New York, NY: National League for Nursing.

Atherton, J. S. (2011). *Learning and teaching: Piaget's developmental theory.* Retrieved August 16, 2013, from http://www.learningandteaching.info/learning/piaget.htm

Benner, P. (1982). From novice to expert. *American Journal of Nursing, 82*(3), 402–407.

Benner, P., Sutphen, M., Leonard, V., & Day, L. (2009). *Book highlights from educating nurses: A call for radical transformation.* Hoboken, NJ: Jossey-Bass Publishers.

Boswell, C., & Cannon, S. (2014). *Introduction to nursing research: Incorporating evidence-based practice* (3rd ed.). Burlington, MA: Jones and Bartlett Learning.

Burman, M. E., Robinson, B., & Hart, A. M. (2013). Linking evidence-based nursing practice and patient-centered care through patient preferences. *Nursing Administration Quarterly, 37*(3), pp. 231–241.

The Cochrane Collaboration. (n.d.). About us. Retrieved August 20, 2013, from http://www.cochrane.org/about-us

Drisko, J. (2012a). Evidence-based practice. Retrieved August 20, 2013, from http://sophia.smith.edu/~jdrisko/evidence_based_practice.htm

Drisko, J. (2012b). What is EBP? Retrieved August 20, 2013, from http://sophia.smith.edu/~jdrisko/what_is_ebp.htm

Encarta World English Dictionary [North American Edition]. (2009). Retrieved March 16, 2010, from http://www.bing.com/Dictionary

Evidence Based Practice and Curriculum. (2011). About evidence based practice. Retrieved July 6, 2013, from http://dese.mo.gov/special-education/three-tiered-models-intervention/evidence-based-practices

Gawlinski, A., & Rutledge, D. (2008). Selecting a model for evidence-based practice changes: A practical approach. *AACN Advanced Critical Care, 19*(3), 291–300.

Hodson-Carlton, K. E. (2009). The learning resource center. In C. M. Schultz (Ed.), *Building a science of nursing education: Foundation for evidence-based teaching–learning* (Chapter 18, pp. 303–321). New York, NY: National League for Nursing.

Holistic Health and Healing. (2012). Complexity theory and nursing: Explanation and application. Retrieved September 13, 2013, from http://maryannehidalgokehoehhh.wordpress.com/2012/02/13/complexity-theory-and-nursing-explanation-and-application/

Joanna Briggs Institute. (2008). Joanna Briggs Institute model of evidence-based health care. Retrieved March 17, 2010, from http://joannabriggs.org/jbi-approach.html#tabbed-nav=JBI-approach

Johns Hopkins Nursing and Evidence-Based Practice. (n.d.). About the Johns Hopkins nursing EBP model. Retrieved March 17, 2010, from http://www.hopkinsmedicine.org/institute_nursing/continuing_education/ebp/ebp_books_consultations.html

Keller, J. (2010). ARCS Motivational Model. Retrieved February 8, 2010, from http://istheory.byu.edu/wiki/Kellers_Motivational_Model

Knowles, M. (1980). *The modern practice of adult education: From pedagogy to andragogy*. Wilton, Connecticut: Association Press.

McClinton, J. (1997). Stetler model of research utilization. Retrieved March 17, 2010, from www.kumc.edu/instruction/nursing/NRSG754/SYLLABUS/stetlermodel.html

McLeod, S. A. (2009). Jean Piaget. Retrieved June 15, 2014, from http://www.simplypsychology.org/piaget.html

Melnyk, B. M. (2013). Editorial, educational programing in undergraduate and graduate academic curricula: Friend or foe to accelerating evidence-based practice? *Worldviews on Evidence-Based Nursing, 10*(4), 185–186.

Melnyk, B. M., & Fineout-Overholt, E. (2005). *Evidence-based practice in nursing and healthcare: A guide to best practice.* Philadelphia, PA: Lippincott Williams & Wilkins.

Mitchell, G. J. (2013). Implications of holding ideas of evidence-based practice in nursing. *Nursing Science Quarterly, 26*(2), 143–151.

Motivation. (1997). In R. Biehler & J. Snowman (Eds.), *Psychology applied to teaching* (Chapter 11, pp. 1–10). Boston, MA: Houghton Mifflin. Retrieved August 20, 2013, from http://www.college.cengage.com/education/pbl/tc/motivate.html

Parse, R. R. (2013). Research as evidence: The many meanings. *Nursing Science Quarterly, 26*(2), 109.

Paul, R., & Elder, L. (2009). Critical thinking: Concepts and tools. Tomales, CA: Foundation for Critical Thinking.

Purvis, N., & Gabb, C. A. (2013). Online learning for professional development. *Nursing Times, 109*(51), 16–18.

Roussel, L., Godfrey, A. J., & Williams, L. (2010). Community resources awareness and networking through advocacy. In J. L. Harris & L. Roussel (Eds.), *Initiating and sustaining the clinical nurse leader role: A practical guide* (Chapter 10, pp. 171–182). Sudbury, MA: Jones and Bartlett Publishers.

Salmond, S. W. (2013). Finding the evidence to support evidence-based practice. *Orthopaedic Nursing, 32*(2), 16–22.

Sweetland, R. (2010). Motivational theory. Retrieved August 20, 2013, from http://www.homeofbob.com/cman/general/motivation/motivatn.html

The Critical Thinking Co. (2005). Critical thinking. Retrieved June 16, 2014, from http://www.criticalthinking.com/company/articles/critical-thinking-definition.jsp

Thompson, C. (2009). Teaching–learning in the cognitive domains. In C. M. Schultz (Ed.), *Building a science of nursing education: Foundation for evidence–based teaching-learning* (Chapter 4, pp. 133–176). New York, NY: National League for Nursing.

Vratny, A., & Shriver, D. (2007). A conceptual model for growing evidence-based practice. *Nursing Administration Quarterly, 31*(2), 162–170.

Chapter 7

Classroom Educational Experiences

Sharon Cannon

CHAPTER OBJECTIVES

At the conclusion of this chapter, the learner will be able to:

1. Trace the path of objectives from the organizational level to the unit level.
2. Identify effective teaching skills for the classroom.
3. Utilize management of classroom strategies.
4. Evaluate students in a classroom educational experience.

KEY TERMS

- 1-minute paper
- Behavioral objective
- Bloom's taxonomy
- Case study
- Classroom assessment
- Classroom management
- Clicker
- Concept-based learning
- Flipped classroom
- Formative evaluation
- Muddiest point
- PDA
- Problem-based learning
- Reflective journaling
- Role play
- Rubric
- Student evaluation
- Summative evaluation

INTRODUCTION

Historically, the traditional approach to teaching has been in the classroom. Though a significant shift occurred with the introduction of distance education, the classroom experience will continue to be a vital venue for teaching, regardless of the discipline/profession. Increased technology for the provision of content to motivate and engage the student in the learning process has impacted how faculty will involve students in the acquisition of knowledge. As a result, classroom experiences for the 21st century will move well beyond the "sage on the stage," lecture-only format (discussed in the chapter titled *The Teaching Experience in Nursing*). The classroom experience will involve much more than the faculty member giving a lecture and students dutifully taking notes. Current trends involve student-centered learning activities that use the classroom to more actively engage the student.

Evidence-based teaching (EBT) has emerged from growing demands of students for involvement in the educational process. In light of economic changes, a diverse audience of learners exists. No longer do all learners come straight from high school. Many are seeking a second career or deciding that perhaps now that their children are in school, they can go back to college and pursue their dream of becoming a nurse. The diverse audience of learners, along with technological advances, requires innovation/creative approaches in the classroom. Consequently, faculty will need to examine closely the course/unit objectives, teaching strategies, and management of the classroom experience. Together, these aspects culminate in evaluating the students' progress toward successfully acquiring the knowledge necessary. To accomplish such goals, faculty will need to acquire sophisticated skills useful in the classroom. Thus, the focus of this chapter is on providing multiple options for faculty to use in the classroom educational experience.

BEHAVIORAL OBJECTIVES

The essence of EBT is deeply embedded in **behavioral objectives**. The initial aspect of teaching requires a close look at behavioral objectives for the course being taught. It is important to realize that those objectives are part of a greater picture. To grasp the complexity of objectives, faculty must look further to the college/university, school, and program objectives (**Figure 7–1**). Obviously, course objectives are just one of the building blocks for the whole educational experience. Course objectives are broken

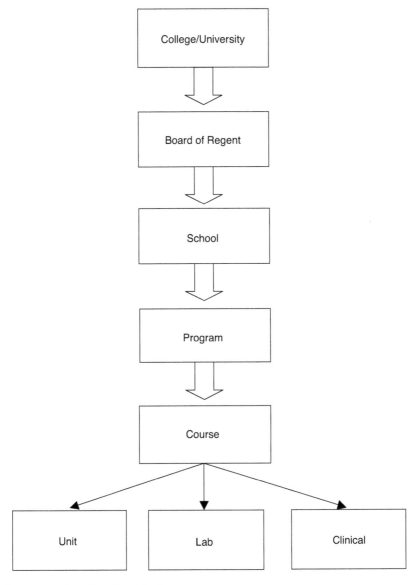

Figure 7-1 Flow sheet for objectives.

down further into unit objectives. All of these objectives will eventually be evaluated throughout the educational process (see the *Program Evaluation* chapter). Ultimately, the measure of success is reflected by students who complete all of the requirements by meeting objectives for graduation.

Perhaps, at this point, a distinction between a goal and an objective is necessary, as we hear a lot about goals related to schools and programs. Often a goal is thought to be an objective, and vice-versa. Some controversy exists, as others believe that goals and objectives are separate. A goal may be considered a broad statement of what is to be achieved. An objective is more specific and determines what is to be accomplished and by whom (Wingate, 2008). An example of a goal that is separated from an objective is, "The goal is to provide students with knowledge regarding genomics." A related objective would be, "To provide genomics information in medical/surgical nursing in the Foundation of Nursing course offered in the first semester of the junior year and the Professional Nursing course taught in the last semester of the senior year." For this chapter, goals are considered as broad and objectives as specific.

As mentioned earlier, course objectives are often broken down to unit objectives to manage the presentation of content; they are also broken down from simple to complex levels of content. Regardless of whether the objectives are based on unit or course content, all objectives must be measureable. Remember, objectives specify what and when content is to be learned. For instance, an objective that states, "The learner will understand fluid and electrolyte balance" is not measurable. The verb "understand" is broad, not specific, and has no criteria for measuring achievement. Instead, the faculty must spell out what behavior the student must display for comprehension about fluid and electrolyte balance. An example might be, "The student will be able to differentiate the results of too much fluid and not enough potassium." This example is more specific and states the mechanism to indicate how the objective will be met. An important point to remember is that course and unit objectives are interrelated and drive the design of the educational experience.

To measure an objective, as stated before, the faculty must determine what behavior the student is to display. Thus, behavioral objectives are required. The seminal work on behavioral objectives began in 1956 when Dr. Benjamin Bloom published his taxonomy of educational objectives in cooperation with a group of educational psychologists, including his mentor Ralph W. Tyler (Eisner, 2000). **Bloom's taxonomy** is considered the gold standard and hallmark of behavioral objectives and is divided into six levels of learning: recall, grasp, apply, analyze, synthesize, and judge. In addition, there are three domains where learning takes place: affective (feeling), cognitive (thinking), and psychomotor (acting). Bloom also thought the environment was important as well as the arrangement of how learning was to be promoted. It must be noted at this point that a controversy exists regarding the use of outcomes and competencies (Caputi, 2010). A more current emphasis in nursing education suggests that behavioral objectives are prescriptive and are unable to elicit more complex outcomes for higher levels of learning. This chapter offers faculty the opportunity to clarify their own opinions. Generally, faculty members are perceived to have control over the curriculum. Thus, it is extremely important for faculty to decide whether to use behavioral objectives, outcomes/competencies, or a modified approach to the design of the program and courses. Regardless of the faculty members' choices, it is important to consider that behavioral objectives are still very highly regarded and are used in most educational venues.

Bloom's taxonomy is widely utilized by nurse educators today in the development, implementation, and evaluation of objectives in the classroom environment. Entire textbooks have been written about the use of Bloom's taxonomy, the details of which are beyond the scope of this chapter. However, all faculty members are highly recommended to study his work so that the behavioral objectives they use are measureable, involve the levels of learning, and are in the appropriate domain. Without this understanding, faculty will be unable to effectively teach and evaluate student outcomes, regardless of the learning environment, as behavioral objectives exist for more than the classroom (i.e., lab/simulation and clinical settings).

One final discussion of behavioral objectives encompasses the use of **rubrics**. Stevens and Levi (2013) suggest that a rubric lists specific levels of performance to be assigned a grade. Behavioral objectives lend themselves well to use of rubrics, ensuring that students are aware of the specific behavior necessary to demonstrate knowledge acquisition, as reflected by a grade.

TEACHING STRATEGIES

Once the behavioral objectives have been determined for the course, unit, and environment, faculty must begin to address the content to be taught. A word of caution must be given here. Faculty cannot teach everything there is to know; nor is it appropriate to try doing so. Time is also a factor. Each course has only so much time allowed for the content to be presented. The type of program (undergraduate or graduate), level of the student learner (junior, senior, or generational category), and physical environment (classroom, online, lab, or clinical) must also be considered. Trying to teach everything can be frustrating for both faculty and students and, needless to say, impossible to accomplish in the given time constraints, regardless of the setting. It is essential that faculty focus on what the student needs to know rather than what would be nice for the student to know in the time allowed. Rushing through content will not always allow students to master content and ultimately will overwhelm the student. Bloom recognized that speed is not the issue, especially to achieve measurable educational objectives and goals. Time to reflect, analyze, and synthesize are important (Eisner, 2000).

Now that objectives have been made measurable and content has been specified, delivery methods must be determined. Whether to lecture or not to lecture may be the question. Traditionally, the lecture format has been the standard. With the advent of adult learning and motivational theories of learning along with advanced technology (see the chapter titled *The Teaching Experience in Nursing*), teaching strategies have become diverse. In fact, some faculty members perceive the available strategies to be an open field and use multiple approaches for teaching in the classroom.

Since the lecture strategy is probably the most widely used, let's look at what options an effective lecture mode should incorporate. Generally, experienced faculty start by dividing content into units and then outlining each unit to be taught. The next step is finding references for the specific content and capitalizing on the expertise of the faculty who will be lecturing. Following that step is the need to determine what resources may be used. For example, faculty may choose to use PowerPoint presentations, videos, or CD recordings, or a combination of these media. Questions and discussion time will also need to be added. Other items to be considered for the classroom include the use of personal digital assistants (PDAs), clickers, case studies, concept-based or problem-based learning, 1-minute papers and muddiest points, the flipped classroom, and role play, each of which is discussed later in this chapter.

Recognizing that different generations of students are in the class, a variety of approaches may be necessary to facilitate each student's grasp of the content being presented. Using a variety of approaches in the classroom plays an important part in motivating students, stimulating thoughts/ideas, and making content (which can be very dry and technical at times) more interesting and applicable to the students' experiences. All of these points should be addressed before you prepare to teach in a classroom. Remember that there is absolutely nothing more boring than for a faculty member to stand in front of a class and read his or her lecture notes. Motivating, engaging, and energizing students in the learning process is essential to achieve the objectives for the unit and the course. As Bloom indicated, the learning process is more than recalling information. Nursing faculty who are engaged in eliciting critical thinking must provide opportunities for higher levels of learning in dynamic teaching approaches. Selecting critical-thinking activities will require faculty to choose the best teaching strategy and to be adept in utilizing a variety of technological approaches.

MANAGING THE CLASSROOM ENVIRONMENT

In **classroom management**, two primary considerations must be addressed. The first is to manage the size of the class. Obviously, strategies used for teaching 30 students will differ greatly from those used when teaching 100-plus students. The greater the size of the class, the more difficult it is to ensure that all students actively participate in class activities. The second consideration is the number of faculty to teach the course.

Sometimes with very large classes only one faculty member may present content, or a teaching assistant might help. In other classes, guest speakers may participate, or several faculty members may be assigned to assist with content. The faculty members assigned primary responsibility must realize the advantages and disadvantages of small versus large class size in managing the class.

Once the objectives have been established and the teaching modalities selected, faculty must determine how to manage the classroom. Coyle-Rogers (2008) suggests that the classroom has a physical and psychological environment that impacts the relationship between the faculty and students. Creating a positive, supportive, respectful, and diverse environment leads to maximum communication and influences learning outcomes. Coyle-Rogers (2008) notes seating arrangements, the setting of expectations, faculty and student preparation, and teacher strategies such as eye contact, tone of voice, personality, and even physical appearance/demeanor as important considerations. Other aspects include room size, temperature, audio equipment, props, handouts, and overall organization of content and activities. Faculty must promote participation from at least a majority of students, with all being engaged as the ultimate goal. Creating a positive environment is powerful and requires faculty to coordinate complex strategies to facilitate learning.

Wingate (2008) looks more closely at classroom management. She starts by examining pre-lecture nerves, which many novice and experienced faculty experience. Not everyone desires being in the spotlight, and some may feel anxious before standing in front of a room full of students who may be younger, older, or the same age as the faculty. Loving the subject you teach and being prepared may alleviate some anxiety. Worthy to note is that though you may present as an authority on the subject, you do not need to have all the answers. It is okay and even preferable to say "I don't know" as long as you state "I'll find out" or prompt the class to find resources providing the answer. Obviously, you cannot reply "I don't know" to every question, but you can also be a role model to students when you explore options for learning for yourself and others. Students are less apt to "bluff" their way through a situation where "knowing" impacts the patient's outcome. Master teachers often express they would rather have a student/nurse say "I don't know but I'll find out" than cause harm to a patient.

Another aspect of classroom management is getting students to pay attention. This can be a daunting task. With computers, smart phones, and students talking to one another, the noise levels and lack of attentiveness become almost chaotic. Most schools have policies regarding cell/smart phones, so faculty should become familiar with and enforce such policies in the classroom. As for students conversing with one another, faculty may have to confront the problem individuals, which becomes extremely uncomfortable for everyone. Some ideas to counteract the discomfort are to randomly assign seats so that offending students are not grouped together. You can also stop talking and wait for students to stop talking, suggest they write notes to each other, ask for them to be courteous to their classmates, stand next to those talking, or simply ask the individuals to share their comments with the class.

If you notice the students aren't being attentive, you might change the tone of your voice, make sure the audio equipment is working, walk around, or change the pace of the lecture. Another suggestion is to be aware of how long students have been sitting. If you are giving a 3-hour lecture, you need to allow for at least one or two 10- to 15-minute breaks. Sometimes just having students stand and stretch, even though it is not break time, helps them to focus. Remember that classes were originally designed for 50 minutes because that is about the maximum length of a student's attention span.

Another aspect to address is the name/title you wish to be called and whether students prefer to be addressed by their first or last name. Working these details out allows for respect to be a two-way street and shows concern so that students know you care about them. Some doctorally prepared faculty wish for students to address them as Dr. (last name). Others don't want to be that formal. By the same token, older students may prefer that you use their last name. Moreover, some students may wish to be called by a name other than the one on your class roster—a middle name or nickname, for instance. The idea is to promote an environment that is courteous, respectful, and yet comfortable for both faculty and students.

Getting students to answer correctly, especially with difficult concepts, can be a challenge. It is extremely important not to embarrass a student. So if the student answers incorrectly, you might rephrase the question or give an example of what kind of response you expect. Perhaps you can allow the students to use a **PDA** or the Internet to find the answer if PDAs or computers are accessible, and then allow the students to report back to the class with the correct information. Again, be sure you are supportive and have laid the groundwork so that it is okay to be wrong as long as the correct information is sought and obtained.

Games and **role playing** create a more participative learning experience that can be incorporated into lectures. Along with **case studies** and **problem-based learning** (or **concept-based learning**), they are ways to promote critical thinking and collaborative learning. A game of Jeopardy, a crossword puzzle, and Trivial Pursuit are ideas that have elicited class participation. Faculty who wish to incorporate games or establish roles for students to play should search the literature for ideas. Some faculty members even create their own games and use them very effectively.

Paring down content is essential for managing the classroom. Herinckx, Munkvoid, Winter, and Tanner (2014) suggest the selection of key concepts for promotion of intense learning through a learner-centered approach.

The **flipped classroom** is another concept-based strategy that promotes a learner-/student-centered environment. The "flipped" classroom allows for content to be taught online and for the classroom to then be used to immerse the content in case scenarios, providing students the opportunity to critically think and problem solve. For example, if the online content is about oxygenation, students may use the classroom to practice nursing care for a patient with chronic obstructive pulmonary disease.

In the flipped classroom, students can access content at their own pace by recordings (e.g., podcasts), PowerPoint presentations, and videos through use of online technology. The classroom then becomes a vehicle for specific exercises (e.g., case studies, role play, games) to clarify and further illustrate concepts. This type of classroom allows for instant feedback and can decrease student frustration when the student is unable to complete an assignment (Knewton, n.d.). The flipped classroom also promotes teamwork, group participation, and peer acceptance.

As can be seen, lecturing and managing the classroom require much thought and preparation. The traditional lecture has gone far beyond faculty presenting content and students taking notes. The "sage on the stage" model is still present, but alternatives are available to engage students in the learning process. To make sure you have been successful, the next step is to perform a classroom assessment. It is not enough to be creative, innovative, or even entertaining if classroom instruction and student learning do not take place.

CLASSROOM ASSESSMENT

Rowles (2009) recommended using the definition of Angels (1994, p. 5) to define **classroom assessment** as consisting "of small scale assessments conducted continuously in the college classroom by discipline-based teachers to determine what students are learning in that class" (p. 262). McDonald (2014) states, "Classroom assessment is a formal process that involves a deliberate effort to gain information about a student's status in relation to course content and objectives" (p. 1). A classroom assessment promotes learning as the class progresses and the faculty member uses techniques to facilitate learning. Thus, you will encounter CATs (classroom assessment techniques) in the literature. CATs are formative in nature. **Formative evaluations** are the ongoing, periodic, and routine assessments done throughout a course (for more information on formative evaluation, see the *Program Evaluation* chapter). CATs provide immediate feedback that faculty can use to determine if they are on track and students are comprehending content. This information can then allow opportunities for faculty to reflect on and change their teaching where appropriate. In addition, students can be more interactive and discover their own individual gaps in knowledge, affirm the knowledge they have gained, or clarify areas that are unclear. Examples of CATs are the 1-minute paper, muddiest points, and clickers. The **1-minute paper** requires students to write a maximum of a half a page in 5 minutes to answer one question: What was the most important thing you learned today? The **muddiest point** may also be done as a 1-minute paper where the student has 5 minutes to write a half-page paper on the most confusing point. **Clickers** are considered to be a type of audience response system (ARS). Faculty members poll student responses to a specific question. Students respond using a remote control device. The program tabulates the responses, and the faculty member then provides feedback to students. Using CATs allows faculty to improve teaching and learning activities while the course is in progress. This allows for adjustments during the course rather than after the course has been completed and provides for more positive outcomes for both faculty and students.

STUDENT EVALUATION

The ultimate determination of the successful classroom delivery modality is through **student evaluation**. Multiple approaches are available to assess whether students learn content provided throughout the classroom experience. The first thoughts that come to mind are those related to tests/

examinations. A test provides a means for students to correct misinformation and identify specific gaps in knowledge. Tests also provide faculty with the tools to measure student progress, identify unclear areas of content, and evaluate desired outcomes for learning. Tests are closely connected to course objectives, which require faculty to be precise about content, time frame, and teaching/learning strategies for course content mastery. Consequently, tests must align with course objectives, be reliable (consistently produce the same results), and be valid (actually/accurately measure the content). Many schools of nursing and even the National Council of State Boards of Nursing establish a blueprint to provide a plan for selecting items for a test. Often the test blueprint is provided to students to assist them in studying and preparing for the exam.

There are a wide variety of options for formatting a test, including multiple choice, true/false, matching, fill in the blank, open ended, and essays. Experienced faculty members often use a variety of these formats to gain a more comprehensive view of students' progress. Test and measurement courses are highly recommended, especially for novice faculty, to obtain greater proficiency and confidence regarding the usage of various test formats and the level and/or domain of learning, such as comprehension, recall, or skill acquisition. Each testing format has a place in the evaluation of student progress.

Regardless of the test format, tests may be formative or summative. Tests used throughout the course are considered formative, usually concentrating on partial content such as a unit. Final comprehensive exams are considered **summative evaluations**, because they measure content presented over the entire course. Whether formative or summative, tests enable students to become adept at taking tests, which also assists with taking standardized tests used for progression through the program, graduation, and ultimately the NCLEX exam to practice nursing.

With advances in technology and changing trends in nursing education, other options for evaluating students are available. Sheldon (2008, p. 287) provides a menu of methods available for measuring student learning:

- Portfolios
- Group projects
- Role play
- Case studies
- Concept maps
- Concept papers
- **Reflective journaling**
- Research critiques

- Socratic questions
- Videotaping

Selection of the method of evaluation depends on multiple criteria: size of the class, number of faculty teaching, setting (classroom, lab, or clinical), types of students (older/younger generation), resources (technology), and nature of the course content, to name a few. As mentioned previously, rubrics are tools that clearly specify for the student the level of learning that is to be evaluated. The faculty also have a description of expectations (Stevens & Levi, 2013). As a result, rubrics are useful tools for evaluation of students, whether formative or summative. Faculty must be knowledgeable about evaluation methods to select the most appropriate type of assessment.

The prior discussion has examined formative evaluation of students throughout a course. The final step of student evaluation involves summative evaluation. Summative evaluation is "done at the end of the semester or course to provide the final judgment as to whether or not the student has achieved the educational goals" (Oermann, Saewert, Charasika, & Yarbrough, 2009, p. 353). Grades accumulated in the formative evaluation must now culminate in a final grade. Some courses, especially clinical or lab courses, are a pass/fail. Most courses taught in the classroom assign grades based on a scale of A, B, C, D, or F. Depending on the faculty selection, the final grade earned by the student may be a compilation of the formative grades, a comprehensive exam, a paper, and/or a case study. Faculty must remember to be fair, consistent, and clear about the evaluation resulting in any grade assigned. If there are several faculty members teaching the course and responsible for a group of students within the course, interrater reliability must be established to maintain consistency, eliminate bias, and assure fairness for all students in the class. Students and faculty alike are often anxious about grading outcomes. Assuring consistency and fairness across the board can alleviate at least some of the stress associated with grades. Faculty and students want positive results from the evaluation process to eliminate biases.

Having mechanisms in place to ensure impartial grading and guidance throughout the course assists the student in achieving the course requirements. Unfortunately, reality is that not all students will be able to accomplish what is required. It would be wonderful if all students were to pass, but that is not always possible. Faculty will need to thoroughly review student evaluations of the course, test results, interrater reliability, peer reviews by other faculty who might teach the course, and appropriateness of objectives, teaching strategies, and resources used.

SUMMARY THOUGHTS

The classroom educational experience is a dynamic, complex venue. An orchestra conductor has multiple musicians to manage just one single harmonious note as part of a total musical score. Faculty in the classroom environment must "orchestrate" the multiple aspects of teaching a course. Developing objectives, designing content presentation strategies, and evaluating student/course outcomes are indeed difficult. Advancements in technology and emerging trends in nursing education obligate nurse educators to adapt to changes that will be required in the new healthcare reform legislation. Traditional approaches to classroom teaching are being challenged to meet the demands of students, programs, employers of nurses, and the public. In fact, Benner, Sutphen, Leonard, and Day (2010) have called for a "radical transformation" in the classroom connected with the clinical setting through integrative teaching of knowledge, skills, and ethics.

The classroom experience may be the traditional lecture format. However, in today's nursing education milieu, lecture is not, and should not be, the only approach for acquisition of knowledge and skills. Many options are available to enhance student participation and performance in the classroom.

Linking course objectives to educational strategies and evaluating students and the course are essential for managing the course. Ultimately, the classroom educational experience is an adaptable forum and an exciting environment for teaching and learning. Evaluations provide evidence of effective teaching/learning in the classroom experience. Through evaluations, faculty who teach in that environment gain confidence that the acquisition of knowledge has occurred, producing positive outcomes for students.

The classroom educational experience is a viable format for EBT. Faculty who use evidence for teaching/learning to guide delivery of content in the classroom can achieve successful outcomes for students and programs by employing diverse teaching strategies and using formative and summative evaluations. Feedback from multiple sources from students and peers enable faculty to effectively manage and evaluate the classroom experience.

SUMMARY POINTS

1. Classroom experiences for the 21st century will move beyond the "sage on the stage," lecture-only format.
2. Evidence-based teaching (EBT) has emerged from growing demands of students for involvement in the educational process.

3. EBT is deeply embedded in behavioral objectives.
4. An objective is specific and determines what is to be accomplished and by whom (Wingate, 2008). Objectives measure the behavior the student is to display.
5. A goal is a broad statement of what is to be achieved.
6. Recent literature reveals that controversy exists regarding the use of behavioral objectives versus outcomes and competencies (Caputi, 2010).
7. Institutions (universities/colleges), schools of nursing, nursing programs, and courses all have objectives that flow and are related to each other.
8. Course objectives can be broken down into unit objectives as well as lab and clinical objectives, where appropriate. Dr. Benjamin Bloom published his taxonomy of educational objectives in 1956. This taxonomy is used widely by nurse educators.
9. Multiple aspects impact the presentation of content to be taught.
10. A wide range of teaching/learning methods is available, such as PDAs, clickers, case studies/problem-based learning, muddiest points, and role playing.
11. Managing the classroom experience involves attention to class size, physical/psychological aspects, faculty preparation, student participation, attendance, respect for faculty and students, and games/role playing.
12. Classroom assessment techniques (CATs) are considered formative evaluations implemented throughout the course. Examples of CATs are 1-minute papers, muddiest points, clickers, and examinations.
13. Student evaluations are both formative and summative.
14. Testing comes in several forms (e.g., multiple choice, true/false, matching, fill in the blanks, open ended, and essay).
15. With the advancement of technology and trends in nursing education, other options for evaluating students are available.
16. The final steps of evaluation of students include the individual performance of each student as well as student evaluations of the course.
17. The classroom educational experience is a dynamic, complex venue.
18. Benner, Sutphen, Leonard, and Day (2010) have called for a "radical transformation" of nursing education.
19. The classroom educational experience is an adaptable forum and an exciting environment for teaching and learning.
20. EBT can be accomplished in the classroom environment.

TIPS FOR NURSE EDUCATORS

1. Develop behavioral objectives that can be measured.
2. Use Bloom's taxonomy to determine the level, type, and domain for learning to be achieved.
3. Focus on specific content to be covered in the time allotted.
4. Explore all options for delivery of content so that different generations of students will participate.
5. Consider class size, number of faculty teaching, and resources available.
6. Utilize effective classroom management techniques.
7. Analyze CATs for formative evaluation to identify gaps in knowledge, affirm knowledge gained, and clarify confusing/contradicting content.
8. Synthesize formative and summative student/course evaluations for trends and use the data (evidence) to improve the course taught in a classroom educational experience.

MULTIPLE CHOICE QUESTIONS

1. In the 21st century, lecture will:
   A. be the only delivery format.
   B. be delivered only by the "sage on the stage."
   C. **involve more than faculty lecturing with students taking notes.**
   D. be obsolete.

   Rationale:
   In the 21st century, classroom experiences will move beyond the "sage on the stage" and involve more than faculty lecturing with students dutifully taking notes, instead using technological advancements and more interactive activities to facilitate student learning.

2. Evidence-based teaching has emerged due to:
   A. **student demands, economic changes, and a diverse audience of learners.**
   B. the abundance of nursing education research to provide data for effective teaching.
   C. the fact that classroom educational experiences have not been effective.
   D. parental concerns that their child is not receiving the best education.

Rationale:
Evidence-based teaching has emerged from growing demands of students for involvement in the educational process. In light of economic changes, a diverse audience of learners exists.

3. Objectives measure what _____ the student is to display.
   A. personality
   B. **behavior**
   C. attitude
   D. understanding

Rationale:
To measure an objective, the faculty must determine what behavior is to be displayed by students.

4. A goal is considered to be:
   A. narrow.
   B. specific.
   C. timely.
   D. **broad.**

Rationale:
A goal may be considered as a broad statement of what is to be achieved.

5. When determining content to be taught, faculty must consider:
   A. personal preferences, physical environment, and time.
   B. **type of program, time allotted, and levels of the students.**
   C. speed of delivery, personality of students, and size of the podium.
   D. personal preferences, size of the podium, and levels of the students.

Rationale:
Time is a factor. The type of program (undergraduate or graduate), level of the learner (junior, senior, or generational category), and physical environment (classroom, online, lab, or clinical) must also be considered.

6. Instructional methodology for the educational classroom experience may include:
   A. **lecture, PowerPoint slides, videos, and/or CD recordings.**
   B. lecture, PowerPoint slides, and/or chats.
   C. chats, discussion board messages, and/or animated cartoons.
   D. note taking, chats, and/or guest lecturers.

Rationale:
Faculty may choose to use lecture, PowerPoint slides, videos, and/or CD recordings, or a combination of these.

7. To be effective lecturers, faculty members should:
   A. read from their notes.
   B. ignore room size.
   C. speak in a quiet/low tone of voice.
   D. **use a variety of approaches.**

   Rationale:
   Using a variety of approaches may be necessary to facilitate a student's grasp of the content being presented.

8. Attendance requirements for a class should involve:
   A. the student's preference.
   B. the faculty's preference.
   C. **the school's/program's policy.**
   D. none of the above.

   Rationale:
   Faculty need to be sure of the school's/program's policy regarding attendance.

9. Critical thinking or problem solving can be:
   A. **accomplished through games and role playing.**
   B. accomplished through recall and memorization.
   C. dull and boring.
   D. impossible to achieve in the classroom.

   Rationale:
   Games and role playing create a more participative learning experience that can be incorporated into lecture. They are ways to promote critical thinking or solutions to problems posed as case studies.

10. Classroom assessment techniques (CATs) are:
    A. summative.
    B. final.
    C. useless.
    D. **formative.**

    Rationale:
    CATs are formative in nature.

11. Student evaluations may consist of:
    A. tests.
    B. portfolios.
    C. journals.
    D. **all of the above.**

    Rationale:
    Multiple approaches are available to assess whether students learn content provided through the classroom experience.

12. Final course grades are based on:
    A. comprehensive exams only.
    B. **a compilation of formative grades.**
    C. administrator decisions.
    D. student requests.

    Rationale:
    Depending on the faculty selection, the final grade earned by the student may be a compilation of formative grades, a comprehensive exam, papers, and/or case study discussions.

13. Bias in grading when several faculty are involved can be eliminated by:
    A. **interrater reliability.**
    B. faculty popularity.
    C. student popularity.
    D. none of the above.

    Rationale:
    If there are several faculty teaching the course who are responsible for a group of students within the course, interrater reliability must be established to maintain consistency, eliminate bias, and assure fairness for all students in the class.

14. The classroom educational experience is:
    A. rigid and set in stone.
    B. loose and free in requirements.
    C. **adaptable and exciting.**
    D. dull and boring.

    Rationale:
    Ultimately, the classroom educational experience is an adaptable forum and an exciting environment for teaching and learning.

DISCUSSION QUESTIONS

1. You have been assigned to teach a nursing research course in a newly established undergraduate nursing program. How will you develop the course objectives?

   Considerations:
   · What are the program objectives?
   · How many objectives does the course need to have?
   · Will you use Bloom's taxonomy or an outcome and competency approach?

- What behaviors/indicators will students need to display?
- How will you measure each objective?

2. You have been assigned the lead instructor role for team teaching a Foundations in Nursing class composed of 130 students. How will you manage the course?

   Considerations:
   - How many other faculty will teach?
   - What is the expertise/clinical background of each faculty member?
   - What responsibility does each faculty have (e.g., grading, simulation/lab, clinical)?
   - Which teaching strategies will be chosen?
   - What formative/summative evaluations will be used?

3. You want to engage students in learning activities that do not involve lecture. What will you need to know to plan activities?

   Considerations:
   - What generational types of learners do you have?
   - What learning activities fit the content to be taught?
   - What learning activities are you comfortable providing?

REFERENCES

Benner, P., Sutphen, M., Leonard, V., & Day, L. (2010). *Educating nurses: A call for radical transformation.* San Francisco, CA: Jossey-Bass.

Caputi, L. (2010). Curriculum design and development. In L. Caputi (Ed.), *Teaching nursing: The art and science* (pp. 367–394). Glen Ellyn, IL: College of DuPage Press.

Coyle-Rogers, P. G. (2008). The power of the classroom climate. In B. K. Penn (Ed.), *Mastering the teaching role: A guide for nurse educators* (pp. 119–131). Philadelphia, PA: F.A. Davis.

Eisner, E. W. (2000). Benjamin Bloom. *Prospects: The quarterly review of comparative education, XX*(3). Paris, UNESCO: International Bureau of Education.

Herinckx, H., Munkvold, J. P., Winter, E., & Tanner, C. A. (2014). A measure to evaluate classroom teaching practices in nursing. *Nursing Education Perspectives, 35*(1), 30–36.

Knewton, Inc. (n.d.). Flipped classroom: The flipped classroom infographic. Retrieved February 11, 2014, from http://www.knewton.com/flipped-classroom/

McDonald, M. (2014). *The nurse educator's guide to assessing learning outcomes* (3rd ed.). Burlington, MA: Jones and Bartlett Learning.

Oermann, M. H., Saewert, K. J., Charasika, M., & Yarbrough, S. S. (2009). Assessment and grading practices in schools of nursing: National survey findings part II. *Nursing Education Perspectives, 30*(6), 352–357.

Rowles, C. J. (2009). Improving teaching and learning: Classroom assessment techniques. In D. M. Billings & J. A. Halstead (Eds.), *Teaching in nursing: A guide for faculty* (3rd ed., pp. 262–267). St. Louis, MO: Saunders Elsevier.

Sheldon, D. P. (2008). Beyond testing: Other ways to evaluation learning. In B. K. Penn (Ed.), *Mastering the teaching role: A guide for nurse educators* (pp. 287–298). Philadelphia, PA: F.A. Davis.

Stevens, D. D., & Levi, J. (2013). *Introduction to rubrics* (2nd ed.). Sterling, VA: Stylus.

Wingate, A. (2008). Managing the modern classroom. In B. K. Penn (Ed.), *Mastering the teaching role: A guide for nurse educators* (pp. 133–152). Philadelphia, PA: F.A. Davis.

Chapter 8

Online Educational Experiences

Carol Boswell

Chapter Objectives

At the conclusion of this chapter, the learner will be able to:

1. Compare different types of teaching strategies that are effective within an online educational experience.
2. Contrast aspects related to the delivery of online learning.
3. Discuss operational technology utilized in online teaching settings.
4. Examine strategies associated with evaluations resulting from online delivery of the educational process.

Key Terms

- Asynchronous activity
- Computer-based instruction
- Deep-dive brainstorming
- Distance learner
- E-book
- Email
- Emoticon
- Engaged learning
- Face-to-face
- Hybrid course
- Mobile learning
- Netiquette rule
- Online course
- Podcast lecture
- Scaffolding
- Synchronous activity
- Technology
- Web-based instruction

INTRODUCTION

With the changing demographics related to health care, the need and expectation to engage in innovative methods of education become increasingly significant. According to a 2013 report from the U.S. Department of Health and Human Services (DHHS) titled "The U.S. Nursing Workforce: Trends in Supply and Education—Results in Brief" (2013), the percentage of registered nurses (RNs) employed full time increased from 58.4% (2004) to 63.2% (2008). This increasing percentage of RNs working full time may be attributed to the economic issues confronting the United States, but it must be noted that these data were collected prior to 2008. The economic recession happened in 2008, with the beginning effects of the downturn occurring for several years prior to this crash. Some of the speculation within the nursing community has centered on the idea that nurses who had anticipated retiring have remained in the workforce at this point due to family economic conditions. During this same time period (2004–2008), the number of nurses with an associate's degree (AD) rose from 42.9% to 45.4% (DHHS, 2010). The number of nurses with an AD reached 60% in 2011 (DHHS, 2013). In comparison, the number of first-time test takers holding a bachelor's degree at the time of testing more than doubled from 2001 to 2011 (DHHS, 2013). As noted in "The U.S. Nursing Workforce" report, the number of RNs receiving a post-licensure bachelor degree has increased a staggering 86% between 2010 and 2013 (DHHS, 2013). Another concerning statistic, this one identified in the DHHS report titled "National Sample Survey of Registered Nurses," is that the share of nurses who are under the age of 40 currently is 29.5%, which is a slight increase from prior years (DHHS, 2010), but still low. The statistics suggest that "among nurses 55 and older, 76,915 intend to leave the nursing profession within 3 years; another 54,539 intend to leave their current nursing job and are unsure if they will remain in nursing afterward" (DHHS, 2010, p. 10). With just these statistical considerations, the need to develop and implement creative ways to further education for the next generations of nurses takes on increasing importance.

One of the primary arguments for the move to higher levels of learning within health care is found in the "Future of Nursing: Leading Change, Advancing Health" document (Institute of Medicine, 2010). This report, based on a thorough review of the evidence, identifies four key messages related to the role of nurses within the transformed healthcare system.

Two key aspects from these four directly impact nursing education and online delivery. The nursing profession recognizes the value of achieving higher levels of education and training through the championing of seamless academic progression, increasing the proportion of RNs at the baccalaureate level to 80% by 2020, and doubling the doctorally prepared nurses (Institute of Medicine, 2010). Each of the aspects is effectively promoted and advanced through the active use of online educational techniques.

Nurses who are prepared at the AD level are working more, thus they cannot (or will not) take off work to attend traditionally offered RN-BSN programs. According to the Tri-Council for Nursing (2010), "A more highly educated nursing profession is no longer a preferred future; it is a necessary future in order to meet the nursing needs of the nation and to deliver effective and safe care" (p. 1). With the push toward Magnet or Pathway to Excellence status by hospitals, the advancement of RNs from the AD level to the BSN level of education is strongly desired. Even with this cry to increase the educational preparation levels of RNs, agencies are focused on strictly controlling costs. Academic institutions are also confronted with the demand to reduce costs. Another complicating aspect to this picture is the finding by AMN Healthcare (2013) that "less than half of RNs with an associate degree or diploma will pursue additional education in nursing; however, younger and mid-career nurses are more likely to pursue advanced education in nursing" (p. 4). Thus, educational programs must carefully consider workload, cost, and validation of the importance of further education as the curricula are considered and delivered. To persuade this generation of nurses to further their education, innovative and engaging programs of study are required.

As a result, dynamic online educational opportunities are viewed as an innovative, cost-effective approach (**Table 8–1**). Connors (2008) notes, "Today's students approach academics with a set purpose: a desire for efficiency in learning, a perception of what they need to learn and, most important, a planned set of outcomes" (p. 164). Generation X and Millennial cohorts want a learning environment that is accessible, flexible, learner-centered, and meshed with their lifestyle and commitments. Noel-Levitz (2011), a higher-education consulting group, reports that approximately 87% of currently enrolled students are engaged in online instruction. Designers of programs of study need to carefully consider the manner in which the courses are presented and managed. Faculty members must take care to ensure that the students can stay true to their need to be individuals and open to fun.

Table 8-1 Strengths Associated with Online Learning by Students

- The process is interactive and reinforces class content.
- Online learning allows students the opportunity to apply theory to practice.
- Nursing curriculum can be developed to use a combination of required and optional assignments.
- Online learning accommodates the different learning styles when set up appropriately.

Source: Adapted from Noel-Levitz. (2006). *National online learner priorities report.* Braintree, MA: Author; and Leski, J. (2009). Nursing students and faculty perceptions of computer-based instruction at a 2-year college. *Journal of Nursing Education, 48*(2), 91–95.

As the concept of evidence-based practice (EBP) is applied to the field of online teaching, thought must be given to what is involved in the process and how it is to be achieved. Burnett (2013) framed EBP around the idea of the ABCs:

A = Ask the question
B = Books and literature review
C = Consider the evidence
D = Develop and apply
E = Evaluate
F = Facilitate

Each of these aspects should be interwoven into the management of the educational setting. As online courses and programs are envisioned, these aspects must be utilized to incorporate the best practices within online education. The online delivery method must be challenged and confirmed as a realistic and rational method for providing health education. Not all topics can effectively be delivered in this format. Care must be given to ensure that only those topics that can be presented within an online delivery method are provided in this manner. For some students and with some topics, face-to-face is the most realistic and practical learning method. Instructors must critically evaluate each concept and topic to convey it in the best process available.

As the movement toward online educational tactics is considered, care must be given to the evidence available concerning the optimal techniques necessary to be effective and successful. Draves (2000) makes a good point that "learning is not purely a cognitive process, but . . . also involves the emotions and even the spirit" (p. 10). This chapter endeavors to present key aspects related to online teaching. These aspects can be thoroughly considered in making decisions related to online delivery methods.

TYPES OF TEACHING STRATEGIES

Several terms related to online education need to be defined to establish a foundation on which to build a body of understanding about the technique. According to Connors (2008), "Distance education is organized education that occurs when the teacher and the learner are not in the same physical space at the same time" (p. 163). Thus, the term *distance education* is basically self-explanatory. Bastable (2014) lists examples of distance learning as online courses (discussed later in the chapter), correspondence courses, independent study, and videoconferencing. Whenever the teacher and the students (learners) are not in the same location, this term is applicable. Draves (2000) describes the characteristics of online learning as follows: "Content is delivered differently, learners have to initiate learning and actively go get it, a learner has to figure out what you want to learn, it takes self-direction, learning online is work, and it is outcome and results oriented" (p. 30). Every aspect within the delivery of the material is changed, thus providing challenges for the faculty member to ensure that each student receives the needed direction to be successful.

Palloff and Pratt (1999) bring up a very important aspect in regard to distance education when they champion the idea that consideration must be directed toward the development of community for the participants to facilitate the learning environment. The learners who elect to engage in the educational process from a distance, or **distance learners**, are frequently compelled to do it as a result of time, geographic, financial, or other constraints that restrict their ability to attend traditional classes. The distance learning environment is viewed as convenient, accessible, and flexible. Bangert and Easterby (2008) state that "the flexibility and convenience offered by Internet-based nursing programs has been an important strategy for addressing the critical shortage of baccalaureate and advanced registered nurse practitioners" (p. 54S). Distance education is viewed as a resourceful and professional alternate for acquiring an advanced degree during these economic times, as it eliminates travel to a traditional classroom setting. Distance education is also coming to the forefront due to the surge of members from the Generation X and Millennial generations, who are technologically advanced.

A second key term central to distance learning is **technology**. Within the realm of online delivery methodology, any venue or device that allows students and faculty members to engage in the learning process from unique locations can be used. While the computer and Internet tend to be the most frequently utilized aspects, other devices are being incorporated as technology grows and develops. The Internet tends to be the only access point, but multiple devices are now being used in place of the computer. Cell/ smart phones, teleconferencing, and e-readers are just a few of the devices that are becoming increasingly important in the world of online education.

Another term used within online learning is **engaged learning**. According to Conrad and Donaldson (2004), "Engaged learning is focused on the learner, whose role is integral to the generation of new knowledge" (p. 5). Engaged learning requires the learner to become directly involved in the entire learning process. The learner is an active participant in the process instead of the passive participant, which can occur within the traditional education setting. Each member within an online learning environment must connect to the material presented.

Other terms used within online education include face-to-face, hybrid courses, synchronous activities, asynchronous activities, web-based instruction, online courses, computer-based instruction, e-books, rubrics, and netiquette rules, each of which is discussed next. As each of these concepts is pulled together, an inclusive view of aspects within online educational experiences can be developed.

Face-to-face is the term applied to traditional classroom experiences. This term is used to depict the opportunity to be one-on-one with the students. With face-to-face educational experiences, faculty members are able to incorporate all of the senses in the process of educating the individual. Both nonverbal and verbal communication activities are utilized within the process. The instructor watches the interactions occurring between class members and many other activities occurring within the classroom. Being able to see the members in the class allows the instructor to assess when and if individuals are upset or frustrated, or when they are reacting positively. Nonverbal communication takes on a different flavor with online teaching. In contrast to the traditional classroom, online classes do not provide opportunities to view student interactions. As a result, faculty members must be attuned to the written messages that are being delivered. It is important to learn to read between the lines but also to correctly interpret the message. Frequently checking with students to confirm the interpretations of the communications is important.

Emoticons, or symbols that convey feelings, allow some aspects of nonverbal communication to come into play. As use of online education and texting has increased with the technologically advanced generations, multiple signs and abbreviations have been developed that take the place of nonverbal communication. Examples of such emoticons and abbreviations are ☺, :-<, LOL (laugh out loud), BFF (best friends forever), and so forth. Typographical distinctions (e.g., italics, all-capital lettering, colors) and punctuation marks (e.g., !, !!!, !?) can also be used to convey emotions. Within each course, students need to be careful, as some faculty members do not allow the use of these nonverbal communication graphics. New abbreviations and graphics constantly are added to the online communication, which allows individuals to see the nonverbal feelings of the other participants. But within the online community, this process is limited. Participants must willingly engage in the documenting of their nonverbal communication, whereas in the classroom, the members of the classroom can look around and view the nonverbal communication of their classmates. In the face-to-face environment, the participants do not have to wait for colleagues to engage in documenting their nonverbal feelings—such communication is readily apparent. Within the online community, participants can remain neutral if desired. If a peer does not convey such information deliberately, the primary indication that a problem is developing may be noted only by the decrease in communication connectiveness by that individual.

With the growing expectations for reaching the Institute of Medicine's goal of 80% of RNs being prepared at the baccalaureate level, many programs are considering using hybrid delivery methods. This educational process combines face-to-face delivery with online delivery. **Hybrid courses** are viewed as combining the effectiveness and flexibility of the online delivery method with the traditional method of education. According to Sowan and Jenkins (2013), several barriers to applying this process exist. Faculty are resistant to the changes within the classroom environment due to perceived lack of preparation in how to convert material from the face-to-face process into the online environment. Another alleged barrier encountered is the lack of time to complete this conversion in an orderly and organized manner. From the work done by Sowan and Jenkins (2013), the principle challenge is the need for clear and concise instructions regarding the expectations and management of the hybrid delivery method.

Web-based instruction is any activity/course that is provided via the Internet; thus **online course** is a synonymous term. Lowenstein and Bradshaw (2004, p. 210) denote the different ways to provide web-based instruction as:

- totally web-based asynchronous (no face-to-face or real-time interaction),
- totally web-based synchronous (no face-to-face interaction but class meets online in real time),
- partially web-based with some face-to-face class meetings (plus asynchronous or synchronous class interactions), or
- a traditional class with supplemental web-based components (emails, forums, chat rooms, class content).

Each of these different methods allows for the individualization of the course. A faculty member can elect to use different levels of web-based instruction within a course presentation. The determination of the manner in which the course is delivered should be based on the needs of the student, content to be delivered, mission of the course/program, and expectations of the learning community. Lowenstein and Bradshaw (2004) postulate that "participation in any form of distance learning requires students to be self-directed and able to function in an environment with limited faculty feedback and lacking face-to-face interaction" (p. 213). Students who engage in distance learning opportunities must understand that the responsibility for learning does fall upon themselves because they don't have the classroom to use for passive learning. Web-based instruction requires active learning and engagement in the learning process by the individual student.

Synchronous activities are planned activities in which all of the members are expected to be online and/or connected at the same time. These activities include chat room discussions, webinar activities, teleconferencing experiences, and so forth. Individuals are assigned to complete the educational proceedings online with the other designated members at a designated time. Synchronous activities provide opportunities for a group to interact to address a topic. Another strength of this type of activity is the ability to cover the material one time with the opportunity to field questions and concerns. A weakness with using synchronous activities is the limitation that many Internet services and platforms cannot manage large classes at one time. Another weakness involves the need for the instructor to be prepared to upload comments and remarks in a timely and organized manner during the designated structured learning time.

The opposite of such activities is **asynchronous activities**. Asynchronous activities are those encounters that are conducted independently of other learners. Within this process, the learner can address the activity within the course at a time convenient for the individual. Asynchronous activities are done usually within a time period but do not require the direct attention of others. Discussion (bulletin) boards are an example of this type of activity. Assignments are made for students to post a specific number of messages within a designated period. The student can determine when during that designated period to complete the assignment. The assignments/postings are not done at the same time for all of the participants. The requirement is for the activity to be successfully completed during the assigned period. Other examples of asynchronous activities can be podcast sessions and voice-over lectures. Both of these learning experiences provide a file for the students to access at their convenience to hear and/or see content presented by the instructor. Any course activity that does not require the cohort to be together in the course shell at the same time but can be done at the convenience of the participant is asynchronous in nature.

Computer-based instruction (CBI) is a term used to denote any activities conducted on a computer for the acquisition of knowledge. From evidence, Leski (2009) notes that CBI:

- pertains to specific content areas,
- presents realistic demands on participants,
- transpires in a setting with nominal disruption,
- is time bound,
- enhances learning under specified key circumstances,
- hinders learning under specific central situations,
- varies in application depending on a diversity of concerns, and
- facilitates nursing education in specific spheres.

CBI is functional for some areas but inappropriate for other areas. Topics that require hands-on management pose difficulty when considered for presentation via a computer-based delivery methodology. As simulation experiences have developed, many new methods for addressing "hands-on" activities within a computer-based venue have been explored. Within a discussion of best practices in teaching and learning, the idea of virtual learning environments has been considered (Felver et al., 2010). While web-based technology is viewed as aiding in learner-centered education, encouraging independent learning, and fostering deep learning, the research evidence does not support the virtual learning environment as better than other forms of learning. CBI is viewed as one tool to be used appropriately within the learning environment.

E-books are gaining in attention and utilization within the learning process. E-books are presented on an electronic device and do not require the purchase of hard copies or printed textbooks. Several advantages can be considered as a result of using e-books. In reviewing their own experience along with other faculty members' experiences regarding e-books, Williams and Dittmer (2009) state that "the bundled e-book package was handier to use than several books, and students felt that the e-book information gave them extra confidence" (p. 224). The computer-based delivery of books allows for a quick turnaround when updates are needed. The cost of the books is reduced because less production time and resources are required. The environment is also saved because the books do not require printing, thus alleviating the need to destroy our trees. In addition, students can access the books for resources when in a clinical setting. As stated by Williams and Dittmer (2009), "It is important for educators and librarians to take note of the different information retrieval styles of new generations of learners" (p. 224). Since the books are accessed via the computer, smart phones, e-readers, or other electronic devices, a question can be quickly researched to determine up-to-date information when making critical decisions. As another incentive to use e-books, many publishing companies are developing customized textbooks for use within programs of study. Instructors and schools can pull from selected books within the publisher's library to construct a learning packet that directly meets the course expectations.

Rubrics, discussed in the *Classroom Educational Experiences* chapter, can be used in any classroom delivery venue and are becoming a valuable assessment method for the online program. According to Stevens and Levi (2013), "A rubric is a scoring tool that lays out the specific expectations for an assignment" (p. 3). This grading tool requires the establishment of the different dimensions within the assignment along with the scale level designations. These scale level designations are frequently worded along the lines of "mastery," "partial mastery," "progressing," and "emerging" (Stevens & Levi, 2013, p. 7). Online delivery is incorporating the rubric concept into its platform to make these grading tools more accessible. By being integrated within the courses, faculty members can rapidly and consistently grade assignments.

A final term to consider in regard to online courses is **netiquette rules**. As the Internet has developed and expanded, users have agreed upon certain concepts and methods for engaging in proper online communication. These rules/recommendations cover the use of capital letters (to be avoided in most situations), proper use of the computer, management of **emails**, and so forth. Netiquette is viewed as the behaviors that reflect being civilized on the computer, similar to etiquette in a face-to-face setting.

GENERAL ASPECTS IN DELIVERY OF ONLINE EDUCATION

According to Chickering and Gamson (1987), effective management of the undergraduate educational experience requires the encouraging of connection concerning students and faculty, cultivating teamwork among students, advancing vigorous learning, providing timely feedback, articulating quality expectations, and recognizing distinct techniques of learning. Within any educational setting, the need to present an effective and successful environment that encourages and showcases learning is of paramount importance.

Dreon (2013) applied each of Chickering and Gamson's principles to the online classroom. Connection within the online environment requires thought and attention. The availability of the instructor must be effectively communicated so that the students can be in contact as needed. Online education should not be a glorified independent study course. Collaboration and interaction between the members of the course are imperative for successful learning. Fostering the discussion and sharing of ideas allows for the connectiveness that comes when learning is facilitated. Learning must be an active process. Each assignment and interaction should have a practical foundation within the healthcare arena. Busywork is not an option. Prompt feedback is always a key to effective teaching. While some faculty and students think that online participants are available 24/7, this total availability is unrealistic. Specific parameters for feedback are important. Teachers need to be very careful about providing the guidelines for feedback. If communications are available only between 8 AM and 5 PM, students should be clearly instructed of this fact. Chickering and Gamson's ideals for quality of learning apply to the online venue. High expectations for learning are paramount in all learning environments. Students must understand that the quality of work does not change based on the delivery method. Communicating these high expectations is critical. Within this online environment, respect for the diversity of the students along with the methods for learning requires thought and attention. Using all of the different learning methods is practical and necessary to engage the diverse learning community.

As education moves forward with online delivery, several aspects are essential to consider. Chickering and Gamson (1987) identified the areas of shared purposes, positive support by the administration, appropriate funding for the online delivery, policies and procedures that address the process of online delivery, and support for faculty members' development as they learn to conduct online education as keys for successful management of the online processes. Another area to carefully address when endeavoring to connect the resources, students, and faculty members is the need for technological support on a 24/7 basis for both the students and faculty members. Everyone within the educational setting needs to be on target in achieving quality outcomes in the different aspects of the process.

As academic facilities consider providing online education, one initial aspect is the formation of the learning community. Since students are not sitting in the room with their colleagues and the faculty member, attention to methods for allowing the individuals within the course to connect as a learning community is essential. According to Palloff and Pratt (1999),

"The keys to the creation of a learning community and successful facilitation online are simple—honesty, responsiveness, relevance, respect, openness, and empowerment" (p. 20). Taking the time to plan how to unite the different members in the course cohort is a critical foundation for the development of discussion and interactions. Since the individuals don't have the advantage of sitting in a room together, the development of a comfort level with the different individuals must take place through the use of communication skills (**Table 8–2**). Bastable (2014) discusses the expectation that online courses need to facilitate learning activities and resources supporting teacher–learner and learner–learner interactions. Each aspect within the course must be painstakingly considered as to how it will lend itself to the formation of a learning community. As faculty endeavor to challenge students to learn, the concept of "just-in-time learning" surfaces. According to Sambataro (2000), this learning system provides the education to individuals when and where they need it. Thus, it investigates innovative venues to deliver the material to the individuals when they need it, not when the class period is scheduled. Waiting to learn becomes a thing of the past. The student and faculty are challenged to provide pioneering and novel approaches for gaining the knowledge needed to address the situation presenting itself for consideration.

Two aspects that tend to be linked together within the learning environment are **scaffolding** and **deep-dive brainstorming**. According to Alber (2014), scaffolding is the process of breaking down the key concepts into chunks to allow for the comprehension of each chunk as it relates to the

Table 8–2 Top Challenges Associated with Online Learning by Students

- Maintaining the quality of the instructional delivery for courses
- Staying attuned to the needs of the student cohort
- Delivering timely and positive feedback to the students
- Allowing enough time for deliberation and consideration by students of the content needed for the assignments
- Allowing time for grading by faculty
- Addressing issues with trust and freedom of expression when assigned reflective journaling
- Ensuring faculty responsiveness
- Clearly defining student assignments within the syllabus

Source: Adapted from Noel-Levitz. (2011). *National online learner priorities report.* Braintree, MA: Author; and Langley, M. E., & Brown, S. T. (2010). Perceptions of the use of reflective learning journals in online graduate nursing education. *Nursing Education Perspectives, 31*(1), 12–17.

whole. By providing manageable segments within a complicated topic, the student can gain understanding of each step within the larger picture. Scaffolding allows the instructor to provide the content in small, functional units from simple to complex. Alber (2014) lists six strategies for use in scaffolding learning segments: (1) allowing the students to show their foundation, (2) tapping into prior knowledge, (3) providing time to talk about new ideas and information, (4) assigning vocabulary before the learning begins, (5) using visual aids (more than just computer slide programs), and (6) asking questions at intervals to provide for review and contemplation of the material. These strategies can be easily incorporated into the online environment to provide a smooth flow of knowledge acquisition. The deep-dive brainstorming technique is viewed as another strategy within the scaffolding framework. According to RapidBi (2007), deep diving is a "technique to rapidly immerse a group or team into a situation for problem solving or idea creation" (para 1). Within an online environment, the idea of deep diving allows students to suggest ideas, concepts, and thoughts within a short time via a discussion board, blog area, or other medium. By encouraging the participants to brainstorm about a topic, innovative techniques and concepts can be identified and explored.

Dorin (2009) states, "Online classes require a time commitment that's similar to that of classes in a traditional university—minus the commute!" (p. 35). Each aspect of the course reflects the openness of the presentation. Since accessing the course is flexible and convenient, the incorporation of assignments needs to flow from the beginning to the end. With online courses breaking out of the mold used for face-to-face classes, such courses need to justify the number of semester credit hours awarded with the work to be completed. Given that the courses depend on self-learning, assignments usually require readings, participation, and one other type of assignment per week. The assignments could involve papers, PowerPoint presentations, tests, or tutorials. The activities can entail actions accomplished individually or within teams.

Conrad and Donaldson (2004) suggest that "to determine whether a classroom-based activity is adaptable to the online environment, the activity must first be examined to see that it meets the learning outcomes of the online course" (p. 17). Learning objectives are the underpinning for the educational experience; thus, every activity to be incorporated into a course needs to be scrutinized to determine its functionality. Most face-to-face activities can be modified for use within the online delivery venue. Brainstorming is one type of activity that can be modified into an online assignment. When adapting this activity, the online "shout out" phrase would be the quick listing of key ideas within the subject line; everyone can quickly identify themes without having to open the documents. Other activities successfully used in face-to-face settings must be analyzed to see how they could be adapted for use in an online delivery venue.

Loyola (2010) looks at online education from the focus of outcome-based education. Outcome-based education "is a paradigm shift from passive traditional learning to an active, learner-centered, result-oriented approach to learning" (Loyola, 2010, p. 19). While any type of education can provide outcome-based education, online delivery is ripe for providing learning experiences that require the active participation of the learner. In regard to education being results-oriented, any educational experience must address the results to be obtained. To be effective, the teacher should determine the results expected from the engagement in the learning process. Loyola (2010) recommends that the faculty member establish an educational milieu that is appealing, exciting, motivating, stimulating, and sustainable. The educator is responsible for the outcomes and conclusions resulting from the learning experience. Another aspect of teaching online relates to being able to effectively summarize. As Loyola (2010) states, "The learner must delete some information (trivial and redundant), substitute some information, and keep some information" (p. 23). This process of summarizing within an online course mandates that the participant scrutinize and dissect the content to a moderately multifaceted and meaningful degree. Superficial scrutiny of the material presented does not allow for the full acquisition of the content to be assimilated from the course. Within online delivery, this process of scrutinizing the information falls to the participants, rather than relying on the summary to be provided by the instructor during the class period. This process of driving the participant to dig deeper and analyze the different components within a topic encourages the participants to synthesize the material. It becomes a part of the student's knowledge bases. One final aspect is the need to focus attention during online education toward appropriate use of recognition and praise that indicates a higher level of learning. According to Loyola (2010), "Effective recognition needs to be positive and sincere in nature, immediately connected to performance, and specific about what is being praised" (p. 23). Since a faculty member is not directly with the students, the need for recognition and immediacy is increased. Face-to-face delivery allows the faculty member to watch the verbal and nonverbal communication and engage accordingly. An online format does not allow this expediency related to encouragement and recognition. Faculty members need to contemplate when and how to provide recognition and encouragement that is timely and directed.

Draves (2000) suggests online education can outshine classroom learning because students can study and develop throughout the duration of the ultimate learning period, learn at their own speed, concentrate on identifiable and detailed content fields, check their progress on a regular and planned schedule, and network effectively with the instructor. Online delivery of educational experiences places a lot of the responsibility squarely on the learner. By making learners responsible for the acquisition of the material, the faculty member can focus on the delivery of the material. The delivery methods are very important, as they are the process by which the learner engages and acquires the information (**Table 8–3**). Draves (2000) states a key aspect: "The heart and soul of an online course will be the interaction between the participants and teacher, as well as the interaction among the participants themselves" (p. 12). The faculty member must establish multiple venues for granting access to peers and faculty. Since the delivery is online and not face-to-face, every opportunity for engaging the participants (students and faculty) must be provided and encouraged. The opportunities to engage with peers and the faculty connect the individuals together in the learning process and aid in networking the members of the cohort involved in the online sessions.

One of the key aspects embedded in an online delivery system is the need to have effective communication. Hanna, Glowacki-Dudka, and Conceicao-Runlee (2000) describe the learning community as "a group of people who have come together to form a culture of learning in which everyone is involved in a collective effort of understanding" (p. 14). The development of this learning community requires that attention be given to the development and management of the communication between the members of the community. Online sessions move rapidly and require each member of the cohort to be self-disciplined and engaged. When members are not committed to the learning process, their delays can adversely affect the rest of the cohort. Discussion within the course requires that all members hold up their part of the bargain, which is to add their "two cents" to the discussion. When individuals do not add their thoughts and comments, other students have nothing to respond to as the discussion progresses. Each participant must take an active role in the conversation for the outcome to be effective.

In recent years, the idea of academic integrity for online courses has come to the forefront. Since students are not directly visible to the instructors, concerns related to who is doing the work are critical. Several new technologies have been developed to aid in the process of addressing academic integrity. Morgan and Hart (2013) discuss a study completed that required students to participate in an academic integrity intervention. This

Table 8–3 Suggestions for Planning and Conducting Online Courses

- Course content and delivery must be prepared in advance.
- Students must be willing and encouraged to ask questions as needed.
- All aspects of the course should promote dialogue between the participants in the course—both students and faculty members.
- Participants within each course should be encouraged to examine their own learning process at regular intervals.
- Each online course should have at least three central components—subject matter, exchange, and appraisal.
- Using between 5 and 10 units/modules provides adequate division for a course.
- "A rough measurement for reading time is 20 pages an hour for nonfiction, 10 pages an hour for extremely technical information, and 40 pages an hour for fiction" (Draves, 2000, p. 79).
- Faculty members must learn to "chunk" materials because reading long narratives does not effectively encourage engagement and learning.
- Bullets and narratives within an online document should be kept short. Approximately 6 to 8 lines of copy is a rule of thumb.
- "The one-minute assessment allows you to ask questions electronically and collect answers anonymously (if you have a program that allows learners to send responses anonymously)" (Hanna et al., 2000, p. 46).
- "A bulletin board, chat room, or threaded discussion can be developed for use by a specific class. Choice of communication method also depends on the need for group interaction, peer-to-peer interaction, or student-to-instructor interaction" (Lowenstein & Bradshaw, 2004, p. 199).
- "There is a skill to asking the 'right questions' to improve higher-level thinking. 'How' and 'why' questions usually require more analysis than 'who,' 'what,' 'when,' or 'where' questions" (Loyola, 2010, p. 27)
- The learners must participate in the class at least every other day to ensure connectedness.
- Instructional proficiency requires time management and boundary setting while constructing an online learning community.
- Fair use of materials within an online course involves an understanding of copyright law, which allows for regulated inclusion of copyrighted material without the owner's permission. A 10% rule advocates the use of 10% or less of a complete material as reasonable use.
- "Students who were assigned to facilitate commented that they learned more when they facilitated discussions than those for which they were not assigned that role" (Dell et al., 2010, para. 4).

Source: Adapted from Dell, C. A., Low, C., & Wilker, J. F. (2010). Comparing student achievement in online and face-to-face class formats. *Journal of Online Learning and Teaching* 6(1). Retrieved November 7, 2013, from http://jolt.merlot.org/vol6no1/dell_0310.htm; Draves, W. A. (2000). *Teaching online.* River Falls, WI: LERN Books; Hanna, D. E., Glowacki-Dudka, M., & Conceicao-Runlee, S. (2000). *147 practical tips for teaching online groups: Essentials of web-based education.* Madison, WI: Atwood Publishing; Lowenstein, A. J., & Bradshaw, M. J. (2004). *Fuszard's innovative teaching strategies in nursing* (3rd ed.). Sudbury, MA: Jones and Bartlett Publishers; and Loyola, S. (2010). Evidence-based teaching guidelines: Transforming knowledge into practice for better outcomes in healthcare. *Critical Care Nursing Quarterly, 33*(1), 19–32.

study investigated the changes in awareness related to academic integrity by those engaged in a planned intervention addressing key aspects of academic integrity. Morgan and Hart (2013) found that the results of this study mirrored the prior study finding that online RN-BSN students were less likely to self-report cheating within assignments. The results from this study supported findings from other studies reflecting that academic dishonesty in nursing schools is an ongoing concern. The study by Morgan and Hart (2013) does recommend the use of interventions to nurture a philosophy of integrity, thus pressuring students to engage in ethical classroom behaviors. When planning courses and assignments, instructors should be mindful of focussing on a positive viewpoint related to academic integrity. Consideration should be given to carefully planning the types of computer tools that will be used to aid in the reinforcement and endorsement of academic integrity.

With the push by the Institute of Medicine's "Future of Nursing" report (2010) to have 80% of RNs prepared at the BSN level, schools are increasing online class size and adding additional sections of the courses. While instructors tend to view 20 to 24 as the acceptable size of an online course, enrollments of up to 100 can be found in a section. Evidence related to acceptable sizes of online courses is not clearly delineated at this time. Class size must be carefully considered when a facility begins the movement toward online education, and a limit for each section should be rationally determined. This determination of online class size should be revisited on a regular basis.

Another challenge in meeting the demand for BSN-level education is the increasing number of sections. With an increasing number of sections, concerns about curriculum drift become important. With multiple sections, care and attention to holding the curriculum consistent to the programmatic objectives are critical. With multiple sections, part-time faculty are being used. These part-time faculty are experts within the areas of instruction and are actively involved in professional environments; however, they are not always as familiar with the department's global objectives or procedures. Concerns about maintaining the focus of the curriculum while still allowing some academic freedom is an area that must be addressed by the faculty members involved in the process.

TECHNOLOGY IN THE CLASSROOM

Conrad and Donaldson (2004) suggest that "lecture is effective for knowledge transmission, but if it is the primary strategy used in the online environment, the course becomes a digital correspondence course with potential problems of learner isolation and high dropout rate" (p. 6). Care must be given to the utilization of technology so that the online delivery is not a digital correspondence course but an exciting, innovative learning environment. The learning outcome must be the "focus of the activity, not the technological tool used to implement the activity" (Conrad & Donaldson, 2004, p. 17). When the tool becomes the key aspect, the content then becomes a secondary aspect of the course, which should not occur. The content needs to be the primary focus.

Connors (2008) states that "in the past 5 years, the number of merging and emerging technologies supported by the Web has increased enormously, making it difficult for faculty members to keep up with the latest advances" (p. 164). New applications of technology are being introduced into the classroom setting continually. Multiple individuals compare this movement and the resulting expectations for the faculty member as converting from the "sage on the stage" to the "guide on the side." Faculty members are being required to change from delivering the material to facilitating the search for information. Teaching by the "spur of the moment" is not easily applied to the online delivery methodology. Faculty members have to set up the learning environment so that the students are challenged to seek out information and apply that knowledge in multiple processes and situations. Connors (2008) explains this process by saying, "The instructor needs to provide learning experiences that require active learning interaction or collaboration among students, and timely feedback" (p. 167). The formulation of interactive, pedagogically sound opportunities to engage in critical thinking and active decision making is of paramount importance for the success of the learning process. Each of the different technologies must be carefully and effectively incorporated at appropriate times to foster best practices and effective outcomes for the learning environment.

Another new concept being utilized in the online environment is **podcast lectures**. The term associated with the podcast concept is **mobile learning** or M-learning. Podcast sessions are media files (e.g., MP3 files) provided for individuals to access as needed for playback on a diverse group of mobile instruments such as computers and portable media players. Research completed by Abate (2013) reports retention and application of lecture content as a result of accessing the material through the use of podcast segments. Students voiced support for the accessing of podcast sessions to review and retain key materials presented through the virtual environment.

Bleich (2009) suggested that "successful adaptation to Web-based instruction requires competence in modularizing concepts and topics, strategies that engage active learning, and assignments that validate both individual and group attainment of course objectives" (p. 63). Care must be taken by the faculty member to ensure that the adaptation of any course, content, or learning assignment strives to address the expected outcome for the process (**Table 8–4**). Over and over, the message is clear that "active learning" is the key for online success. The participants must be stimulated to enthusiastically and dynamically engage with the material presented to assimilate the data into the thinking process. As Bleich (2009) states, "Being facile with the tools embedded within a technology teaching-learning platform requires work but enlivens learning opportunities and student engagement" (p. 63). Using technology just to be able to boast about the tools used does not correlate to effective teaching. Competent and resourceful instruction mandates that learning be accomplished.

Table 8–4   Recommendations for Successful Online Teaching

- The quality of the instructional delivery for courses needs to be excellent.
- Faculty members should be attuned to the needs of the student cohort.
- Feedback for all course assignments must be provided to the students in a timely and positive manner.
- Program and course content should be appropriate for the investment required to obtain the degree.
- Activities incorporated within the program of study should reflect innovation and uniqueness and should excite the desire to learn.
- The institution, program, and faculty members must provide timely and appropriate management of requests made by the student cohort.
- Faculty members should provide understandable and comprehensible student assignments within the syllabus.
- Convenient registration should be provided for each online course.
- Care must be given to ensure that instructional materials address appropriate course content.
- Programmatic requirements must be unambiguous, realistic, and practical.
- Financial aspects must be equitable and practical.
- Evaluation processes used within the course delivery should be obvious and rational.
- Mechanisms must be in place to help the student access books and other resources needed for courses.
- The convenience factor should be evident in all aspects of the program.
- Faculty members should be mindful of individuals' work schedules along with the reputation of the institution.

Source: Adapted from Noel-Levitz. (2011). *National online learner priorities report.* Braintree, MA: Author; and Langley, M. E., & Brown, S. T. (2010). Perceptions of the use of reflective learning journals in online graduate nursing education. *Nursing Education Perspectives, 31*(1), 12–17.

Berger, Topp, Davis, Jones, and Stewart (2009) summarized part of the work that was reported in a 2002 study as indicating that participants realized higher grades in online courses; however, the amount of learning was actually related to the enthusiasm and expectations held by the individual student. Online learning is not appropriate for each and every learner. The learner must have the motivation and determination to embrace the learning process. The commitment to the acquisition of knowledge is essential to the success of the individual in the online setting.

Online tools do not increase teaching and learning. The tools are just that—means to an end. Effective use of the tools can potentiate the learning process. Lowenstein and Bradshaw (2004) note, "A tool's effectiveness is determined by the manner in which it is integrated into a course to support the objectives and to create a community of learners" (p. 216). The faculty member's ability to use the tools effectively and efficiently to transfer content is the outcome desired by using a tool.

Since participants can access the tools 24 hours a day, 7 days a week, faculty members should enlighten them as to any limits established for faculty input, such as the condition that faculty will not be available 24/7 to respond to student requests. By setting out the limits, frustrations on both sides (students and faculty members) can be reduced. Without the limits, engagement expectations can become overwhelming and unmanageable. Faculty members need to carefully consider "how accessible" they are willing to be given the 24/7 environment of the online delivery mechanism. Adequate communication must take place while ensuring that continuous communication is not required.

According to Kyong-Jee and Bonk (2006), "Confusion swells as higher education explores dozens of e-learning technologies (for example, electronic books, simulations, text messaging, podcasting, wikis, blogs), with new ones seeming to emerge each week" (para. 1). With each passing day, new applications of electronic tools are being considered and put to the test within online classes. Some of this utilization has resulted in frustrations. These new applications of the technology tools challenge the education community at a time of budgetary retrenchment and rethinking. The added costs resulting from the acquisition of the new tools and training for the faculty members to be able to use the tools place a burden on the educational community. Care must be given to the best utilization and incorporation of innovative tools into the learning environment so that the goal continues to be the acquisition of learning and knowledge, not the integration of "bells and whistles." Too many bells and whistles without appropriately focusing on the learning can result in bored students who drop courses because the delivery of content is not enriched and engaging.

Jaschik (2009) conducted a meta-analysis of research related to online education. This analysis found that "using technology to give students control of their interactions' has a positive effect on student learning" (Jaschik, 2009, para. 8). Within this study, the inclusion of technology tools was determined to be an advantage for engaging the students in a positive manner. The study further determined that "students who took all or part of their instruction online performed better, on average, than those taking the same course through face-to-face instruction" (Jaschik, 2009, para. 2). Although online learning tools seemed to demonstrate a strong correlation for success, the results did not support the superiority of the online delivery application as a method of instruction. According to Jaschik, (2009) "This report correctly recognizes that online learning and blended learning are growing components of higher education and, employed properly, can play a significant role in promoting student learning" (para. 15). The research included within the meta-analysis sustained the idea of utilizing the methods that best address the content provided and result in successful learning. The linking of instructional methodology and content is the ultimate mechanism for ensuring effectiveness in the learning process.

EVALUATION

Bangert and Easterby (2008) affirm that student evaluations of teaching note that "teaching is a complex, multidimensional task that comprises distinct instructional acts" (p. 59S). The process of student evaluation is very complex. Inserting the online delivery technologies adds to the complexity of the process. The evaluation process within online delivery methods must focus on the student materials and not the tools used. Tools are techniques that are outside of the control of the student. Care must be given to ensuring that the assessment of the student is based upon those aspects that are controllable by the student. Included in this consideration is the timing of the assessment. The turning in of assignments has always been compromised by the excuses that students can use. Faculty members need to carefully consider their expectations given the procrastinating student and the potential that Internet access may be compromised. Lateness and/or inability to submit assignments due to the availability of the Internet for whatever reason are areas that each faculty member should consider and address within a course. The availability of Internet access adds to the complexity of the evaluation process. According to Loyola (2010), "The bottom line is that well-designed and well-implemented educational programs determine the effectiveness" (p. 21). Educational institutions must carefully consider the issue of Internet access as well. When students are unable to access the courses in a timely manner for whatever reason, the evaluation and effectiveness of the online program will be impacted. Whether the online delivery platform, Internet portal, or information technology support are the challenge, the quality and functionality of the program will be questioned.

Hanna et al. (2000) explain that as the students partake in an interactive online course, they promptly appreciate that the class is with them all the time. They are compelled to engage with the cohort and react to the materials provided more than is expected in a face-to-face class. The evaluation of the student is based upon this documentation of the engagement within the content of the course. Students cannot sit back and wait—they must actively and appropriately interject their ideas and thoughts into the course to be successful.

Accrediting organizations are concerned at this point about the ability of institutions to find avenues for assuring that the student registered for the course is completing the work assigned. When online testing is done, the question of who is actually taking the test is raised. For online testing, security pieces must be put into place to ensure that the student registered for the course is doing the actual testing. The institution must develop those guidelines to help make sure that the student registered and receiving the course grade has done the actual work for the course.

Noel-Levitz (2011) states that institutions should identify the issues that are pertinent to students, such as (1) their communication with faculty, along with the assistance received from staff and administrators; (2) the resources afforded to the students; (3) the guidelines in place; and (4) students' general opinions about the usefulness of the learning experience. Educational environments that use online methodologies need to understand the experiences both within and outside of the educational context that best contribute to the student's successful completion. Evaluation of the process must address all aspects to guarantee that the student is being heard. Noel-Levitz (2011) suggests that research reflects that when there is agreement about the expectations and reality of the learning environment, students are more likely to persist in school, resulting in student success and dependability. Although these aspects are difficult to assess with evaluation tools, mechanisms need to be considered that can address the expectations and realities of the educational experience.

SUMMARY THOUGHTS

A study reported by Dell, Low, and Wilker (2010) highlights several aspects within online education. This study found that in the United States, over 20% of all higher education students had taken at least one online course in the fall of 2007. This movement of students toward online education continues to encourage faculty members to access and utilize online aspects within the educational process. According to Dell et al. (2010), "Online instructors should focus on providing high quality instruction for online learners. Interaction among the learners and with the instructor is important in face-to-face and online formats" (para. 2). This finding further supports the idea that it is the engagement with the students that results in success rather than the methodology. The methodology is used to access the students but is only the means to success. The faculty member's relationship with the students is the foundation for success or lack of success. Dell et al. (2010) determine that for online courses, the "design of the learning environment should include tools to help students with time management, pacing their work load, deadlines that facilitate the completion of their assignments, and appropriate learning strategies" (Conclusion, para. 5). Since the students are not in the classroom or directly accessible, the online delivery must address key aspects to keep the students moving in the correct direction for success. The study further supports the ideas discussed in this chapter when it states, "It is important for the instructor to facilitate higher level thinking skills, reflection, and promote problem solving through interactive, problem-based activities" (Dell et al., 2010, Conclusion, para. 5). Faculty members must expect and demand quality interactions and engagement in the learning process. Online courses require the student to strive for excellence in the management of the learning environment. The acquisition of knowledge rests with the student, but is stimulated by the faculty member.

SUMMARY POINTS

1. During 2004–2008, the number of nurses with an associate's degree (AD) rose from 42.9% to 45.4% (DHHS, 2010). This number of nurses with an AD reached 60% in 2011 (DHHS, 2013).
2. The statistics reflect that "among nurses 55 and older, 76,915 intend to leave the nursing profession within 3 years; another 54,539 intend to leave their current nursing job and are unsure if they will remain in nursing afterward" (DHHS, 2010, p. 10).

3. As a result of these dynamics, online educational opportunities are viewed as an innovative, cost-effective approach.
4. Generation X and Millennial cohorts want a learning environment that is accessible, flexible, learner-centered, and meshed with their lifestyle and commitments.
5. Whenever the teacher and the students (learners) are not in the same location, the term *distance education* is applicable.
6. Palloff and Pratt (1999) bring up a very important aspect in regard to distance education when they champion the idea that consideration must be directed toward the development of a community for the participants to facilitate the learning environment.
7. The learners who elect to engage in the educational process from a distance are frequently compelled to do so as a result of time, geographic, financial, or other constraints that restrict their ability to attend traditional classes. The distance learning environment is viewed as convenient, accessible, and flexible.
8. Distance education is viewed as a resourceful and professional alternate for acquiring an advanced degree during economic times that may restrict traveling to a traditional classroom setting.
9. Within the realm of online delivery methodology, any venue or device that allows students and faculty members to engage in the learning process from unique locations can be used.
10. Engaged learning necessitates that the learner become directly involved in the entire learning process.
11. Online class participants must engage in the documenting of their nonverbal behavior, whereas in the classroom, learners can simply look around and view the nonverbal communication of their peers. In the face-to-face environment, participants do not have to wait for classmates to engage in documenting their nonverbal feelings.
12. In addition to online and face-to-face delivery of content, another method to consider is the hybrid method, which involves both online and face-to-face interactions within the framework.
13. Web-based instruction is any activity/course that is provided via the Internet, also denoted as an online course.
14. The determination of the manner in which the course is delivered should be based on the needs of the student, content to be delivered, mission of the course/program, and expectations of the learning community.
15. The assigned individuals are compelled to be online with the other designated members at the same time for any synchronous activity.

16. Asynchronous activities are viewed as those encounters that are conducted independently of others. Within this process, the learner can address the activity within the course at a time convenient for the individual. Asynchronous activities are done usually within a time period but do not require the direct attention of others.

17. E-books are gaining in attention and utilization within the learning process. They are viewed on a computer and do not require the purchase of hard copies or printed textbooks.

18. Rubrics are being incorporated into online delivery to provide consistency in the grading process.

19. According to Chickering and Gamson (1987), effective management of the undergraduate educational experience requires the encouraging of connection concerning students and faculty, cultivating teamwork among students, advancing vigorous learning, providing timely feedback, articulating quality expectations, and recognizing distinct techniques of learning; such concerns are similar in an online environment.

20. Since students are not sitting in the room with their colleagues and the faculty member, attention to methods for allowing the individuals within the course to connect as a learning community is of paramount importance.

21. Superficial scrutiny of the material presented does not allow for the full acquisition of the content to be assimilated from the course.

22. Online delivery of the educational experience places a lot of responsibility squarely on the learner.

23. Scaffolding and deep-dive brainstorming are two techniques being used to move from simple to complex issues and to produce increased participation from members of the learning community.

24. Care must be given to the utilization of technology so that the online delivery is not a digital correspondence course but an exciting, innovative learning environment.

25. Over and over, the message is clear that "active learning" is the key for online success. The participants must be stimulated to enthusiastically and dynamically engage with the material presented to assimilate the data into the thinking process. Using technology just to be able to boast about the tools used does not correlate to effective teaching.

26. Online learning is not appropriate for each and every learner.

27. New applications of technology tools challenge the education community at a time of budgetary retrenchment and rethinking. The

added cost resulting from the acquisition of the new tools and training for the faculty members to be able to use the tools places a burden on the educational community.

28. Care must be given to ensure that the assessment of students is based on aspects that are controlled by the student.

29. The availability of Internet access adds to the complexity of the evaluation process.

30. When students are unable to access the courses in a timely manner for whatever reason, the evaluation and effectiveness of the online program will be impacted.

TIPS FOR NURSE EDUCATORS

1. The learners who elect to engage in the educational process from a distance are frequently compelled to do so as a result of time, geographic, financial, or other constraints that restrict their ability to attend traditional classes.

2. While the computer and Internet tend to be the most frequently utilized aspects for online delivery, other devices are being incorporated as technology grows and develops.

3. Within the online community, the participants can remain neutral if desired. If a peer does not engage, the primary indication that a problem is developing may only be decreased by that individual.

4. Web-based instruction requires active learning and engagement in the learning process by the individual student.

5. Within asynchronous activities, the learner can address the activity within the course at a time convenient for the individual. Asynchronous activities are done usually within a time period but do not require the direct attention of others.

6. E-books allow for quick turnaround when updates are needed. Since the books are accessed via the computer, smart phones, or other electronic devices, a question can be quickly researched to determine up-to-date information when making critical decisions.

7. Rules/recommendations for online communication, called netiquette, include the use of capital letters, proper use of the computer, management of emails, and so forth.

8. Taking the time to plan how to unite the different members in the course cohort is a critical foundation for the development of

discussion and interactions. Since the individuals don't have the advantage of sitting in a room together, the development of a comfort level with the different individuals must take place through the use of communication skills.

9. Learning objectives are the underpinning for the educational experience; thus, every activity to be incorporated into a course needs to be scrutinized to determine its functionality.
10. To be effective, the teacher should determine the results expected from the engagement in the learning process.
11. The process of summarizing within an online course mandates that the participant scrutinize and dissect the content to a moderately multifaceted and meaningful degree.
12. Since a faculty member is not directly with the students, the need for recognition and immediacy is increased. Faculty members need to contemplate when and how to provide recognition and encouragement that is timely and directed.
13. Online sessions move rapidly and require each member of the cohort to be self-directed and engaged.
14. When the technological tools become the key aspect, the content becomes a secondary aspect of the course, which should not occur.
15. Faculty members within an online delivery process are charged with facilitating the search for the information, not the delivery of the material.
16. Faculty members have to set up the learning environment so that the students are challenged to seek out information and apply that knowledge in multiple processes and situations.
17. Care must be taken by the faculty member to ensure that the online adaptation of any course, content, or learning assignment strives to address the expected outcome for the process.
18. Lateness and/or inability to submit assignments due to the availability of the Internet for whatever reason are areas that each faculty member should consider and address within a course.
19. Students cannot sit back and wait—they must actively and appropriately interject their ideas and thoughts into the course to be successful.
20. The faculty member's relationship with students is the foundation for success or lack of success.
21. Since the students are not in the classroom or directly accessible, the online delivery must address key aspects to keep the students moving in the correct direction for success.

MULTIPLE CHOICE QUESTIONS

1. Generation X and the Millennial generations expect a learning process that is:
   A. flexible, teacher-centered, and open to lifestyles.
   B. **flexible, learner-centered, and committed to different lifestyles.**
   C. rigid, learner-centered, and committed to specific learning processes.
   D. rigid, teacher-centered, and committed to different lifestyles.

   Rationale:
   Generation X and Millennial cohorts want a learning environment that is accessible, flexible, learner-centered, and meshed with their lifestyle and commitments.

2. Examples of distance learning opportunities include:
   A. **online courses, correspondence courses, and independent studies.**
   B. online courses, videoconferencing, and regular courses.
   C. correspondence courses only.
   D. online courses only.

   Rationale:
   Bastable (2014) lists examples of distance learning as online courses, correspondence courses, independent study, and videoconferencing. Whenever the teacher and the students (learners) are not in the same location, this term is applicable.

3. Some of the reasons that students elect to participate in distance education opportunities are:
   A. time, geographic, and financial liberties.
   B. convenience, accessibility, and rigidity.
   C. **time restrictions, flexibility, and geographic considerations.**
   D. commitment to excellence, rigidity, and structure.

   Rationale:
   The learners who elect to engage in the educational process from a distance are frequently compelled to do so as a result of time, geographic, financial, or other constraints that restrict their ability to attend traditional classes. The distance learning environment is viewed as convenient, accessible, and flexible.

4. Engaged learning requires the learner to:

A. be a passive learner.
B. follow the lead of the faculty member.
C. engage as needed.
D. **become directly involved in the learning process.**

Rationale:
According to Conrad and Donaldson (2004), "Engaged learning is focused on the learner, whose role is integral to the generation of new knowledge" (p. 5). Engaged learning necessitates that the learner become directly involved in the entire learning process. The learner is an active participant in the process. Lowenstein and Bradshaw (2004) postulate that "participation in any form of distance learning requires students to be self-directed and able to function in an environment with limited faculty feedback and lacking face-to-face interaction" (p. 213). Students who engage in distance learning opportunities must understand that the responsibility for learning falls upon them, as they don't have the classroom to use for passive learning.

5. Synchronous activities are those activities within an online course that require:
A. **all members of the cohort to be online at the same time.**
B. a few members of the cohort to be online at the same time.
C. engagement in the activity at a time conducive for the participant.
D. engagement in the activity at the same time by the cohort only.

Rationale:
Synchronous activities are those planned activities in which all of the members are expected to be online and/or connected at the same time.

6. Asynchronous activities within an online course are those that require activities to be posted:
A. at a time convenient for the faculty member.
B. at a time convenient for the cohort.
C. **at a time convenient for the learner.**
D. all at the same time.

Rationale:
Asynchronous activities are viewed as those encounters that are conducted independently of others. Within this process, the learner can address the activity within the course at a time convenient for the individual. Asynchronous activities are done usually within a time period but do not require the direct attention of others.

7. Topics that are harder to address via a computer-based delivery methodology are those that:
   A. are stand-alone topics.
   B. **require hands-on management.**
   C. require faculty in attendance.
   D. are complex.

   Rationale:
   Computer-based instruction is functional for some areas but inappropriate for other areas. Those topics that require hands-on management pose difficulty when considered for presentation via a computer-based delivery methodology.

8. Bundled e-book packages have the advantage of:
   A. **allowing quick turnaround when updates are needed.**
   B. requiring students to be technologically savvy.
   C. restricting access to the package when not at school.
   D. allowing anyone to change the package as needed to update it.

   Rationale:
   E-books are gaining in attention and utilization within the learning process. They are viewed on a computer and do not require the purchase of hard copies or printed textbooks. The computer-based delivery of the books allows for quick turnaround when updates are needed.

9. Netiquette rules and recommendations are considered as methods for ensuring:
   A. assertive management of the online communication.
   B. passive engagement with fellow students.
   C. **civilized interactions with individuals on the Internet.**
   D. control within a classroom setting.

   Rationale:
   Netiquette rules and recommendations include the use of capital letters, proper use of the computer, management of emails, and so forth. Netiquette is viewed as the behaviors that reflect being civilized on the computer.

10. To ensure connection between faculty members and students, the educational experience should:
    A. discourage vigorous learning, as it will disrupt the learning process.
    B. **recognize specific techniques of learning to facilitate the process.**

C. articulate the expectations for individual work, not team activities, within the process.
D. hold feedback until the end of the process to allow the student to be creative.

Rationale:
Chickering and Gamson (1987) state that effective management of the undergraduate educational experience requires the encouragement of connection concerning students and faculty, cultivating teamwork among students, advancing vigorous learning, providing timely feedback, articulating quality expectations, and recognizing distinct techniques of learning. Online learning environments must include these aspects as well.

11. Characteristics that need to be evidenced when attempting to engage and facilitate online courses are:
    A. directness, truthfulness, rigidity, and disregard.
    B. disrespect, relevance, openness, and empowerment.
    C. duplicity, sensitivity, openness, and empowerment.
    D. **honesty, responsiveness, openness, and empowerment.**

Rationale:
According to Palloff and Pratt (1999), "The keys to the creation of a learning community and successful facilitation online are simple—honesty, responsiveness, relevance, respect, openness, and empowerment" (p. 20). Taking the time to plan how to unite the different members in the course cohort is a critical foundation for the development of discussion and interactions.

12. Online delivery does not have the advantage of the classroom as a method for developing comfort levels within the cohort. What method is paramount for use within the online delivery mechanisms for establishing a comfort level with the members of the class?
    A. Multiple assignments.
    B. Use of hands-on assignments.
    C. **Use of communication skills.**
    D. Assignments that require ongoing communication.

Rationale:
Taking the time to plan how to unite the different members in the course cohort is a critical foundation for the development of discussion and interactions. Since the individuals don't have the advantage of sitting in a room together, the development of a comfort

level with the different individuals must take place through the use of communication skills.

13. Engagement of the learner in the educational process necessitates that the faculty member find ways to encourage:
    A. **networking for the members of the class.**
    B. individualization of the learning process.
    C. independence from the other members of the class.
    D. collaboration with the faculty member.

Rationale:
The faculty member must establish multiple venues for granting access to peers and faculty. Since the delivery is online and not face-to-face, every opportunity for engaging the participants (students and faculty) must be provided and encouraged. The opportunities to engage with peers and the faculty connect the individuals together in the learning process and aid in networking the members of the cohort involved in the online sessions.

14. The key focus for any online course should be the:
    A. process.
    B. technological tools.
    C. **content.**
    D. individuals in the course.

Rationale:
When technological tools become the key aspect, the content becomes a secondary aspect of the course, which should not occur. The content needs to be the primary focus.

15. The design of the learning environment for an online course should address:
    A. **time management, workload pace, deadlines, and appropriate learning strategies.**
    B. scheduling of outside assignments, teaching strategies, and workload.
    C. scheduling of all aspects of the student's time and pacing of outside endeavors.
    D. time management, self-confidence, and building of respect.

Rationale:
Dell et al. (2010) determine that for online courses, the "design of the learning environment should include tools to help students with time management, pacing their work load, deadlines that facilitate the completion of their assignments, and appropriate learning

strategies" (Conclusion, para. 5). Since the students are not in the classroom or directly accessible, the online delivery must address key aspects to keep the students moving in the correct direction for success. The study further supports the ideas discussed in this chapter when it states, "It is important for the instructor to facilitate higher level thinking skills, reflection, and promote problem solving through interactive, problem-based activities" (Dell et al., 2010, Conclusion, para. 5).

DISCUSSION QUESTIONS

1. In an online delivery format, what type of strategies would a faculty member need to consider to ensure that the learning environment is at an optimum level for the students?
   Considerations:
   Carefully look at the recommendations for successful online teaching provided in Table 8–4 as you look for these strategies. These items will help to stimulate your thoughts as to ways you can effectively facilitate the online environment. In your thoughts, consider the different teaching ideas such as e-books, podcasts, etc., to determine which of these strategies would work best with your topic of presentation.
2. From the list of suggestions provided concerning planning and conducting online courses, select three to four of the suggestions and discuss how each could be used in improving a course currently taught or being prepared for teaching.
   Considerations:
   Use Table 8–3 (Suggestions for Planning and Conducting Online Courses) as you carefully and thoughtfully determine the optimum strategies for use in your course. Different topics require different strategies to address the material being presented. Take the content into consideration as the strategies are reviewed.
3. Develop a scaffolding assignment for a course topic, and discuss the barriers and challenges encountered as you organized this assignment.
   Considerations:
   Alber (2014) presents six strategies to consider when contemplating the use of scaffolding techniques within a course. Look at these strategies as you consider this question. Include the ideas presented related to "deep-diving" within the considerations.

4. List the pros and cons that you see in regard to online, hybrid, and face-to-face delivery of materials.

Considerations:

Consider making a list of the pros and cons for each of these delivery methods from the readings provided within this chapter. Each delivery method is functional and appropriate in multiple settings. Carefully considering the good aspects along with the challenges ensures that the selection of the method for delivery related to a topic is effective.

REFERENCES

Abate, K. S. (2013). The effect of podcast lectures on nursing students' knowledge retention and application. *Nursing Education Perspectives, 34*(3), 182–185.

Alber, R. (2014). *Six scaffolding strategies to use with your students.* Retrieved June 28, 2014, from http://www.edutopia.org/blog/scaffolding-lessons-six-strategies-rebecca-alber

AMN Healthcare. (2013). *2013 survey of registered nurses: Generation gap grows as healthcare transforms.* San Diego, CA: Author.

Bangert, A. W., & Easterby, L. (2008). Designing and delivering effective online nursing courses with the Evolve electronic classroom. *CIN: Computers, Informatics, Nursing, 26*(2), 99–105.

Bastable, S. B. (2014). *Nurse as educator: Principles of teaching and learning for nursing practice* (4th ed.). Burlington, MA: Jones and Bartlett Learning.

Berger, J., Topp, R., Davis, L., Jones, J., & Stewart, L. (2009, May/June). Comparison of web-based and face-to-face training concerning patient education within a hospital system. *Journal for Nurses in Staff Development,* 127–132.

Bleich, M. F. (2009). Technology: An imperative for teaching in the age of digital natives. *Journal of Nursing Education, 48*(2), 63.

Burnett, A. (2013). From our readers: ABC's of evidence-based practice. *American Nurse Today, 8*(4), 1.

Chickering, A. W., & Gamson, Z. F. (1987, March). Seven principles for good practice in undergraduate education. *The American Association for Higher Education Bulletin.*

Connors, H. R. (2008). Beyond the classroom: Considering distance education approaches. In B. K. Penn (Ed.), *Mastering the teaching role: A guide for nurse educators* (pp. 163–175). Philadelphia, PA: F.A. Davis.

Conrad, R., & Donaldson, J. A. (2004) *Engaging the online learner: Activities and resources for creative instruction.* San Francisco, CA: Jossey-Bass Publishers.

Dell, C. A., Low, C., & Wilker, J. F. (2010). Comparing student achievement in online and face-to-face class formats. *Journal of Online Learning and Teaching, 6*(1). Retrieved November 7, 2013, from http://jolt.merlot.org/vol6no1/dell_0310.htm

Dorin, M. D. (2009, February). Cyber-instructor? Consider becoming an online educator. *Nursing Management*, 34–37.

Draves, W. A. (2000). *Teaching online*. River Falls, WI: LERN Books.

Dreon, O. (2013). Applying the seven principles for good practice to the online classroom. *Faculty Focus*. Retrieved December 7, 2013, from http://www.facultyfocus.com/articles/online-education/applying-the-seven-principles-for-good-practice-to-the-online-classroom/

Felver, L., Gaines, B., Heims, M., Lasater, K., Laustsen, G., Lynch, M., Mathews, L.R., . . . Tanner, C., (2010). *Best practices in teaching and learning in nursing education*. New York, NY: National League for Nursing.

Hanna, D. E., Glowacki-Dudka, M., & Conceicao-Runlee, S. (2000). *147 practical tips for teaching online groups: Essentials of web-based education*. Madison, WI: Atwood Publishing.

Institute of Medicine. (2010). *The future of nursing: Leading change, advancing health*. Washington DC: National Academy of Sciences.

Jaschik, S. (2009). The evidence on online education. Retrieved June 28, 2014, from http://www.insidehighered.com/news/2009/06/29/online#sthash.0DAxshfi.dpbs

Kyong-Jee, K., & Bonk, C. J. (2006). The future of online teaching and learning in higher education: The survey says . . . . *EDUCAUSE Quarterly, 29*(4). Retrieved November 7, 2013, from http://www.educause.edu/node/157426.?time=1291863108

Langley, M. E., & Brown, S. T. (2010). Perceptions of the use of reflective learning journals in online graduate nursing education. *Nursing Education Perspectives, 31*(1), 12–17.

Leski, J. (2009). Nursing students and faculty perceptions of computer-based instruction at a 2-year college. *Journal of Nursing Education, 48*(2), 91–95.

Lowenstein, A. J., & Bradshaw, M. J. (2004). *Fuszard's innovative teaching strategies in nursing* (3rd ed.). Sudbury, MA: Jones and Bartlett Publishers.

Loyola, S. (2010). Evidence-based teaching guidelines: Transforming knowledge into practice for better outcomes in healthcare. *Critical Care Nursing Quarterly, 33*(1), 19–32.

Morgan, L., & Hart, L. (2013). Promoting academic integrity in an online RN-BSN program. *Nursing Education Perspectives, 34*(4), 240–247.

Noel-Levitz. (2011). *National online learner priorities report*. Braintree, MA: Author.

Palloff, R. M., & Pratt, K. (1999). *Building learning communities in cyberspace: Effective strategies for the online classroom*. San Francisco, CA: Jossey-Bass Publishers.

RapidBi. (2007). *Deep dive brainstorming technique, an innovative process for organizational development*. Retrieved December 7, 2013, from http://rapidbi.com/deepdivebrainstormingorganizationaldevelopment/

Sambataro, M. (2000). Just-in-time learning. Retrieved December 7, 2013, from http://www.computerworld.com/s/article/44312/Just_in_Time_Learning?pageNumber=1

Sowan, A. K., & Jenkins, L. S. (2013). Use of the seven principles of effective teaching to design and deliver an interactive hybrid nursing research course. *Nursing Education Perspectives, 34*(5), 315–322.

Stevens, D. D., & Levi, A. J. (2013). *Introduction to rubrics* (2nd ed.). Sterling, VA: Stylus Publishing.

Tri-Council for Nursing. (2010). *Educational advancement of registered nurses: A consensus position.* Washington, DC: Author.

U.S. Department of Health and Human Services, Health Resources and Services Administration. (2010). *The registered nurse population: Initial findings from the 2008 national sample survey of registered nurses.* Washington, DC: Author.

U.S. Department of Health and Human Services, Health Resources and Services Administration. (2013). *The U.S. nursing workforce: Trends in supply and education—Results in brief.* Washington, DC: Author.

Williams, M. G., & Dittmer, A. (2009). Textbooks on tap: Using electronic books housed in handheld devices in nursing clinical courses. *Nursing Education Perspectives, 30*(4), 220–225.

Chapter 9

Clinical Educational Experiences

Joyce Miller and Carol Boswell

CHAPTER OBJECTIVES

At the conclusion of this chapter, the learner will be able to:

1. Discuss the differences and similarities between clinical judgment, clinical reasoning, and clinical decision making.
2. Explain the uses of high-fidelity simulation, low-fidelity simulation, static manikins, and Objective Structured Clinical Examinations.
3. Examine the evidence related to clinical simulation.
4. Discuss methodologies that educators, preceptors, and coaches can use to incorporate evidence-based activities in clinical or simulation-based settings.
5. Identify a variety of venues for student evaluations in the clinical or simulation setting from the perspective of educator, preceptor, or coach.

KEY TERMS

- Clinical decision making
- Clinical judgment
- Clinical reasoning
- Coaching
- Cognitive knowledge acquisition
- Debriefing
- Experiential learning
- High-fidelity simulation

- Low-fidelity simulation
- Moderate-fidelity simulation
- Objective Structured Clinical Examination
- Preceptor
- Self-confidence
- Self-efficacy
- Static manikin

INTRODUCTION

As nursing education moves forward into the next decade, the concepts of evidence-based teaching and clinical competency that can be acquired using simulation and other resources have taken on new meaning and importance. The acknowledgement of innovative opportunities to bring the skills and applications to the students must be embraced and embedded into the educational process as we advance the profession of nursing. New and innovative means of providing clinical and simulation experiences have been researched to manage the growing problem confronting many schools of nursing across the country. Adams and Valiga (2009) submit that the challenge within the current healthcare environment is to provide students with a full and efficient variety of clinical learning opportunities while dealing with the restrictions encountered by fewer clinical resources. As the challenge of fewer clinical settings—resulting in increasing problems when trying to locate clinical sites—becomes a reality, the concept of simulation becomes progressively more imperative within the educational environment (Adams & Valiga, 2009; Bambino, Washburn, & Perkins, 2009; Letvak, 2008). This chapter examines the provision of clinical learning opportunities. With the number of schools proliferating due to the current and anticipated future nursing workforce shortage, clinical placements are becoming scarce. As a result, many schools and state boards of nursing are considering the option of clinical simulation experiences as a partial alternative to face-to-face clinical involvement.

Letvak (2008) suggests that an ideal clinical setting is one that presents encounters that are applicable, pertinent, and timely for the content being presented within the courses and that offers opportunities to reinforce and practice the skills already acquired. So no matter in what location the clinical experience is provided or what resources are used, the ultimate criterion for the learning process is the acquisition of skills in a timely manner while also supporting and confirming skills already learned.

Jeffries (2008) defines evidence-based teaching as "using 'best evidence' to select, develop, and implement educational strategies and conducting research to further define educational practice" (slide 14). For this text, evidence-based teaching (EBT) is a dynamic, holistic system using educational principles validated by evidence to support, maintain, and promote a new level of knowledge for a learner in a variety of settings. EBT must strive to locate the best evidence instead of depending on the patterns used over the decades. Jeffries (2008) goes on to list three reasons why EBT is important: (1) integrating pedagogical research results helps in the development of a foundational body of knowledge related to healthcare education,

(2) utilizing teaching strategies that have been identified by evidence allows for stability within learning outcomes, and (3) incorporating evidence-based instructional tactics provides a means for replication, refinement, and establishment of "best practices." These three motivations for moving toward EBT provide a foundation for the effective incorporation of evidence and the establishment of excellence within nursing education. As stated by Adams and Valiga (2009):

> Excellence means striving to be the very best you can be in everything you do—not because some . . . 'authority' figure [demands it], but because you can't imagine functioning in any other way. It means setting high standards for yourself and the groups in which you are involved, holding yourself to those standards despite challenges or pressures to reduce or lower them, and not being satisfied with anything less than the very best. (p. 3)

Within every endeavor in the educational process, excellence should be the goal for the development of an effective nursing profession.

Holland, Landry, Mountain, Middlebrooks, Heim, and Missildine (2013) identify simulated environments as a means to encourage realism, collaborative scholarship, involved participation, and improved clinical reasoning proficiency. Today's nursing graduate is expected to (1) effectively manage patients presenting with increased acuity levels, (2) carefully investigate and embrace the expanding role of the modern nurse, (3) successfully collaborate within an interprofessional environment, (4) competently utilize innovative technology, and (5) resourcefully work with limited resources. Each and every nurse must step into the role of being a fully functional nurse who understands the changing healthcare setting. As new technology is integrated into the workplace, nurses at all levels are expected to understand and successfully assimilate the technology to improve health care. Through the use of simulation and other clinical experiences, success in this effort can be assured.

INSTRUCTIONAL SETTINGS

Clinical experiences are a mainstay within nursing educational activities. Since nursing is viewed to be both an art and a science, the "hands-on" aspect is highly valued within all nursing programs. Clinical experiences allow the practical application of the information covered during the didactic aspects of the program. Clinical sites can include acute care agencies, secondary schools, day cares, senior centers, home health agencies, hospice settings, mobile clinics, physician and/or nurse practitioner managed clinics, industrial health clinics, and community agencies. By using the material provided with actual and/or simulated clients, students are better able to understand and effectively use the information as they work to apply safe nursing care. The instructional settings used for these clinical experiences can be a variety of agencies and resources. Any location where individuals are seen and encountered can be a potential clinical site. Clinical experiences are really the interactions with people, not the physical settings where these interactions might happen. As a result, faculty members have to be constantly open to new and innovative locations that may meet student and course needs. The basic driving force related to clinical experiences is the course objectives. The course objectives are those concepts and skills that need to be attained during a given clinical engagement. Faculty members within selected courses need to be persistently searching for appropriate agencies and settings where the objectives for that course can be attained.

As faculty members identify potential clinical agencies or sites, the nursing program has the responsibility for establishing a relationship with the designated group. According to Misener (2008), this responsibility must be shared by faculty, the dean's office, and the central administration for locating clinical facilities. Frequently, the actual clinical contract or affiliation agreement is developed and maintained through the dean's office and the central administration for the clinical agreements. The central administration is accountable for ensuring that any contract/agreement is in compliance with all university rules and regulations. The dean assumes the responsibility for assuring that the areas covered in the contracts/agreements comply with the partnership. The resulting relationship needs to be symbiotic and synergistic and must address the mission of the university and the clinical agency. The partnerships should always reflect a "win-win" situation for the groups involved in the joint venture. Faculty members are accountable for maintaining the different aspects related to a clinical association. Both the university and the agency are expected to preserve an infrastructure that supports the aspects covered by the agreement. Documentation of the preceptor and site affiliation process is an important key to the success of the collaboration from both an administrative and a clinical standpoint. One key aspect that is essential to the successful management of clinical affiliations is communication. All parties involved in the educational process must be committed to maintaining and augmenting the partnership as the clinical experiences move forward. It takes everyone's involvement and commitment to effectively communicate needs, successes, and barriers.

According to Letvak (2008), factors that are important within the selection and management of clinical sites are:

- Course objectives
- Consistency between the agency's and the school of nursing's philosophy
- Maintenance of a high standard of care
- Reasonability of commute distance for students
- Provision of adequate parking and safety when students are traveling between parking lot and agency
- Availability of food service or storage for students to bring their own food
- Accessibility to conference or meeting space
- Commitment and positive interactions by agency staff with students

With the changing environment of health care and academia, other areas that also need to be considered when selecting clinical experiences are directly related to the type of clinical experiences required. Computer access is an increasingly important consideration. Another area for consideration is the availability of current textbooks and resources for the students to use as they endeavor to provide safe and effective health care to clients.

SIMULATION

One such way to provide and support the acquisition of clinical skills and competency is the use of simulation, which has taken on new importance with the restrictions placed on clinical resources. As increasing enrollments, nursing shortages, agency accreditation requirements, and current scares within the media about problems within the healthcare arena place a toll on healthcare agencies, clinical resources are becoming harder and harder to attain. Navigating the highly competitive clinical preceptor acquisition of clinical site experiences has become significant. Jeffries (2009) asserts that "clinical simulation offers students rich, authentic clinical experiences in a safe, nonthreatening environment" (p. 71). Through the use of simulation, students are provided the opportunities to try out new skills prior to performing them on real patients (Bambino et al., 2009; Cato, Lasater, & Peeples, 2009; Jeffries, 2009; Smith & Roehrs, 2009). With the complexities of the inpatient population, simulation activities allow the students to acquire knowledge with situations prior to being placed in that setting. By having the opportunities to work through problems with the use of a device, students and faculty members can provide educational materials, evaluate the different options, and incorporate research while in a safe, nonthreatening environment. Simulation experiences through utilization of **Objective Structured Clinical Examinations** (OSCEs) have emerged as a gold standard of health professional assessments within many medical disciplines (Guraya, Alzobydi, & Salman, 2010). Marwaha (2011) reports that the aim of an OSCE is to "examine skills and ability at the 'shows how' level." These experiences simulate realistic clinical scenarios and can be used for skills, competencies, and evaluation.

Standardized patients (SPs) have traditionally been used in simulation centers for advance practice nurse practitioner students. However, use of SPs for undergraduate students is gaining momentum. SPs provide human contact in a safe environment for students to gain assessment and communication skills for planning patient care. SPs receive extensive training and work with students and faculty members to evaluate student progress. The sessions are video recorded and allow faculty members and SPs to target areas for improvement through review of the videos and debriefing.

Let's clarify some words and concepts frequently used within the world of simulation. The first term that needs to be considered is **experiential learning**. Experiential learning implies that the learning is done by a person or through a program/activity structured by others (Neill, 2005). Within this form of learning, the emphasis is placed on active participation by all members involved (Dreifuerst, 2009). Within the context of the different generational cohorts discussed elsewhere in this text, experiential learning is seen as a valuable way to engage members and to incorporate the use of group/cohort work. As individuals take an active part in the learning process, genuine, meaningful, and long-lasting learning occurs.

Two additional terms to become familiar with are **self-efficacy** and **self-confidence**. Van Wagner (n.d.) postulates that self-efficacy is directly related to Bandura's work on social cognitive theory. Self-efficacy is viewed as an individual's conviction in his or her capacity to thrive in a given situation. Self-confidence goes along the same lines. It is understood to be a certainty in the capacity, credibility, or dependability of a person. As a person develops self-efficacy and self-confidence, he or she becomes adept at confronting challenges successfully, seeking learning opportunities, developing commitment to the learning process, and recovering promptly from obstacles and disappointments. Successful management of simulation activities is viewed as a means to improve self-efficacy within the student. As a result, the student is better able to move forward successfully within the educational environment.

According to Dreifuerst (2009), "Mastery of critical thinking, clinical decision making, and clinical judgment is a milestone of professional development as a nurse moves from being a novice to becoming an expert clinician" (p. 109). Critical thinking is defined and discussed in the *Overview of Evidence-Based Practice* chapter. **Clinical decision making** works with critical thinking through the use of nursing knowledge, proficiency, and viewpoints to ascertain an appropriate action and/or response. **Clinical reasoning** then takes the critical thinking and clinical decision making together with additional cognitive elements to see beyond the obvious solutions to innovative management of the clinical situation. Holland et al. (2013) characterize clinical reasoning as "using formal and informal thinking to evaluate information and take action" (p. 269). **Clinical judgment** is established by identification of the dynamic transitions by individuals across time as they react to health concerns and associated treatment (Benner, 1984). Each of these clinical aspects is somewhat of a staircase to higher levels of utilization within the clinical setting. As individuals gain confidence, the information used within the decision-making process is increased, thus allowing for more complex management of the client situation. A final aspect within this process is **cognitive knowledge acquisition**. Cognitive learning is understood to incorporate listening to, watching, touching, and experiencing the world around us (ThinkQuest Team, n.d.). As our brains manipulate the physical objects and events encountered, the information is processed and formulated into retrievable memories. Cognitive knowledge acquisition is considered to be an active process of learning that engages and stimulates the individual to view items from many different perspectives instead of as one-dimensional objects.

Let's move to the differences within the process of simulation. Some of the terms used are *static manikin, low-fidelity simulation, moderate-fidelity simulation,* and *high-fidelity simulation*. **Static manikins** are those partial task trainers that are used to practice specific skills, such as ear or prostate manikins (Simulation Innovation and Resource Center, n.d.). Static manikins can be at either the low-fidelity or moderate-fidelity level. **Low-fidelity simulation** (LFS) experiences are those opportunities for the students to engage in case studies, role playing, or group activities that are specific to a narrow skill process. Static manikins at this level would be restricted to one narrow task practice, such as the ear or prostate manikins. According to Adams and Valiga (2009), "High fidelity and medium [moderate] fidelity simulators are life-like mannequins, referred to as human patient simulators that are programmed to mimic the responses of a human being" (p. 100). **Moderate-fidelity simulation** (MFS) includes those models that are two-dimensional in their focus on the experience being learned, such as IV arms. This level does encourage problem solving within the management of the manikin case study. Spunt and Covington (2008) assert, "High-fidelity simulation offers the most realistic clinical experience possible, short of caring for a real patient, and may involve advanced equipment that interacts with the learner" (p. 234). With **high-fidelity simulation** (HFS), the case presentations can be complicated and in-depth; Harvey simulators are an example. Dillon, Noble, and Kaplan (2009) relate that the HFS process provides incomparable opportunities that allow the students to practice skills within a safe and controlled environment. They also recommend HFS activities because they allow the presentation of clinical experiences that may not be as frequently encountered within the healthcare setting. Spunt and Covington (2008) sum up the use of simulators as enabling "the student to experience simple or complex, stable or unpredictable clinical situations before encountering real ones in the clinical setting" (p. 234). Because the situation is controlled by the faculty members involved, the depth of the clinical situation with the incorporation of key knowledge points can be managed and addressed during the simulation experience prior to the student confronting the aspects within a real-world setting. Depending on the clinical opportunities available at different sites, some skills and tasks may not be readily available for all of the students to manage. The simulation process is well positioned to address these skills and tasks for the entire cohort. Of importance to any simulation experience is the debriefing process to improve understanding, whether as a cognitive or a technical process. Outcomes of learning can be met either in face-to-face conferences or in an online setting (Oermann & Gaberson, 2014). The faculty member must carefully consider the best venue for meeting the needs of the students.

An understanding of each of these terms is necessary for synthesizing the evidence related to simulation. Each of these different aspects is directly related to the effective utilization of this teaching strategy within the clinical arena. Adams and Valiga (2009) state that simulation and simulated case scenarios are an effective means for appraising and examining clinical skills, critical thinking, and clinical judgments within the context of recreating the healthcare needs from a client's viewpoint. Tagliareni (2009) states, "Throughout our history, nurse educators have used simulation to teach basic skills, to promote mastery of tasks in the clinical lab, and to replicate practice situation" (p. 69). Simulation has become the hope for the future within nursing education. With the many challenges confronting nursing education and the call to change the way that nursing is being taught, simulation is viewed as a lifeline that is appropriate for addressing these concerns and challenges. Smith (2009) relates that HFS activities within skills labs are predominantly used to ensure the learning of skills and tasks. Smith (2009) goes on to say that the use of HFS activities within a simulated clinical setting incorporates the solving of problems, encourages teamwork, facilitates a better understanding of complex disease problems, and augments decision making and critical thinking. At this point, let's look at what a few of the experts say about simulation. The concepts put forth by the experts are based on research evidence and practical application evidence.

One of the theoretical frameworks utilized within simulation is the situated cognitive theory. According to Holland et al. (2013), this framework addresses contextual learning, which is common in simulation. This theory holds that learning is contingent on the situation where it occurs. As a result, learning is improved when the setting, such as in simulation, mirrors the clinical environment. Holland et al. (2013) explain that "the development of communities of practice, individuals with a common interest who learn through practice and participation, is considered essential to situated learning" (p. 270). This idea supports the expectations within the simulation milieu. Spunt and Covington (2008) provide a well-rounded look at the ideas included within clinical simulation activities. One of the advantages of the use of this teaching strategy is that the learner must be self-directed because the environment is interactive. The learner is called on to engage and advance the scenario at a speed reflective of individual needs and knowledge. Another advantage of the use of simulation is the opportunity for faculty members to be able to provide missing experiences that have not been provided within the actual clinical setting or that can't be done by all of the members of the cohort. By using the clinical simulation option, those clinical scenarios can be provided to each member of the cohort without having to locate the experience within the authentic clinical setting. Thus, the students can benefit from the learning without having to be stressed to locate a patient with that disease or equipment. As has already been discussed, clinical simulation provides opportunities for the students to apply their didactic knowledge and problem-solving skills, critical-thinking abilities, and time management skills. Because the clinical simulation activities allow time for the students to think about time management and aspects of care, skills in managing time effectively in the busy world of health care and appropriate delegation can be contemplated and determined in a safe environment. Spunt and Covington (2008) continue to acknowledge that due to the safe environment provided by the clinical simulation setting, the students learn faster because they do not perceive personal threats and barriers. From the evidence, clinical simulations are valued from the first undergraduate semester through to the graduate program with specialized clinical applications and all the way to the doctoral research programs. Simulations allow faculty members to adjust variations based upon the current healthcare arena and the learning needs of the participants. As new and innovative changes are encountered in the workplace, changes can be made to the scenarios to address these changes. Also, as political changes occur, such as in national healthcare policy, these aspects can be incorporated into the scenario to allow for the currency of the educational process. Spunt and Covington (2008) acknowledge the positive benefit of the clinical simulation related to reflective opportunities. Students and faculty members can reflect on the processes utilized within the scenarios to advance the profession of nursing.

Smith and Roehrs (2009) provide several key thoughts related to the evidence associated with the use of clinical situations. Historically, nursing education has employed a variety of simulation activities for clinical experiences, involving static manikins, task trainers, case studies, and role playing. Although these types of activities offer advantages depending on the objectives and cost constraints of the institution, Smith and Roehrs (2009) contend that "they do not provide students with a realistic context for performing nursing skills or the opportunity to learn to perform a skill while interacting with a patient" (p. 74). The use of HFS provides these extra benefits within a simulation activity. For a clinical simulation to be effective, the evidence shows that the designing of the scenario should embrace five related aspects:

- clear objectives and information,
- support during the simulation,
- a suitable problem to solve,
- time for guided reflection/feedback, and
- fidelity or realism of the experience.

The research done by Smith and Roehrs (2009) suggests that "having clear objectives and an appropriate problem to solve requires special consideration by nurse education when designing an HFS experience" (p. 77). Faculty members must embrace the idea that clinical simulations require the pre-session work of planning and management of the learning expectations. Each scenario and engagement should be carefully deliberated upon to identify and clarify the objectives and problems to be confronted within the scenario. Though some areas of the clinical process will be unique based upon the decisions made by the students, the foundational expectations for the learning session must be carefully and thoroughly planned and incorporated into the learning packet for the session.

Another source of evidence related to clinical simulations is provided by Bambino et al. (2009). They identified three themes related to areas that were supported and addressed via this teaching strategy. The initial theme related to communication, both verbal and nonverbal. According to Bambino et al. (2009), "Participants [in the study] indicated that they learned the importance of communicating with significant others as well as the patient" (p. 81). The second premise was associated with the confidence gained in the areas of psychomotor skills and patient interactions. Through the use of clinical simulation activities, students thought they gained confidence by "letting them know what to expect and giving them experiences in working through assessments and problem solving" (Bambino et al., 2009, p. 81). The final idea was associated with clinical judgment. Prioritizing assessment skills, determining when and how to intervene, and identifying aspects concerning abnormal physical assessment findings were facets of clinical judgment that were thought to be improved from engaging in these clinical scenarios. The work done by Bambino et al. (2009) also identified that the aspect within clinical skills that is missing in traditional skill lab experiences is the context of the process. Clinical simulation allows for an improved addressing of the context of the material, skills, and goals for the session. The complexities of context within a clinical simulation activity require the students to be able to reprioritize and modify rules and situations based upon the needs of the client and the healthcare assessments. Bambino et al. (2009) concluded that "simulation can introduce novice students to the process of being able to perceive characteristics and aspects of patient care situations that may alter the manner in which nursing care is provided" (p. 79). By utilizing the clinical simulation process, students' self-efficacy and self-confidence were strengthened. Students were found to be able to work through patient encounters with increasing complexities of patient care to provide nursing care that was safe, resulting in reduced errors in clinical judgment and fewer potential harmful situations for living clients.

Holland et al. (2013) explain a strategy employed with students to weave learning through the use of simulation, SPs, and virtual communities. Many virtual communities are being developed and tested. Two current options are The Neighborhood and Second Life. The Neighborhood is a virtual community that is accessible online. Within the community, storylines are developed using the unfolding case study concepts. This process allows for faculty and students to engage in an environment offering opportunities to develop self-confidence and knowledge within a safe setting. Second Life (2014) claims to be "a 3D world where everyone you see is a real person and every place you visit is built by people just like you" (para 1). Second Life provides a three-dimensional world for interacting around a learning situation. This format allows the faculty member to develop a complete unfolding case study moving from community to inpatient back to community with multiple family interaction opportunities along with the interdisciplinary aspects.

Further evidence is provided by Hoadley (2009) for the use of clinical simulation. It is recommended that "with the use of HFS, nurses can improve skill versatility and increase self-confidence" (p. 95). This development of self-confidence is an outcome of amplified internalization of the content provided and improved satisfaction with the learning environment. A final benefit advanced by Hoadley (2009) is that "the incorporation of experiential learning and reflection/debriefing enhances knowledge by developing one or both of the following behaviors: retention and transferences" (p. 92). This research study further supports the idea that the "hands-on" experiences created by clinical simulation opportunities allow students to better grasp the complexity of nursing care provision. Students emerge with confidence in being able to direct the complex care of clients after having been exposed to these types of client situations in the less threatening environment of clinical simulation.

The research work completed by Elfrink, Nininger, Rohig, and Lee (2009) provides additional EBT considerations. According to Elfrink et al. (2009), "Best practices for simulation design in nursing education incorporate learner support in the form of hints, cues, or direction, offered before, during and after simulation experiences" (p. 83). Faculty members must be attentive to the use of hints, cues, and direction. These aspects must be inserted habitually within the scenario, not as a one-time-only occurrence. As faculty members consider the generational aspects of learners, this point becomes even more important. By providing the hints, cues, and directions throughout the scenario, the generational cohort can see the expertise held by the faculty members and develop respect for the knowledge base and authority residing within the faculty members. The work of Elfrink et al. (2009) produced two aspects that need to be carefully considered. Within this study, students found videotaping the simulation experience to be very stressful and unproductive. The students related that they were distracted by the worry related to the taping. Faculty members viewed the videotape as helpful for the debriefing sessions. Students, on the other hand, found the use of the videotape during the debriefing sessions to be negative. Another concern that they raised was the negativity resulting from having to repeat the simulation. Repeating the same simulation was seen as more busywork than productive learning time. From this study, the students suggested that the content and management of the debriefing session be strengthened instead of repeating any simulation experience, and that videotapes not be used to review the experience. A positive aspect that resulted from this research study was the recommendation of using planning sessions. According to Elfrink et al. (2009), "A large number of students felt that a planning session following the patient hand-off and report would be a productive step toward lessening anxiety, placing a particular student 'on the spot' and facilitating 'where to start'" (p. 85). This idea of planning sessions concurs with the generational aspects related to Generation X that support group engagement. It allows the group to work through the anticipated scenario to be prepared for what is expected. The student group would still need to deal with the unexpected complexities that emerge during the scenario. The preplanning allows for teamwork and an interactive, collaborative process. Elfrink et al. (2009) concluded that "promoting an environment of collaborative learning has the potential to increase ownership in the entire simulation experience" (p. 86). This evidence strongly supports and upholds the evidence noted about the strengths and challenges presented by the different generational cohorts. The incorporation of teamwork and collaboration is directly supportive of the characteristics within these different generational groups.

Kim and Shin (2013a, 2013b) offer a glimpse at the use of simulation with an obstetrical focus. This project used a pretest/posttest design when looking at the outcomes of using simulation scenarios with obstetrical nursing challenges incorporating a computerized birthing simulator. The study used the concept of self-confidence as the framework to demonstrate the effects of the simulator with the student population (N = 138). The results did support the use of simulation to develop self-confidence within nursing students through the use of scenarios and simulation-based training.

Dillon et al. (2009) provide additional evidence related to the appropriateness of clinical simulation by noting that "receiving immediate feedback, without the possibility of causing patient harm, allows students to develop a repertoire of possible solutions" (p. 87). Feedback without the threat of penalty supports the characteristics seen within the generational cohorts. As an experiential learning technique and strategy, simulation promotes the cohort to associate the applicable concepts, employ suitable theories in clinical practice, and determine satisfactory clinical decisions. From the work done by this team of researchers, simulation was found to endorse the skills of communication, teamwork, delegation, priority setting, and leadership.

The work done by Cato et al. (2009) turns the research toward the aspect of **debriefing** within the clinical simulation process. The evidence found within this study further supported the idea that the clinical simulation process was instrumental in developing the students' clinical judgment and critical-thinking skills. The process of the clinical simulation endeavor frequently takes the path of one group interacting directly in the scenario while another group serves as reviewers of the process. Following the completion of the scenario, the entire group comes together for a debriefing process. Cato et al. (2009) state that the "debriefing that follows each scenario focuses on the team's care of the patient, including safe practice, priority setting, continuous assessment, communication, resource management, and leadership" (p. 106). From their work, the debriefing session is the opportunity for the faculty to develop and support the ability of the student to "think like a nurse." It is during these sessions that the positive aspects of the interactions must be recognized and developed.

Dreifuerst (2009) completed extensive work examining the debriefing process. The evidence relates the debriefing session as "the process whereby faculty and students reexamine the clinical encounter," which "fosters the development of clinical reasoning and judgment skills through reflective learning processes" (p. 109). It is during this session that the faculty members embrace the opportunity to support and develop the student cohort in a positive manner. Dreifuerst (2009) established five objectives for the debriefing process:

1. identification of the different perceptions and attitudes that have occurred;
2. linking the exercise to specific theory or content and skill-building techniques;
3. development of a common set of experiences for further thought;
4. opportunity to receive feedback on the nature of one's involvement, behavior, and decision making; and
5. reestablishment of the desired classroom climate, such as regaining trust, comfort, and purposefulness. (p. 110)

Faculty members need to carefully consider these five aspects as they strive to come to grips with the idea of debriefing. The debriefing session should be provided to facilitate the students' best learning opportunity. As a result, faculty members need to understand how important this part of the learning process is. Dreifuerst (2009) found that the attributes of reflection, emotion, reception, integration, and assimilation were the defining attributes of simulation debriefing. When these five attributes are carefully considered by the faculty, the debriefing sessions can be an effective teaching/learning situation. Reflection is viewed as an occasion to retrace the experience. During this aspect, the group takes the time to come to an agreement about what actually happened during the experience. It is a listing of the different processes that occurred—a timeline of the case. Next, the connected emotions and emotional release are important to verbalize. As students engage in the scenario, emotions become an integral part of the process. Emotions related to past experiences may be encountered by some of the students. Emotions related to the process may also be encountered as each member assumes a role within the scenario. The debriefing process should address these emotions and allow the student group to work through them. Reception, or openness to feedback, is a crucial aspect of learning. Simulation experiences embrace cognitive, affective, and psychomotor skills. All of the participants should be expected to provide feedback on those skills from their viewpoints. During the debriefing session, the views of each person should be acknowledged and considered to provide an inclusive view of the experience. According to Dreifuerst (2009), "Integration of the simulation experience and the facilitated reflection into a conceptual framework is one of the most challenging and least common attributes of debriefing" (p. 111). This process of bringing all of the parts together to enable the student to understand the complexity of healthcare delivery is important. According to Dreifuerst (2009), the components of the simulation experience "link the experience to the curriculum, guide the facilitation of the debriefing discussion, and provide structure for evaluating the experience" (p. 113). When conducting the debriefing, each student and each learning objective along with the multicomplexity of the clinical scenario should be carefully and completely discussed to allow for the development of a firm foundation of nursing knowledge. The debriefing is viewed as a fundamental and essential component within the clinical simulation experience. It closes the loop on the learning process and allows the students to connect the different pieces, both negative and positive, into a learning opportunity.

Rudolph, Foldy, Robinson, Kendall, Taylor, and Simon (2013) challenged the idea of task-versus-relationship dilemma within the debriefing process. Debriefing can be viewed as a mechanism for clarifying, codifying, and translating learning into guidelines for use throughout future practice (Rudolph et al., 2013). Within this case study project, the idea emerged that faculty members struggled with the idea of a task-versus-relationship dilemma when providing constructive feedback during the debriefing sessions. Faculty members were viewed as apprehensive and concerned about negatively impacting their relationship with students by providing judgmental reviews following simulation activities. As a result of this perceived negativity related to providing judgemental reviews, faculty members may bias the comments provided. This study looked at a retrospective analysis of a difficulty debriefing session using a two-column case approach. The discussion addressed recommendations for faculty members to incorporate, resulting in "accurate, specific and timely feedback about task performance without demoralizing the learner" (p. 314). Allowing faculty members to learn how to deliver effective feedback in debriefing sessions is critical to the learning process.

The final piece of evidence presented here is focused on the faculty member and was presented by Dillard, Sideras, Ryan, Hodson-Carlton, Lasater, and Siktberg (2009). An urgent need was identified that faculty members require faculty development opportunities related to the development of the new pedagogical skills necessary for the management of the complex pieces of technology involved in HFS. To expect faculty members to already have the skills needed to effectively organize, manage, and facilitate clinical simulation experiences is inappropriate. The skill set needed to be applicable to this type of clinical experience requires the faculty members to update their knowledge and thought processes. Because the faculty-to-student ratios utilized within the clinical settings do not consistently allow faculty members time to adequately observe the students as they attempt to make clinical judgments, clinical simulation experiences are viewed as a means to overcome this deficiency by allowing sufficient time to observe each student's clinical judgment process. Dillard et al. (2009) found that "HFS allows for a more comprehensive evaluation of the development of students' clinical judgment as well as recognition of gaps in their understanding of clinical practice" (p. 100). HFS and other clinical simulations focus on the outcomes. As a result, faculty members have to convert their thought processes for clinical experiences to the idea of outcomes. This conversion of thought compels the faculty members to reconceptualize the pedagogy of teaching as it relates to simulation implementation and linking learning from simulation opportunities to clinical practice. According to Dillard et al. (2009), "No standardized curriculum has yet been developed for simulation use" (p. 103). In addition to the lack of a standardized curriculum, a consistent technique for appraising student learning in simulation is also nonexistent. Thus, the evaluation aspect of simulation experiences needs to be carefully and thoughtfully discussed and envisioned.

Evidence is present for the incorporation of clinical simulation as a means for addressing the clinical knowledge needed to conduct health care. Ongoing research is also being done to further clarify the roles and expectations needed to effectively conduct the acquisition of nursing knowledge related to the clinical setting.

TYPES OF CLINICAL STRATEGIES

Many nurses and other healthcare providers have not actively incorporated research findings into clinical practice settings. In fact, until recently, many nurses were aware of research but had not shifted the research into their practice. Evidence-based practice (EBP) through research utilization has become a major goal within schools of nursing. Research utilization is the process by which research is put into practice. The types of research utilized include instrumental, conceptual, persuasive, and overall (Squires, Estabrooks, Gustavsson, & Wallin, 2011). EBP involves (1) best evidence from a thorough search and critical appraisal of all studies, (2) context, (3) healthcare resources, (4) patient status and individual circumstances, and (5) the client's values and preferences for his or her care.

Educators, **preceptors**, and **coaches** can adapt the following steps to incorporate EBP into their specific clinical settings: (1) Formulate a clinical question to be researched; (2) systematically search for relevant research/ evidence that either supports or disputes the specific clinical practice; (3) evaluate the relevance, quality, and application to the practice setting; (4) determine the evidence-based decision through consideration of the research/evidence compiled; (5) couple the research/evidence with the practitioners' clinical experiences and expertise and resources; (6) apply to the patient's clinical status and preferences that support the specific action; (7) implement the change within the practice setting; and (8) evaluate the outcome of the clinical change through systematic EBP (DiCenso, Cullum, Ciliska, & Guyatt, 2004). The difference between a preceptor and a coach is the responsibility for the learning situation. Traditionally in undergraduate programs, preceptors are assigned one or two students whom they oversee during a specific time period (usually 1 day or 1 week). Some accelerated baccalaureate programs use the coach concept. A coach takes the responsibility for a designated student over a longer period with increased attention to the learning opportunities. A coach may work with the designated student for the entire semester or even entire education program. One exception to the normal definitions related to coach and preceptor can be found in graduate courses where preceptors oversee graduate students throughout the program. Within the graduate-level preceptor process, the preceptor can be responsible for the student for over 300 clinical hours and four semesters. The decision to use the term *coach* versus *preceptor* may depend on the type of program, model, and institutional faculty. Clinical reasoning strategies to provide guidance for specific student clinical questions should be prioritized through the evidence-based process for both the hospital bedside and community clinical office settings. One such process for clinical reasoning applies EBP analysis through case studies. When students recognize the process of incorporating EBP within their settings, optimal provision of healthcare services will occur.

Traditionally, clinical faculties have utilized care plans, care maps, case studies, simulation activities, comprehensive clinical reflection papers, and clinical logs to evaluate students' growth. Today, a large portion of clinical activities use preceptors or coaches to facilitate growth as (1) a "hands-on" approach that includes teaching microskills, (2) observation of their skill sets by being observed or shadowed by their students, (3) provision of mini-lectures on skills and clinical processes, (4) mentoring of students through clinical projects, and, finally, (5) "learning" vicariously through their students' research on projects and papers. Through utilization of a mixture of methods, education will likely be more enjoyable and effective to facilitate realistic and maximum clinical growth for the student (DiCenso et al., 2004). Hands-on approaches will provide solid interventional strategies through clinical reasoning that is based on routinely incorporating current evidence and guidelines.

Conducting clinical experiences at the undergraduate setting requires more face-to-face time with clinical faculty members. Since these students are novice healthcare providers, both time and energy must be given to ensure that they develop the foundation needed to provide safe and practical health care. The faculty member's energy and focus should be directed toward providing appropriate and adequate clinical opportunities for each student to develop clinical expertise while ensuring that critical-thinking opportunities are presented. Care must be taken in relation to the clinical experience as to which skills, tasks, and/or opportunities must be provided to ensure that the students are competent following the conclusion of the clinical process. Each and every student will not be afforded the same exact opportunities, so the drive is to determine which aspects must be provided at which level and setting. Another aspect of the clinical experience relates to the thought process being developed. Determinations of the types of assignments are needed to reflect and ensure that the students develop the appropriate clinical decision-making skills. Most daily teaching should include the combination of (1) precepting using "microskills," (2) being observed or shadowed by the student, (3) observing the student, (4) giving "mini-lectures," (5) mentoring student projects with application of evidence-based clinical practice guidelines and research studies, and (6) learning together with the student as both the preceptor/coach and student search the Internet, clinical resources, evidence-based guidelines, or texts for answers to clinical questions. These clinical decision-making skills can then be incorporated into other clinical settings.

Teaching while practicing on busy days can be challenging, but the reality is that every day is a busy day. Effective preceptors and coaches prepare ahead for the day and include specific strategies for success. Prior to the beginning of the rotation, it is helpful to actually meet the student and determine his or her objectives, goals, learning style, and past experiences prior to this experience. All members in the practice setting need to meet the student and discuss the clinical strategies. To ensure optimal success for the student and the agency, scheduling of patients, understanding of experiences desired, examination room availability, a documentation area, and planning for the student to have access to patient records are necessary (DiCenso et al., 2004). To facilitate immersion of students in the clinical setting, an identified workspace should be arranged for the students to use their texts, references, and computers and to access the Internet, enabling the optimal evidence-based learning experience for the student. As healthcare complexities increase along with the number of patients having medical care access through the Affordable Care Act, a more complex system of patient treatment for healthcare issues will emerge. Student utilization of online access such as a 5-minute online consult will bring evidence into specific clinical practice experiences. Golway (2008) reports that the focus of the 2008 Accreditation Symposium for American Nursing Credentialing Center was to question if evidenced-based approaches were guiding teaching in nursing. Their recommendation was to adopt the evidence-based approach to teach by these four steps: (1) Question your own teaching practices, (2) search for evidence to answer questions, (3) decide if findings are applicable to your own teaching situation, and (4) use evidence to guide teaching. Ideally, the student workspace would emulate the workspace provided for the preceptor/coach to facilitate immersion of the students to maximize clinical learning and application of both teaching and student EBP activities.

Clinical expertise, teaching style, and philosophy of patient care should be covered by the preceptor. This process should focus on the actual services provided within the specific clinical setting. Coverage of the agency's mission, patients served, standards, and guidelines that the site has incorporated facilitates clinical practitioner roles as well as expected student behaviors. Prior to clinical activities, students should be introduced to the organization of the clinic, including the reception area, patient/staff restrooms, laboratory, clinical rooms, procedure rooms, staff offices, and library resource rooms. This introduction will facilitate student familiarity prior to the first day of the clinical experiences, resulting in reduction in stress for the preceptor, clinical staff, the student.

Daily clinical schedules should be provided for the student when arriving for clinical experiences, and a short post-clinical reflection at the end of the experience will identify specific professional growth and challenges on a daily basis. Consideration should be given to request the students to examine one to two clinical case studies based on the specific challenges they have experienced. When students report their research findings, utilization of evidence-based research studies and clinical guidelines should be stressed. As student nurses, preceptors, coaches, and other healthcare providers adapt evidence-based clinical guidelines and research into daily clinical practice settings, current and solid patient care will be provided to their patients.

STUDENT EVALUATION

Teachers and preceptors/coaches share the responsibility of monitoring the progress of students by analyzing specific clinical activities, types of patients seen, complexity of health issues, procedural activities, and application of case studies for provision of solid, evidence-based practice. Evaluation can be done through a variety of venues, including (1) clinical schedules and patients seen; (2) individualized contracts with preceptors/coaches based on their area of expertise; (3) development of specific clinical goals that are measurable and appropriate for the courses being taken; (4) review of written goals by the student, preceptor/coach, and clinical faculty to evaluate the students' growth; (5) clinical performance scores through measurement tools utilized by preceptors/coaches and clinical faculty; (6) successful site visits where students, preceptors/coaches, and faculty meet face-to-face to observe and discuss progress of students; (7) successful clinical performance by students with faculty members through simulation activities such as OSCEs; and (8) final course evaluations by preceptors/coaches and clinical faculty to determine specific competencies obtained during the course of the semester. Opportunities should be provided to students to evaluate the clinical site where they have worked, their preceptors/coaches, the effectiveness of their clinical experience, support from their clinical faculty, and whether the site should be used for future students. Gaberson and Oermann (1999) support the triad of clinical experiences the student, preceptor/coach, and clinical faculty have participated in, and evaluation to determine clinical outcomes. Using multiple individuals to evaluate the setting allows for a clearer analysis of the educational experience.

Evaluation of student complexities includes issues such as the types of patients seen and healthcare complexity, variety of preceptor/coach working hours, goal-specific clinical locations, preceptor/coaching expertise, student work schedules, and family responsibilities. Evaluation of clinical experiences can no longer always be done face-to-face in the classroom setting. As online nursing care programs expand, so too does complexity for student evaluations. Growth of programs from local or regional applicants to state or national program extensions are on the rise. Ongoing evaluation must be done through a mixture of experiences, such as telephone contact, emails, online chat rooms, WebEx sessions, travel to schools for simulation experiences, and face-to-face contact in specific clinical settings. Contact between the preceptor/coach and the clinical faculty is imperative to off-set challenges and enhance learning opportunities the students may have within their clinical setting. When preceptors/coaches provide feedback concerning learner performance, the clinical faculty should offer guidance and recommendations based on their expertise. Challenges can be daunting, time consuming, and expensive for course faculty, preceptors/coaches, colleges, and universities as they guide their students through the various clinical activities.

In hospital settings, clinical evaluations should focus on clinical standards such as professional behavior, professional integrity, patient-centered care, interdisciplinary care, quality improvement, informatics, and patient safety, with EBP as the foundational thread for clinical judgment utilized to guide appropriate clinical decisions. Coaches and faculty members should provide evaluation based on the ability to communicate with patients and families, cultural and health beliefs of patients and families, and specific contributions to coordination of patient care that utilize the nursing process framework within the current evidence guidelines. Whether the clinical experiences are in community settings or hospital settings, the continuous communication between student, preceptor, and faculty is paramount. All care should embrace patient safety issues in terms of safe and effective patient-centered care, provision of care in a timely manner, and identification and reduction of risks to patients.

SUMMARY THOUGHTS

Clinical experiences, whether direct hands-on or simulation-based experiences, must always be a large component of nursing education. The question becomes one of how such experiences can be effectively and efficiently managed. With the Affordable Care Act producing markedly increasing numbers of patients, more schools of nursing and faculty members will be needed. This issue, coupled with students enrolling from farther distances from the school, means access to clinical activities will become more complicated. Though actual care of clients is paramount and should never be completely removed from the educational process, clinical simulation is one way to get the best out of the process during times when availability is compromised. According to Tagliareni (2009), "New technologies and changing patient demographics require our graduates to work quickly, efficiently, and safely, and to think and act in ways that reach far beyond current practice realities" (p. 69). Simulation embraces the undertaking of transforming faculty members' beliefs about how students discover and deliberate while becoming an indispensable teaching/assessment/evaluation strategy in the education of nurses. Further, simulation experiences afford a safe environment for active student learning with direct faculty feedback.

With appropriate clinical strategies and evaluation methodologies, most nurses with extensive clinical experiences can and do serve as excellent preceptors/coaches. Utilization of evidence-based educational strategies includes (1) continuous preplanning, (2) provision of student time with patients, (3) facilitation of challenging patient case presentations, and (4) post-clinical discussion times. Students, preceptors, and coaches will readily be able to recognize each student's clinical growth and challenges (Burns, Beauchesne, Ryan-Krause, & Sawin, 2008). Preceptors and coaches are and will continue to be the front line for training the future generations of nurses through access to clinical sites, patients, expert mentoring, and sharing of clinical experiences to facilitate students' clinical growth.

SUMMARY POINTS

1. An ideal clinical setting is one that presents encounters that are applicable, pertinent, and timely for the content being presented within the courses and that sanctions persistent reinforcement and practice for the skills already acquired.
2. Evidence-based teaching must strive to locate the best evidence instead of depending on the patterns used over the decades.
3. The ultimate criterion for the learning process within the clinical setting is the acquisition of skills in a timely manner while supporting and confirming skills already learned.
4. With the Affordable Care Act, large numbers of patients will be entering the healthcare arena who previously had no access. This access will require more schools of nursing and faculty support to handle the increasing numbers of students who will need to be educated to provide for these patients.
5. With the complexities of the patient population, simulation activities allow students to acquire knowledge with situations prior to being placed in that setting.
6. By having the opportunities to work through problems with the use of a device, students and faculty members can provide educational

materials, evaluate the different options, and incorporate research/ evidence while in a safe, nonthreatening environment.

7. As individuals take an active part in the learning process, genuine, meaningful, and long-lasting learning occurs. Student reflection after the clinical experiences will provide further growth and expertise.

8. As a person develops self-efficacy and self-confidence, he or she becomes adept at confronting challenges successfully, seeking learning opportunities, developing commitment to the learning process, and recovering promptly from obstacles and disappointments.

9. Because the simulation situation is controlled by the faculty members involved, the depth of the clinical situation with the incorporation of key knowledge points can be managed and addressed during the simulation experience prior to the student confronting the aspects within a real-world setting.

10. Static manikins restrict the learning to one narrow task practice.

11. Moderate-fidelity simulators are those models that are two-dimensional in their focus on the experiences being learned.

12. With high-fidelity simulators, case presentations can be complicated and in-depth.

13. High-fidelity simulations incorporate the resolution of problems, advance teamwork, facilitate a better understanding of complex disease problems, and support decision making and critical thinking.

14. Objective Structured Clinical Examinations (OSCEs) have been developed to provide a range of health tasks based on "real-life" patient complaints and are used for both evaluation of knowledge and development of problem-solving skills. OSCEs involve processes for taking health histories, performing physical examinations, determining diagnostics and labs needed, identifying differential and final diagnoses, forming treatment plans, and providing patient education.

15. Clinical simulation provides opportunities for students to apply their didactic knowledge and problem-solving skills, critical-thinking abilities, and time management skills.

16. Simulation allows the faculty member to adjust variations based upon the current healthcare arena and subsequent evidence available.

17. Simulation has been found to endorse the skills of communication, teamwork, delegation, priority setting, and leadership.

18. Debriefing sessions are a key component within the simulation process. During these sessions, faculty members must help the students

to examine the case and analyze the clinical reasoning and judgment skills used during the process. The students' perceptions must be the driving focus for debriefing.

19. During debriefing, each student and each learning objective along with the multiplicity of the clinical scenario should be carefully and completely discussed to allow for the development of a firm foundation of nursing knowledge.

20. Faculty members require faculty development opportunities related to the development of new pedagogical skills needed to manage the complex pieces of technology involved in HFS.

21. Principles of clinical teaching include the following: (1) Learning is evolutionary and occurs from both a student and preceptor/coach focus; (2) participation, repetition, and reinforcement facilitate student learning; (3) various aspects of clinical experiences increase role satisfaction for students and preceptors/coaches; and (4) use of the most current clinical guidelines and evidence-based studies enhances clinical expertise and provision of care.

22. Both student and preceptor/coach satisfaction will increase through preplanning and ongoing clinical experience planning to facilitate maximum student experiences. Frequent communication between faculty, preceptor, and student is necessary.

23. Utilization of evidence-based clinical teaching will provide mentorship to students and facilitate their use of current clinical guidelines and evidence-based applications for provision of patient care.

TIPS FOR NURSE EDUCATORS

1. Clinical experiences must be carefully planned and organized to gain the utmost positive outcome for the students. The agency, unit, personnel, and objectives for the clinical experience must be thoughtfully considered.

2. Clinical simulation is one strategy for addressing clinical skills and knowledge.

3. High-fidelity simulation requires focused preparation time from both the faculty member and the students.

4. Student planning time should be included in the time allotted for simulation experiences to gain the maximum results from the opportunity.

5. The debriefing session for each clinical encounter should be carefully planned and orchestrated for the optimum outcome. Within

each session, the clinical objectives should be addressed prior to the experience so that students understand where within the course materials the experience is directed.

6. Provision of student work areas within the clinical setting is integral to creating an optimal learning experience. These areas should allow students to readily access computers, learning materials, and the Internet.

7. Access to resources will provide strong learning environments that link didactic and clinical strategies for optimal patient care.

8. Teaching strategy options should include utilization of evidence-based clinical case presentations based on the direct clinical experiences of the day. Both open-ended and direct questioning can facilitate the critical-thinking processes.

9. Student assignments between clinical experiences should facilitate EBP through use of the most recent clinical guidelines and research studies that support the care the students provide to their patients.

MULTIPLE CHOICE QUESTIONS

1. The primary reason for utilizing clinical experiences with students is the:
   A. **timely acquisition of skills and confirmation of previously learned skills.**
   B. management of clinical skills for management of the education experience.
   C. timely acquisition of skills without the need for further follow-up.
   D. supporting and confirming of previously learned skills only.

   Rationale:
   No matter the location of the clinical experience provided or the resources used, the ultimate criterion for the learning process is the acquisition of skills in a timely manner while also supporting and confirming skills already learned.

2. Experiential learning is understood to mean learning that:
   A. is completed within a specific site or location.
   B. **is completed by a person or through a program/activity structured by others.**
   C. is completed by a person without structure from another person.
   D. results from a program that is directed by the individual.

Rationale:

Experiential learning implies that the learning is done by a person or through a program/activity structured by others (Neill, 2005). Within this form of learning the emphasis is placed on active participation by all members involved (Dreifuerst, 2009). As individuals take an active part in the learning process, genuine, meaningful, and long-lasting learning occurs.

3. The simulators referred to as human patient simulators are:
   A. low-fidelity simulators, moderate-fidelity simulators, and high-fidelity simulators.
   B. **moderate-fidelity simulators and high-fidelity simulators.**
   C. static manikins, moderate-fidelity simulators, and high-fidelity simulators.
   D. low-fidelity simulators and high-fidelity simulators.

Rationale:

According to Adams and Valiga (2009), "High fidelity and medium [moderate] fidelity simulators are life-like mannequins, referred to as human patient simulators that are programmed to mimic the responses of a human being" (p. 100). Moderate-fidelity simulators are those models that are two-dimensional in their focus on the experience being learned. This level of simulator encourages problem solving within the management of the manikin case study. Spunt and Covington (2008) note that "high-fidelity simulation offers the most realistic clinical experience possible, short of caring for a real patient, and may involve advanced equipment that interacts with the learner" (p. 234). With the high-fidelity simulators, the case presentations can be complicated and in-depth.

4. Simulation and simulated case scenarios are effective means for appraising and examining:
   A. didactic skills, critical thinking, clinical judgment, time management, delegation, communication skills, and leadership only.
   B. didactic skills, critical thinking, clinical judgment, and leadership only.
   C. **clinical skills, critical thinking, clinical judgment, time management, delegation, communication skills, and leadership.**
   D. clinical skills only.

Rationale:

Adams and Valiga (2009) state that simulation and simulated case scenarios are an effective means for appraising and examining clinical skills, critical thinking, and clinical judgments within the context of re-creating healthcare needs from a client's viewpoint. Cato et al. (2009) state that the "debriefing that follows each scenario focuses on the team's care of the patient, including safe practice, priority setting, continuous assessment, communication, resource management, and leadership" (p. 106). From the work done by the team of Dillon et al. (2009), simulation was found to endorse the skills of communication, teamwork, delegation, priority setting, and leadership.

5. Objective Structured Clinical Examinations (OSCEs) were first developed in 1975 and are utilized for standardized assessment for a range of tasks based on clinical simulation, including:
   A. **comprehensive health histories, physical examinations, diagnostics, plan of care, and patient education.**
   B. didactic skills, critical thinking, clinical judgment, time management, delegation, communication skills, and leadership only.
   C. utilization of static manikins, moderate-fidelity simulators, and high-fidelity simulators only.
   D. communication skills, procedural competence, and contract negotiations.

Rationale:
Larsen and Jeppe-Jensen (2008) indicate that OSCEs are utilized and widely recognized for student learning, particularly with assessment methods. OSCEs were first developed for medical students with a series of standardized assessment stations based on clinical situations. Each student has the same specific tasks to solve, which gives the OSCE a greater degree of objectivity as opposed to standard clinical examinations. This objectivity is enhanced by basing the marking of the performance on specific predetermined criteria agreed upon by the participating examiners beforehand.

6. Research has shown simulations to be effective at:
   A. incorporating the management of problems, discouraging teamwork, facilitating an improved understanding of complex disease problems, and augmenting decision making and critical thinking.
   B. incorporating the solving of problems, encouraging teamwork, restricting understanding of complex disease problems, and augmenting decision making and critical thinking.
   C. incorporating the management of problems, encouraging teamwork, facilitating an improved understanding of only simple

disease problems, and augmenting decision making and critical thinking.

D. **incorporating the solving of problems, encouraging teamwork, facilitating an improved understanding of complex disease problems, and augmenting decision making and critical thinking.**

Rationale:

Smith (2009) relates that HFS activities within skills labs are predominantly used to ensure the learning of skills and tasks. Smith goes on to say that the use of HFS within a simulated clinical setting incorporates the solving of problems, encourages teamwork, facilitates a better understanding of complex disease problems, and augments decision making and critical thinking.

7. One advantage identified with the use of simulations is that it:

A. restricts faculty members from making variations in the case study based upon current healthcare issues and practices.

B. **allows faculty members to make variations in the case study based upon current healthcare issues and practices.**

C. allows students to make variations in the case study based upon current healthcare issues and practices.

D. allows faculty members to hold constant any variations in the case study for consistency.

Rationale:

Simulations allow faculty members to make variations to case studies based upon the current healthcare arena. As new and innovative changes are encountered in the workplace, changes can be made to the scenarios to address them. Also, as political changes occur, such as in the national healthcare policy, these aspects can be incorporated into the scenario to allow for currency of the educational process.

8. As an experiential learning technique and strategy, simulation promotes the cohort to:

A. **associate applicable concepts, employ suitable theories in clinical practice, and determine satisfactory clinical decisions.**

B. associate applicable concepts, contrast suitable theories to clinical practice, and restrict the formation of clinical decisions.

C. associate concepts, employ all theories to clinical practice, and determine some clinical decisions.

D. associate applicable strategies, employ all theories to clinical practice, and determine satisfactory clinical decisions.

Rationale:

As an experiential learning technique and strategy, simulation promotes the cohort to associate the applicable concepts, employ suitable theories in clinical practice, and determine satisfactory clinical decisions. From the work done by Dillon et al. (2009), simulation was found to enhance the skills of communication, teamwork, delegation, priority setting, and leadership.

9. Debriefing sessions used following a simulation period serve as an opportunity for:
   A. faculty members to develop and support the ability of students to "think like a student."
   B. students to develop and support the ability of each other to "think like a nurse."
   C. **faculty members to develop and support the ability of students to "think like a nurse."**
   D. faculty members to develop and support the ability of advanced practice registered nurses to "think like a physician."

Rationale:

Cato et al. (2009) state that the "debriefing that follows each scenario focuses on the team's care of the patient, including safe practice, priority setting, continuous assessment, communication, resource management, and leadership" (p. 106). From their work, the debriefing session is characterized as the opportunity for the faculty to develop and support the ability of the student to "think like a nurse." It is during these sessions that the positive aspects of the interactions must be recognized and developed.

10. The debriefing session should address:
   A. **course objectives, the timeline, resulting emotions, integration of key concepts, self analysis and feedback.**
   B. course objectives only.
   C. problems encountered during the session and what the students should have done.
   D. mistakes identified and areas not addressed.

Rationale:

Dreifuerst (2009) found that the attributes of reflection, emotion, reception, integration, and assimilation were the defining characteristics of simulation debriefing. During the debriefing session, the views of each person should be acknowledged and considered to provide an inclusive view of the experience. This process brings all of the parts together to enable the student to understand that the complexity of healthcare delivery is important. According to Dreifuerst (2009), the attributes "link the experience to the curriculum, guide the facilitation of the debriefing discussion, and provide structure for evaluating the experience" (p. 113). Within the conduction of the debriefing, each student and each learning objective along with the multiplicity of the clinical scenario should be carefully and completely discussed to allow for the development of a firm foundation of nursing knowledge. The debriefing is viewed as a fundamental and essential component within the clinical simulation experience. It closes the loop in the learning process and allows the students to connect the different pieces, both negative and positive, into a learning opportunity.

11. As faculty members move toward the use of clinical simulations, the thought and evaluation processes need to move toward:
    A. faculty development.
    B. **outcomes.**
    C. preplanning.
    D. shortcomings in the curriculum.

    Rationale:
    High-fidelity simulations and other clinical simulations focus on the outcomes. As a result, faculty members have to convert their thought processes for clinical experiences to the idea of outcomes.

12. One strategy preceptors can use to facilitate maximum student learning while maintaining patient loads in clinical settings is:
    A. reducing the client flow for the student's clinical day.
    B. having the student "jump in," with little discussion of student expectations.
    C. **utilizing preplanning and continuous planning prior to student arrival.**
    D. having the student follow the preceptor throughout the entire day.

    Rationale:
    Burns et al. (2008) indicate that to be successful on a busy day, it is essential to preplan the day. This preplanning includes having the student arrive prior to the day of the clinical experience to meet the staff, review student objectives, learn the charting for the clinical setting, and learn the layout of the setting. Doing so will facilitate increased comfort for the preceptor, staff, and student.

13. The recommended evidence-based approach to teaching includes all of the following, *except*:

A. use evidence to guide clinical-based teaching.

B. question your own clinical practice.

C. search for evidence to answer specific clinical questions.

D. **save research activities until after clinical experiences.**

Rationale:

Golway (2008) reports that the focus of the 2008 Accreditation Symposium for American Nursing Credentialing Center was to question if evidence-based approaches were guiding teaching in nursing. Their recommendation was to adopt the evidence-based approach to teach by these four steps: (1) Question your own teaching practices, (2) search for evidence to answer questions, (3) decide if findings are applicable to your own teaching situation, and (4) use evidence to guide teaching.

14. To evaluate the teaching day, the preceptor/coach and student should:

A. provide a written list of concerns prior to leaving for the day.

B. have the clinic staff evaluate the effectiveness of the student.

C. **think briefly about who was seen, what was accomplished, and how the student felt.**

D. ask the patients how the patient encounter went.

Rationale:

Evaluation of the day should occur routinely and focus on who was seen, what was done, how the student felt about the experience, where the student wants to go next in terms of experiences, and why things worked or didn't work. Through critical reflection on the day's experiences, both the preceptor/coach and student can determine the next clinical day's activities.

15. Teaching that incorporates utilization of microskills, shadowing, observation, mini-lectures, mentoring, and use of Internet, clinical resources, evidence-based guidelines, and texts is an effective strategy in:

A. research arenas.

B. evidence-based practice.

C. **classroom activities.**

D. educational projects.

Rationale:

Most daily teaching will include the combination of (1) precepting using "microskills," (2) being observed or shadowed by the student, (3) observing the student, (4) giving "mini-lectures," (5) mentoring student projects with application of evidence-based clinical practice guidelines and research studies, and (6) learning together with the student as both the preceptor/coach and student search the Internet, clinical resources, evidence-based guidelines, or texts for answers to clinical questions.

16. The best use of evidence to guide complex clinical teaching includes:
    A. using clinical experiences of the day to facilitate learning.
    B. lecturing the student about difficult clinical experiences encountered.
    C. **having both the preceptor and student research recommended treatments.**
    D. asking the student to verify specific clinical experiences obtained.

Rationale:

To support a higher level of questioning and stimulate learning, analyze and utilize critical thinking through research that both the preceptor and student work on together. This experience will bring to the table clinical expertise and student questioning of the validity of treatments used.

DISCUSSION QUESTIONS

1. Is a solid, evidence-based approach currently being utilized to guide teaching in nursing?
   Considerations:
   Building from Golway (2008), questions to consider include:
   · Are traditional approaches in clinical teaching effective?
   · Do we question our own teaching practices?
   · Is the teaching technique for searching the evidence appropriate or practical?
   · Are evidence-based guidelines applicable to your own teaching situation?
   · How can you use evidence to guide your teaching?

2. What are the role expectations for the student, faculty, and preceptor?
   Considerations:
   Drawing from Burns et al. (2008), considerations include:
   · Student expectations: student role pressures, including connections between didactic and clinical work.
   · Faculty expectations: identification and securing of appropriate sites/preceptors in a time of preceptor shortage; support of preceptor to facilitate student learning experiences; and cost-effectiveness for nursing schools.

- Preceptor expectations: provision of course objectives for student clinical experiences; understanding of how preceptors can provide informal, collaborative, respectful, and challenging learning environments.

3. There are more nurses in the United States than any other type of healthcare provider, and they deliver preventive care to help seniors manage chronic diseases. What impact will the Affordable Care Act have on nursing, and are nursing schools prepared for that impact?

   Considerations:

   Building from "HRSA Investments in the Nursing Workforce" (U.S. Department of Health and Human Services, n.d.), considerations include the following:

   - How will the increased patient load affect nursing care?
   - How will nursing handle increased enrollments with an aging nursing educator faculty?
   - How will underserved rural and urban areas handle checkups, preventive screenings, vaccines, and other health care with limited healthcare providers?
   - What are the changes in nursing demographics, education levels, employment, scope of practice, and critical roles for nurses and advanced practice nurses that are fundamental in the healthcare delivery system?

4. How can teaching strategies incorporate simulation, standardized patients, and virtual communities to improve education?

   Considerations:

   - How might virtual communities such as The Neighborhood or Second Life facilitate development of simulation case studies toward an all-inclusive library for varied student learning activities?
   - What storylines might be developed and tested to produce an organized method for unfolding case studies?
   - How might faculty engage in a learning environment for students that will offer opportunities to develop self-confidence and knowledge procurement?
   - How might faculty and students identify levels of anxiety within these activities?

REFERENCES

Adams, M. H., & Valiga, T. M. (2009). *Achieving excellence in nursing education*. New York, NY: National League for Nursing.

Bambino, D., Washburn, J., & Perkins, R. (2009). Outcomes of clinical simulation for novice nursing students: Communication, confidence, clinical judgment. *Nursing Education Perspectives, 30*(2), 79–82.

Benner, P. (1984). *From novice to expert.* Menlo Park, CA: Addison-Wesley.

Burns, C., Beauchesne, M., Ryan-Krause, P., & Sawin, K. (2008). Mastering the preceptor role: Challenges of clinical teaching. *Journal of Pediatric Health Care, 20*(3), 172–183.

Cato, M. L., Lasater, K., & Peeples, A. I. (2009). Nursing students' self-assessment of their simulation experiences. *Nursing Education Perspectives, 30*(2), 105–108.

DiCenso, A., Cullum, N., Ciliska, D., & Guyatt, G. (2004). *Evidence-based nursing: A guide to clinical practice.* Philadelphia, PA: Elsevier.

Dillard, N., Sideras, S., Ryan, M., Hodson-Carlton, K., Lasater, K., & Siktberg, L. (2009). A collaborative project to apply and evaluate the clinical judgment model through simulation. *Nursing Education Perspectives, 30*(2), 99–104.

Dillon, P. M., Noble, K. A., & Kaplan, L. (2009). Simulation as a means to foster collaborative interdisciplinary education. *Nursing Education Perspectives, 30*(2), 87–90.

Dreifuerst, K. T. (2009). The essentials of debriefing in simulation learning: A concept analysis. *Nursing Education Perspectives, 30*(2), 109–114.

Elfrink, V. L., Nininger, J., Rohig, L., & Lee, J. (2009). The case for group planning in human patient simulation. *Nursing Education Perspectives, 30*(2), 83–86.

Gaberson, K. B., & Oermann, M. H. (1999). *Clinical teaching strategies in nursing.* New York, NY: Springer.

Golway, J. (2008). Conference report—2008 accreditation symposium: Is an evidence-based approach guiding teaching in nursing? *American Nurses Credentialing Center.* Retrieved June 29, 2014, from http://www.medscape.com /viewarticle/581824

Guraya, S. Y., Alzobydi, A. H., & Salman, S. (2010). Objective Structured Clinical Examinations: Examiners' bias and recommendations to improve its reliability. *Journal of Medicine and Medical Sciences, 1*(7), 269–272.

Hoadley, T. A. (2009). Learning advanced cardiac life support: A comparison study of the effects of low- and high-fidelity simulation. *Nursing Education Perspectives, 30*(2), 91–95.

Holland, B., Landry, K., Mountain, A., Middlebrooks, A., Heim, D., & Missildine, K., (2013). Weaving the tapestry of learning: Simulation, standardized patients, and virtual communities. *Nurse Educator, 38*(6), 269–272.

Jeffries, P. R. (2008). The three E's: Effective, engaging, and evidence-based teaching using simulation. PNEG 2008 Conference.

Jeffries, P. R. (2009). Dreams for the future for clinical simulation. *Nursing Education Perspectives, 30*(2), 71.

Kim, M., & Shin, M. (2013a). Development and evaluation of simulation-based training for obstetrical nursing using human patient simulators. *CIN: Computers, Informatics, Nursing, 31*(2), 76–84.

Kim, M., & Shin, M. (2013b). Objective Structured Clinical Examinations: A guide to development and implementation in orthopaedic residence. *Journal of the American Academy of Orthopaedic Surgeons, 21*(10), 592–600.

Larsen, T., & Jeppe-Jensen, D. (2008). The introduction and perception of an OSCE with an element of self- and peer-assessment. *European Journal of Dental Education, 12*, 2–7.

Letvak, S. (2008). Developing new clinical experiences for students. In B. K. Penn (Ed.), *Mastering the teaching role: A guide for nurse educators* (pp. 191–199). Philadelphia, PA: F.A. Davis.

Marwaha, S. (2011). Objective Structured Clinical Examinations (OSCEs), psychiatry and the clinical assessment of skills and competencies (CASC) same evidence, different judgement. *BMC Psychiatry, 11*(85), 1–6.

Misener, T. (2008). Strategic relationships with clinical agencies. In B. K. Penn (Ed.), *Mastering the teaching role: A guide for nurse educators* (pp. 179–190). Philadelphia, PA: F.A. Davis.

Neill, J. (2005). What is experiential learning? Retrieved June 29, 2014, from http://www.wilderdom.com/experiential/ExperientialLearningWhatIs.html

Oermann, M. H., & Gaberson, K. B. (2014). *Evaluation and testing in nursing education* (4th ed.). New York: Springer.

Rudolph, J. W., Foldy, E. G., Robinson, T., Kendall, S., Taylor, S. S., & Simon, R. (2013). Helping without harming: The instructor's feedback dilemma in debriefing—A case study. *Simulation in Healthcare, 8*(5), 304–316.

Second Life. (2014). What is Second Life? Retrieved June 29, 2014, from http://secondlife.com/whatis/

Simulation Innovation and Resource Center. (n.d.). SIRC glossary—Static manikin. Retrieved December 30, 2009, from http://sirc.nln.org/mod/glossary

Smith, M. M. (2009). Creative clinical solutions: Aligning simulation with authentic clinical experiences. *Nursing Education Perspectives, 30*(2), 126–127.

Smith, S. J., & Roehrs, C. J. (2009). High-fidelity simulation: Factors correlated with nursing student satisfaction and self-confidence. *Nursing Education Perspectives, 30*(2), 74–78.

Spunt, D., & Covington, B. G. (2008). Utilizing clinical simulation. In B. K. Penn (Ed.), *Mastering the teaching role: A guide for nurse educators* (pp. 233–251). Philadelphia, PA: F.A. Davis.

Squires, J. E., Estabrooks, C. A., Gustavsson, P., & Wallin, L. (2011). Individual determinants of research utilization by nurses: A systematic review update. *Implementation Science, 6*(1) 1–20.

Tagliareni, M. E. (2009). Beyond the realities of current practice: Preparing students to provide safe and effective care. *Nursing Education Perspectives, 30*(2), 69.

ThinkQuest Team. (n.d.). Cognitive processes. Retrieved July 25, 2014, from https://archive-it.org/collections/3635?q=Cognitive+processes&page=1&show=ArchivedPages

Van Wagner, K. (n.d.). What is self-efficacy? Retrieved July 25, 2014, from http://psychology.about.com/od/sindex/f/what-is-self-esteem.htm

Chapter 10

Program Evaluation

Patricia Allen, Melinda Mitchell Jones, and Carol Boswell

At the conclusion of this chapter, the learner will be able to:

1. Differentiate the strengths and limitations of different evaluation models.
2. Describe different aspects inherent in the accreditation process.
3. Summarize key characteristics found within a program evaluation process.
4. Discuss crucial facets necessary for effective course evaluation.
5. Recognize significant aspects within the evaluation of faculty members.

KEY TERMS

- Evaluation model
- Formative evaluation
- Gap analysis
- Professional or national accreditation
- Program evaluation
- Regional accreditation
- Regulatory agency
- Summative evaluation

INTRODUCTION

As evidence-based practice (EBP) has gained traction as the standard in the clinical setting, so too is the concept of evidence-based teaching (EBT) gaining traction in identifying educational strategies and methods in nursing education (Spector, 2010). In nursing education, the drive toward quality and excellence must be guided by evidence in the same manner as nursing practice is guided by evidence. The transition to using EBT to propel and empower nursing education is viewed as a natural progression toward excellence. EBP Evidence is the underpinning for excellence in nursing practice, resulting in quality nurses and improved patient outcomes. According to Newhouse and Johnson (2009), "The evaluation of the work context for readiness for EBP is the first step to laying the groundwork to successfully build the structures and processes needed to support decision making by nurses in the organization" (p. 409). By considering the evidence for each aspect within the educational process, the educational community will advance the profession to an exceptional and enhanced delivery of the key components within the process. Because evaluation is a crucial facet within this process, it must be carefully and thoroughly discussed and incorporated into the process of EBT.

Evaluation has an impact on every aspect within the educational process. According to Oermann and Gaberson (2013), evaluation is both the process of systematic collection and interpretation of data gathered from a variety of data sources to assess clinical competence and the product to interpret the decision about whether the student has achieved the course or program outcomes. Systematic continuous evaluation of courses, faculty effectiveness, and achievement of student learning outcomes are all pieces essential to program evaluation (Southern Association of Colleges and Schools, 2010). This process of systematically collecting, analyzing, and interpreting data to aid in the determination of quality educational outcomes is crucial for the establishment and management of effective nursing programs. Every aspect within the educational program is open to evaluation.

Accreditation agencies mandate that each facet of a program be carefully, methodically, and logically appraised to reflect the quality of the programmatic goals and outcomes designated within the program (Council on Higher Education Accreditation, 2012). Within this process, administration, faculty, curriculum, and students are all assessed to determine their unique parts within the advancement of a quality program of study resulting in highly qualified students ready to assume the role of competent entry-level registered nurse. This chapter will provide insight into the many aspects of evaluation as it relates to the educational setting.

EVALUATION MODELS

Evaluation models have been in use by educators for the past 150 years. The first noted evaluation model began when a principal in Boston compared student test scores to gain insight into the test questions and how effective the test was in capturing student knowledge. Next, the U.S. military began to have uniformity policies for all arms manufacturing, and arms were evaluated for adherence to uniformity measures (Stufflebeam, Madaus, & Kellaghan, 2000). It is essential that faculty be able to document change through both formal and informal methods. Crucial to documentation are designing and using evaluative tools and methods to enhance feedback. Though this process of formal and informal methods of evaluation can be traced back 150 years, the push for development of knowledge in the field of evaluation began in earnest during the Lyndon B. Johnson administration with the "Great Society." Through this initiative, the government began pushing for accountability in areas of federal laws for equitable services for the disabled and minorities. Program evaluation continued to grow in the 1970s to hold social organizations accountable for resource use. In the 1980s, evaluation focused on excellence as a method of increasing international competiveness. Finally, in the 1990s, industry engaged in evaluation as a means of improving quality.

Evaluation provides the evidence needed for delivering effective teaching methodologies, curricula, and program development. Strong methods of evaluation are needed to yield accurate evidence for creating, critiquing, and revising current programs. Evaluation is the anchor of the growing "science of quality" that monitors and assures the quality of selected methods, curricula, and programs. Evaluation models are used to help define the characteristic or features of an evaluation, the concepts to be studied, and the processes or methods needed to extract critical data, evidence, and outcomes. A brief review of widely used evaluation models was obtained from Virginia Tech (2009) and includes the following:

- *Connoisseurship evaluation (Eisner, 1976)* involves an expert in the discipline of study estimating the value of a new innovation. Obvious biases and threats to validity can be seen in this approach to evaluation.
- *Goals-oriented/objectives-based (Tyler, 1949)* describes whether or not students have met their goals and objectives, with the results suggesting how to handle a new instructional strategy (i.e., revise, adopt, reject). One shortfall may be that the evaluator may overlook unexpected outcomes or benefits of instruction beyond original goals and objectives. This is one of the earliest models of evaluation used in nursing education. Tyler's model was widely used in nursing education in the 1960s and 1970s.
- *Goals-free evaluation (Scriven, 1972)* supplements inherent weaknesses in a goals-oriented approach by providing an unbiased tracking of

ongoing events. This model uses a checklist beginning with a needs assessment, then noting comparative value, and then assessment of overall value. Evaluators are encouraged to use this checklist with three columns comparing need, comparative value, and overall value.

- *Judicial/adversary evaluation (Worthen, Sanders, & Fitzpatrick, 1997)* focuses on comparing or describing all sides of a program, both strengths and weaknesses. It is compared to the defense and prosecution of a courtroom because the potential for evaluation bias by a single evaluator cannot be ruled out. To deter bias, each "side" has an evaluator to make its case.

- *Kirkpatrick's four-level model (Kirkpatrick, 1998)* describes student reactions to and learning from an event, program, or innovation, as well as perceived or observed changes in performance. The four levels are reaction, learning, behavior, and results. This model is used in training programs.

- *Situated evaluation (Bruce & Rubin, 1993)* is a contextual model for evaluation. Here the characteristics of varying contexts that cause programs to fail or succeed are reviewed. Proponents of situated evaluation argue that educational events, programs, and training are situated within their context of use; therefore, context cannot be overlooked.

- *Stufflebeam's context, input, process, product (CIPP) model (Stufflebeam, 2002)* describes the context in which an innovation occurs, the inputs of the innovation, the formative processes occurring, and the summative products or outcomes. The CIPP model flows from a checklist format where the evaluator reviews multiple components of this feedback loop: contractual agreements, context evaluation, input evaluation, process evaluation, impact evaluation, effectiveness evaluation, transportability evaluation, sustainability evaluation, and meta-evaluation.

- *Logic models* display the sequence of actions describing what the program is and the outcomes of the program, as well as how each step is linked to achieve results. Five core components in this depiction of the program action are inputs, outputs, outcomes, assumptions, and external factors (University of Wisconsin Extension, 2009).

- **Gap analysis** is a tool for comparing "where we are" to "where we want to be." This method of evaluation comes to education from business and economics, where it has been widely used to compare actual corporate performance with potential performance. The gap in performance is identified and the bridge to improve the gap is defined by performance improvement. This gap is the beginning point for a system-wide improvement process. The gap is seen following the analysis of "where you are" as compared to "where you want to be." This is reflected in a predetermined performance number. The gap analysis can facilitate the improvement process if the users understand the dynamics involved in what created the gaps. The process looks at system problems rather than individual or group shortfalls. Once gaps are identified, goals and objectives are aligned to create an improvement plan (Dana, 2004).

Continuous quality improvement (CQI) models, such as the one currently used by the American Association of Colleges of Nursing, in association with Educational Benchmarking, Inc. (AACN/EBI, n.d.), help align program assessment results with professional standards. CQI provides benchmarking to similar institutions or institutions an organization may strive to be like, helps the school to identify where resources are best allocated for improving program quality, and offers research-based results for budget justification (AACN/EBI, n.d.). Continuous assessment of data provides the opportunity for continuous improvement. Many of these CQI programs, such as the AACN/EBI program, are provided through third-party vendors. Another example is the Sloan Consortium, an online resource for educators, which also provides individuals or institutions with tools for program evaluation through the use of the Sloan-C Quality Scorecard. The scorecard is interactive and covers nine pillars of quality education, describes best practices, and identifies key artifacts necessary for ongoing continuous improvement (Sloan Consortium, 2014).

Today, logic models, gap analysis, and CQI programs are widely used methods of program evaluation in nursing education programs in the United States.

ACCREDITATION

The U.S. Department of Education oversees accreditation of schools, colleges, and universities. According to the U.S. Department of Education (2010):

> The goal of accreditation is to ensure that education provided by institutions of higher education meets acceptable levels of quality. Accrediting agencies, which are private educational associations of regional or national scope, develop evaluation criteria and conduct peer evaluations to assess whether or not those criteria are met. Institutions

> and/or programs that request an agency's evaluation and that meet an
> agency's criteria are then "accredited" by that agency. (para. 2)

The goal, stated more basically, is to ensure education provided by higher education institutions meets acceptable levels of quality standards. These standards can be set by regulatory agencies, regional accrediting bodies, and professional accrediting bodies. The outcome for each level of accreditation serves as evidence of a quality unit or institution. Accreditation is important to students, obviously as a sign of quality, but, more important, accreditation is necessary for students attending programs to receive federal dollars to support their education.

Regulatory agencies for nursing programs are generally state nursing boards. The approval obtained by state boards of nursing applies only to the college, school, or department of nursing; this is not an approval process for the entire university or college. State boards of nursing do not directly report to the National Council of State Boards of Nursing (NCSBN) but do fall under the supervision of the state government and, indirectly, the legislature and governor's office. Although state boards are normally closely aligned with the NCSBN, policies, rules, and regulations for schools of nursing seeking state board approval are established by individual state agencies within the authority granted by state legislatures. Approved nursing programs have obtained board of nursing approval through a defined process. This process begins with initial program approval, allowing the program to begin enrollment, and schools follow up with state boards in a process for full approval. Many states require annual reporting by schools of nursing to assure ongoing board of nursing approval. Ongoing program approval requires schools of nursing to meet predetermined benchmarks for National Council Licensure Examination (NCLEX) RN Pass Rates, review of a program's annual report submitted to the board of nursing, the program's compliance as evaluated with a survey visit if deemed necessary by the state board of nursing, and the program's ongoing compliance with state rules.

Regional accreditation is a continuous improvement process involving the entire university or college. Many of the regional accrediting agencies, such as the Southern Association of Colleges and Schools (SACS), engage the college or university to pursue a continuous improvement process of self-evaluation, reflection, and improvement (SACS, 2010). The SACS is aligned with other regional accrediting bodies. These regional bodies are located in the north-central, western, and northeastern states. All of the regional accrediting agencies subscribe to unifying quality standards for education. One of the best examples of a regional accrediting body is the SACS.

The SACS is a regional body for accrediting of degree-granting higher education institutions in defined southern states. The mission of the

SACS (2010) Commission on Colleges is "the enhancement of educational quality throughout the region and . . . to improve the effectiveness of institutions by ensuring that institutions meet standards established by the higher education community that address the needs of society and students" (para. 1). The SACS Commission on Colleges accredits associate degree, bachelor's, master's, and doctoral programs in the regionally aligned states. In addition, the SACS accredits some international sites. To meet accreditation standards defined by the SACS Commission, the college or university must comply with the standards established in *Principles of Accreditation: Foundations for Quality Enhancement* and with the policies and procedures of the Commission on Colleges (SACS, 2010).

Accreditation procedures can be found on the regional accrediting websites. The process varies by accrediting body, but all agencies require a self-study or compliance report, which may be followed by a campus visit. The SACS Commission will then review all materials and deny or approve accreditation for a designated time period. All regional accrediting bodies other than the SACS can be found on the website for the Council for Higher Education Accreditation (CHEA) at www.chea.org/Directories/regional.asp. Seven regional accrediting bodies are recognized by CHEA.

Professional or national accreditation varies by discipline and is a key to defining a quality unit or discipline within a community college, college, and/or university. For nursing, three widely sought professional accrediting agencies are the National League for Nursing Commission on Nursing Education Accreditation (NLN CNEA), the Accreditation Commission for Education in Nursing (ACEN), and the Commission on Collegiate Nursing Education (CCNE). Both the ACEN and the CCNE are recognized by the U.S. Department of Education. The CCNE agency accredits only baccalaureate and higher degree programs in nursing. The NLN CNEA and the ACEN offer accreditation to vocational/practical nursing programs, associate degree, diploma, and bachelor's, master's, and doctoral programs within nursing schools and/or departments. Seeking accreditation for a school of nursing can be costly regardless of the entity selected for accreditation. Additionally, it should be noted that some schools of nursing select to seek and maintain accreditation from multiple accrediting agencies. For each of the accrediting agencies—NLN CNEA, ACEN, and CCNE—continuous self-assessment is the key to assuring quality.

The NLN CNEA is a new accrediting agency. The NLN elected to initiate this process to address gaps identified within the accreditation process. The NLN CNEA is being established with full approval of the U.S Department of Education. While this accrediting agency is currently being envisioned, it is focused on showcasing the uniqueness and innovation of nursing education as it moves into the near future.

ACEN accreditation provides a nongovernmental approach to recognizing quality in educational programs. Accreditation is a voluntary, self-regulatory process. The accredited institutions have met or exceeded standards identified for quality nursing programs. During the accreditation review, resources invested, processes followed, and results obtained are examined. The ACEN is also closely tied to state regulatory agency findings related to NCLEX pass rates and licensing rules and regulations (ACEN, 2013). Standards are well defined and allow schools of nursing to demonstrate quality. Graduation from a school recognized for quality in higher education in the discipline of nursing is required for admission to many graduate programs and for acceptance into many branches of the military.

For ACEN accreditation, six standards are reviewed in the areas of mission, faculty and staff, curriculum, students, resources, and outcomes. Responses to the standards and substandards under each standard are reflected in a report known as the "self-study." The self-study affords each school the opportunity to reflect on where it is going, what is in place to achieve the mission and/or what is needed to get there, and what the outcomes are of current efforts. Additionally, a site visit by ACEN-designated visitors is an important component of the process. Accreditation renewal periods with the ACEN vary by the findings of the evaluators. The end result of self-study is validation of the evidence of delivery of a quality nursing program.

The CCNE is an autonomous agency granting accreditation for baccalaureate, residency, and higher degree programs for validation of quality and integrity. The global mission of the CCNE is to protect the public health (CCNE, 2009). This accreditation is also a voluntary, self-regulatory process for recognizing effective educational practices in nursing education. For CCNE accreditation, four standards are reviewed in the school's self-assessment. These standards are Mission and Governance, Institutional Commitment and Resources, Curriculum and Teaching–Learning Practices, and Aggregate Student and Faculty Outcomes. The first three standards speak to program quality, and the last standard assures program effectiveness. CCNE accreditation can be given to a school of nursing for up to 10 years. Like the self-study, the self-assessment yields evidence for validation of a quality nursing program.

PROGRAM EVALUATION

Program evaluation is an ongoing process in nursing education and requires a framework for evaluation to be adopted by the faculty, definition of standards and outcomes, and a timeline for measurement of achievement. Program evaluation focuses on review and improvement. The need for curriculum revision, resources, and faculty and staff may become apparent during this ongoing review process.

Program evaluation allows educators to facilitate meaningful change while providing feedback. Evaluation is an ongoing process included in all program development stages. There are six general evaluation frameworks:

- An *objectives-oriented framework* measures attainment of identified goals and objectives.
- A *management-oriented framework* gathers data for managerial decisions as a source of evaluation.
- A *consumer-oriented framework* uses the voice of the consumer to evaluate the curricula and instructional products.
- An *expertise-oriented framework* enlists an expert to evaluate the quality of the educational program.
- An *adversary-oriented framework* applies opposing points of view of different evaluators (pro and con) as the central point of the evaluation.
- *Naturalistic- and participant-oriented frameworks* focus on naturalistic inquiry and involvement of participants (stakeholders are a part of what is being evaluated) in determining needs, data collected, and outcomes of the evaluation. (Welch & Reineke, 2003)

Whether you select a framework for evaluation focused on attainment of objectives or a management-oriented framework, all program evaluation gathers evidence for measurement against predetermined outcomes. The framework will provide the steps to outcome attainment. All program evaluation should be systematic and ongoing to be effective. With systematic program evaluation, decisions are based on the evidence rather than assumptions. Program evaluation should have utility; that is, stakeholders should be identified, credible evaluators should be enlisted in the process, appropriate questions and answers should be asked and sought, values should be clarified, the reporting system should be clear, and reporting and dissemination of findings should be timely to obtain the impact or feedback from the evaluation (Centers for Disease Control and Prevention [CDC], 2004). How did the findings of this program evaluation result in changes in the program? Additionally, frameworks for program evaluation should be feasible and reveal and display accurate information. Steps described in a general program evaluation process reflect engaging stakeholders, describing the program, focusing on the evaluation design, gathering credible evidence, justifying conclusions against standards, and providing feedback on findings and lessons learned for stakeholders (CDC, 2004).

COURSE EVALUATION

According to Oermann and Gaberson (2013), planning assessment at the course level allows faculty to be sure data collection methods provide information they need, are consistent when used by a team of teachers and preceptors engaged in the course, and reflect faculty standards. Course evaluations are frequently viewed as stressful and challenging. At times, faculty members question the advantage of having the course evaluation. Though they understand that course evaluations are mandated by accrediting agencies, state boards of nursing, and the institutions, the applicability of the evaluation tends to be the aspect that is questioned. Lowenstein and Bradshaw (2013) note that evaluations are to be performed to provide the foundation for making decisions about the course and/or other aspects related to the course. Because the process is driven by these other entities, the functionality of the course evaluations for the course is frequently questioned by the faculty members involved in the course. What aspects are included on the evaluation? When is the evaluation scheduled to be completed? Is the participation in the evaluation process coerced in some manner? What impact does the course evaluation have on the individual faculty member? So many questions are raised by the process of course evaluations.

As the process of course evaluation and EBT are considered, minimal research evidence can be found related to course evaluation. Textbooks and manuscripts speak to the process and current status of course evaluations but research evidence is not readily accessible. As a result, the evidence to be used falls in the areas of opinions, current practices, and accepted processes.

Wittman-Price, Godshall, and Wilson (2013) provide an overview of the current practices viewed within the evaluation process. The determination of the evaluation process is based upon the faculty members structuring each course syllabus to concentrate on the program objectives. This structuring or mapping process challenges the strengths and weaknesses perceived in each course and across the curriculum. By ascertaining the linkages between the course syllabus, program objectives, and the total curriculum, a systematic course analysis process can be established. To determine learner progress toward the educational outcomes, the faculty members must formulate an effective and useful evaluation process; delineating the data and processes requires a positive teaching and learning process. Two types of course evaluation processes, formative and summative, are recommended.

Formative evaluation is a method of checking in or gathering data to make any needed changes during the planning, development, and implementation of the program (Lowenstein & Bradshaw, 2013). Other terms used for this type of evaluation are *content* or *process evaluation*. Formative evaluation is viewed as the ongoing, periodic, and routine assessment of the progression of the course process (Caputi, 2010; Lowenstein & Bradshaw, 2013). This type of evaluation can take many different forms. Faculty member tend to use this type of assessment to get at the essences of quality of the course. It can be done through the use of one-minute papers, as noted in the *Classroom Educational Experiences* chapter, which asks the students what key item (or items) was effectively covered during a session of the course. A similar formative evaluation is the muddiest point assignment, also discussed in *Classroom Educational Experiences* chapter, which allows the student to list any areas from the content presented that continue to be confusing. Formative evaluations can also be surveys given at key times within the semester to assess the students' perception of the course. According to Caputi (2010), "The purpose of this type of evaluation is to improve the instruction as the course is progressing to ensure students are learning before the end of the term when it is too late to make adjustments" (p. 43). When seeking formative evaluative information, the faculty member initially determines the impetus and stimulus for the data collection process. The questions and/or other data-collecting methods can then converge on gathering the appropriate material being sought.

At times, the formative evaluations could be directed toward the determination of the appropriateness and/or success of a new teaching strategy. On other occasions, the focus for the evaluation could be on the coverage of the content needed within the course. Thus, formative evaluations should be done at intervals and with a purpose. Oermann and Gaberson (2013) view formative evaluation as an educative process that is directed toward supplying feedback to students about their readiness and learning needs to identify strategies to address learning needs. Within formative evaluation, the focus is directed toward the student and assisting the student to be successful in the course. Every effort is made to ensure that appropriate teaching strategies are used to substantiate the effective coverage of the selected material.

According to Bastable (2014), "The purpose of process or formative evaluation is to make adjustments in an educational activity as soon as they are needed" (p. 606). Formative evaluation allows the faculty member or team to make real-time adjustments to the course in progress, whether those adjustments be in personnel, materials, facilities, learning activities, or attitudes. The adjustments need to be viewed as an ongoing course of action to confirm that every aspect of the course is functioning in an appropriate manner. By using this type of evaluation effectively, the faculty member can make changes as needed within the course prior to a negative outcome for the student cohort. Because each student cohort has unique needs and learning expectations, the use of formative evaluation allows for the changes to be made that are appropriate for each student cohort. Does that mean the faculty member needs to be querying the students and changing directions every week? No. It does mean that at intervals, the learning environment should be challenged to verify that the needs of all those involved in the learning are being addressed.

Bastable (2014) establishes that "learner behavior, teacher behavior, learner–teacher interaction, learner response to teaching material and methods, and characteristics of the environment are all aspects of the learning experience within the scope of process evaluation" (p. 608). Because formative evaluations are designed to look at the content and/or purpose, each of these areas needs to be authenticated as effective.

Summative evaluations (also called *outcome evaluations*) are completed at the end of a semester or course to provide the final input as to whether or not the student has achieved the educational outcomes, in effect judging if the student's practice meets established standards for competency (Oermann & Gaberson, 2013). Summative evaluations are used to confirm the overall success of the course, not the individual aspects within the course. Frequently, this evaluation process is uniform for all courses and all programs within the school and university. As a result, the information gained from these summative (outcome) evaluations is based on the content that is general and applicable across courses, programs, and schools. The questions habitually are global in nature. Thus, the applications for modifying individual courses are less apparent.

In addition to the end-of-course surveys that are provided and controlled by the school, another example of summative evaluations is the final examination used within a course. The final assignments within any course are used to determine the success of the course. From these final assignments (such as final examinations or formal papers), the students' performance can be viewed. By examining the course grade analysis, changes can be determined to improve the course. Additionally, schools may select to use standardized testing programs offered nationally by ATI Nursing Education and/or HESI Elsevier, two companies creating content-specific examinations for schools of nursing as well as comprehensive examinations. Use of standardized testing allows schools to benchmark against like programs nationally.

Evaluations are a key component of the educational environment. As faculty members consider the different aspects of this process, the anticipated function of the process and the methods for utilizing the information acquired need to be carefully and thoughtfully considered. Bastable (2014) makes a sound recommendation when noting that evaluation should be built into the program development and never included as an afterthought. The entire evaluation flow must be carefully determined as the program is developed and never patched in at a later date. By painstakingly and meticulously determining the multidimensional aspects imperative to a beneficial evaluation, the results found through the appraisal process can be analyzed and utilized to improve the learning environment. If the resulting information cannot be or is not used to improve the program, course, or methods of the faculty member, it needs to be reviewed and revised. Material not used in this nature is inconsequential to the learning environment. Each piece of data collected should be utilized to move the program forward to the educational goals set by the faculty within the school's mission statement and program objectives.

Within many programs of education, the gap analysis process is used to analyze and organize the results found through the summative end-of-course evaluations. Gap analysis propels a program or process from here to there; however, first faculty must determine the desired outcome. A gap analysis strives to identify two key levels of factors, such as the current understanding held by students and the desired understanding wanted by students. From these two levels, the differences between the two levels are determined, which is viewed as the gap. In the process of collecting and determining the gap analysis, the present and future states are both sought. By comparing the two levels, the areas that need to be addressed in the process can be identified. Schools that employ the gap analysis process for summative evaluation establish the benchmark level that is acceptable for the gap analysis values. Areas in the course that do not meet this benchmark are then expected to be addressed prior to future provisions of that course. If all areas of the summative evaluations meet or exceed the benchmark level established, the faculty member and/or team can feel confident that the course is meeting the needs of the school based on the areas covered within the summative evaluation. Faculty members must carefully examine the outcomes from the gap analysis. For all areas denoted within the analysis, any sporadic events or evidence of a pattern evident in more than one semester must be included in the interpretation of the results.

Most recently, over 700 schools have joined the Quality Matters Program for higher education (www.qualitymatters.org). This program provides a national benchmark to online course design, but can also provide insights for blended instruction for educators currently designing and evaluating courses. One excellent program feature of Quality Matters is the development of an evidence-based rubric for course evaluation. According to the Quality Matters (n.d.) website:

> The Quality Matters Rubric is a set of 8 general standards and 41 specific standards used to evaluate the design of online and blended courses. The Rubric is complete with annotations that explain the application of the standards and the relationship among them. A scoring system and set of online tools facilitate the evaluation by a team of reviewers. (para. 1)

FACULTY EVALUATION

Though summative and formative evaluations include assessment of the faculty member in the process, the faculty member also participates in a separate evaluation process related to the total role of the faculty member. Often the documentation for faculty evaluation is compiled through an online software system such as Digital Measures. The job descriptions, tenure/promotion criteria, and accreditation standards provide the framework that guides the faculty evaluation. Job descriptions are established by the institution to reflect the overall teaching and clinical responsibilities in addition to the general faculty participatory expectations such as committee work, scholarly endeavours, and research/practice undertakings. For most institutions, the faculty members are obliged to document their different activities reflective of the aspects listed on the job descriptions. Commonly, faculty members are asked to establish annual performance goals that indicate those areas on which they anticipate focusing during the upcoming academic year. These annual goals are then used to drive the yearly performance evaluation. One strategy for faculty to use when establishing the annual goals is to investigate which tenure and/or promotion criteria are appropriate to concentrate on for this year. When faculty members use the different criteria established within the tenure and/or promotion guidelines as their annual goals, they receive double "bang for their buck." Doing so meets the annual goal expectations for advancement while moving the faculty member closer to being ready to seek promotion and/or tenure. The guidelines provided in the tenure and promotion documents along with the materials found included on the job description give a clear picture of the institution's expectations for faculty members. These annual goals developed by the individual faculty member are usually reviewed and approved by some member of administration within the school. That person could be a dean, chairperson, associate dean, faculty development designee, or dean-appointed representative. The goals are reviewed to ensure that faculty members are continuing to grow and develop in the role of academician. Once the faculty member has launched the annual goals, a mechanism and/or strategy needs to be established to assemble the needed documents. Throughout the year, the faculty member needs to have a place to put any documents that will be used during the annual evaluation to support the successful completion of the designated goals.

The work documented by Hessler and Humphreys (2008) is directed toward the effective use of student evaluations, particularly by novice faculty. The information provided can be used by all levels of faculty members as they deal with the comments submitted by students. According to Hessler and Humphreys (2008), "Students can provide valuable feedback on instructional techniques and course design but cannot necessarily judge whether the material in the course is current or whether the instructors knows [*sic*] the subject matter" (p. 187). Having an understanding concerning the focus of student evaluations helps faculty members recognize how the material can be used to strengthen skills and applications within the faculty role and the classroom (**Table 10–1**). According to Hessler and Humphreys (2008), studies have found that the grade expected in the course might or might not have a bearing on the outcomes of the evaluation. In one research study they reviewed, it was found that lower expectations of grades correlated to lower evaluations. But in another study, the opposite was true—lower expected grades did not correlate to poorer evaluations. Fairness by the faculty along with a perceived availability of the faculty member frequently results in faculty evaluations that reflect the actual course delivery and teaching environment. Schools have begun to use these evaluations during the annual faculty evaluations and tenure/promotion processes. The summative evaluations developed by the school/university do not address the key component reflected in the job descriptions and the tenure/promotion guidelines. Hessler and Humphreys (2008) raise the concern that the reliability and validity of the student evaluations are not conclusively proven. Yet, they do remain an important aspect within the evaluation process. Another grave aspect that must be considered in relation to these evaluations is the timing of them and any coercion that might be evident. When students are forced to complete the evaluations in order to receive credit for the course, the consequent evaluation results are tainted. Questions must be raised in these situations as to the appropriateness of any results when the results were forced. Care must be given to encouraging the completion of student evaluations without the use of threats (**Table 10–2**).

Table 10-1   Suggestions for Improving Student Evaluation Response Rates

- Arrange evaluations to be accomplished at times when final examinations are not planned or scheduled.
- Make sure students have ample time to complete the evaluation forms.
- Take the time to explain the evaluation process prior to administering the forms.
- As explanations for the evaluation process are provided, ensure that students understand who or what they are to evaluate—course, faculty, curriculum, clinical, etc.
- Clarify the importance and value of comments—both positive and negative in nature—for the improvement of the program.
- Encourage students to provide specific examples related to negative comments and suggestions for improving the course.
- Remember that the student is the consumer of the educational experience.
- Validate that the evaluation tool addresses the aspects that are key to improving the course and/or faculty.
- Work to ensure that the tool is not so global that specific areas of improvement become hard to identify.

Source: Adapted from Hessler, K., & Humphreys, J. (2008). Student evaluations: Advice for novice faculty. *Journal of Nursing Education, 47*(4), 188.

Table 10-2   Recommendations for Faculty to Use When Considering Student Evaluations

- Use the expertise of seasoned faculty at intervals to validate the information documented within student evaluations.
- When using a seasoned faculty member to evaluate teaching abilities, identify key goals for the individual to focus on to guide the comments and recommendations.
- At different times, take advantage of sitting in on proficient faculty members as they conduct the classroom and/or clinical experience.
- Select and utilize at least one faculty mentor.
- Trend the student evaluation data instead of dwelling on one cohort's comments. Trends are key to identifying areas needing improvement.
- Utilize formative summaries to provide a more rounded evaluation of the learning environment instead of depending on one summative evaluation.
- Maintain an open mind and willingness to strive to improve on what is currently used and to incorporate new teaching methods as needed. Don't become stale in your teaching.

Source: Adapted from Hessler, K., & Humphreys, J. (2008). Student evaluations: Advice for novice faculty. *Journal of Nursing Education, 47*(4), 188.

SUMMARY THOUGHTS

Evidence-based evaluation involves many components. By determining the model or framework you would like to use for evaluation, directions for evidence obtainment are identified. All stakeholders must understand and be committed to the model used for evaluation of the data gathered to be valid, reliable, and, most important, meaningful. Although accreditation assures program quality and requires in-depth self-appraisal or self-evaluation, program evaluation should be in place and continuous to ensure program purposes and standards are being met.

SUMMARY POINTS

1. Because evaluation is a crucial aspect of education, it must be carefully and thoroughly discussed and incorporated into the process of evidence-based teaching.
2. Evaluation has an impact on every aspect within the educational process.
3. The process of systematically collecting, analyzing, and interpreting data to aid in the determination of quality educational outcomes is crucial for the establishment and management of effective nursing programs.
4. Accreditation agencies mandate that each facet of a program be carefully, methodically, and logically appraised to reflect the quality of the programmatic goals and outcomes designated within the program.
5. Although faculty members understand that course evaluations are mandated by accrediting agencies, state boards of nursing, and the employing institutions, the applicability of the evaluation tends to be the aspect that is questioned.
6. Textbooks and manuscripts note the process and current status of course evaluations, but research evidence is not readily accessible.
7. By ascertaining the linkages between each course syllabus, program objectives, and the total curriculum, a systematic course analysis process can be established.
8. Formative evaluation is viewed as the ongoing, periodic, and routine assessment of the progression of the course process.
9. When seeking formative evaluation information, the faculty member initially determines the impetus and stimulus for the data collection process.

10. Within formative evaluation, the focus is directed toward the student and assisting the student to be successful in the course.
11. The learning environment should be challenged to verify that the needs of all those involved in the learning are being addressed.
12. Summative evaluations are used to confirm the overall success of the course, not the individual aspects within the course.
13. The information gained from summative (outcome) evaluations is based on the content that is general and applicable across courses, programs, and schools.
14. The entire evaluation flow must be carefully determined as the program is developed, not left to be an afterthought.
15. Each piece of data collected should be utilized to move the program forward to the educational goals set by the faculty within the school's mission statement and program objectives.
16. A gap analysis strives to identify two key levels of factors, such as the current understanding held by students and the desired understanding wanted by students.
17. Areas in the course that do not meet a gap analysis values benchmark are expected to be addressed prior to future provisions of that course. If all areas of the summative evaluations meet or exceed the benchmark level established, the faculty member and/or team can feel confident that the course is meeting the needs of the school based on the areas covered within the summative evaluation.
18. Though summative and formative evaluations include assessment of the faculty members in the process, the faculty member also participates in a separate evaluation process related to the total role of the faculty member.
19. Commonly, faculty members are asked to establish annual performance goals that indicate those areas on which they anticipate focusing during the upcoming academic year.
20. Having an understanding concerning the focus of student evaluations helps faculty members recognize how the material can be used to strengthen skills and applications within the faculty role and the classroom.
21. Evaluation provides the evidence needed for delivering effective teaching methodologies, setting appropriate curricula, and directing program development.
22. Evaluation models are used to help define the characteristics or features of an evaluation, the concepts to be studied, and the processes or methods needed to extract critical data, evidence, and outcomes.

23. Today, logic models, gap analysis, and continuous quality improvement programs are widely used in nursing education programs in the United States.
24. Accrediting agencies are monitored by the Department of Education. Accreditation can be regional, such as SACS accreditation, or professional/national, such as NLN CNEA, ACEN, and CCNE accreditation. Regulatory agencies such as state boards of nursing also provide program approval.
25. Program evaluation is an ongoing process in nursing education and requires a framework for evaluation to be adopted by the faculty, definition of standards and outcomes, and a timeline for measurement of achievement to be set. Program evaluation focuses on review and improvement.

TIPS FOR NURSE EDUCATORS

1. Once the faculty member has launched the annual goals, a mechanism and/or strategy needs to be established to assemble the needed documents.
2. When faculty members use the different criteria established within the tenure and/or promotion guidelines as their annual goals, it meets the annual goal expectations for advancement while moving faculty members closer to being ready to seek promotion and/or tenure.
3. The goals are reviewed to ensure that faculty members are continuing to grow and develop in the role of academician.
4. Throughout the year, the faculty member needs to have a place to file any documents that will be used during the annual evaluation to support the successful completion of the designated goals.
5. Fairness by the faculty along with a perceived availability of the faculty member frequently results in faculty evaluations that reflect the nature presented in the classroom.
6. Care must be given to encouraging the completion of student evaluations without the use of threats.
7. Evaluation provides the evidence needed for delivering effective teaching methodologies, curricula, and program development. Therefore, it is very important that each faculty member buy into the model selected for the nursing unit to use for evaluation.
8. Accreditation can be very costly. Planning for accreditation costs in the annual budget is a very important step for nursing education administrators.

9. Accreditation may have hidden costs, such as the need for outside consultants during the self-study or appraisal process.

10. Some states are now recognizing national/professional accreditation and are not requiring state boards of nursing to make annual site visits or annual reports to the state board of nursing. Check with your state board of nursing to see if this may be the case in your state.

11. Use the self-study/self-appraisal process to recognize the strengths of your program, and realize that this is also a very important time to gather data needed to share with college or university administration about needed resources such as technology, space, or salary alignment for the nursing unit.

MULTIPLE CHOICE QUESTIONS

1. Individuals working in an institution of higher education who need to be evaluated to ensure a quality program of study are the:
   A. **administration, faculty, and students.**
   B. faculty only.
   C. students only.
   D. administration and students only.

   Rationale:
   Within this process, administration, faculty, curriculum, and students are all assessed to determine their unique parts within the advancement of a quality program of study resulting in highly qualified students ready to assume the role of competent entry-level registered nurse.

2. During the establishment of the evaluation process, faculty members work to structure:
   A. the course expectations to the course objectives.
   B. **each individual syllabus to the program objectives.**
   C. the course philosophy to the program mission.
   D. the course objectives to the program objectives.

   Rationale:
   The determination of the evaluation process is based upon the faculty members structuring their syllabi to concentrate on the program objectives. This structuring or mapping process challenges the strengths and weaknesses perceived in each course and across the curriculum.

3. A systematic course analysis process can be established when a linkage is noted between:
   A. total curriculum and school mission.
   B. **the course syllabus, program objectives, and the total curriculum.**
   C. total curriculum and faculty job descriptions.
   D. each individual syllabus, faculty job descriptions, and the school mission.

   Rationale:
   By ascertaining the linkages between each individual syllabus, program objectives, and the total curriculum, a systematic course analysis process can be established. Sewell et al. (2008) state that "support for the scholarship of teaching and learning by academic leadership is crucial to a successful program outcome process" (p. 100S). By identifying the "data-driven incremental multidimensional processes and procedures that positively impact the teaching and learning process" (Sewell et al., 2008, p. 100S), the faculty members can formulate an effective and useful evaluation process.

4. Formative evaluations strive to gather data to make decisions during the:
   A. planning and development stages of the curriculum.
   B. planning stage only.
   C. implementation stage only.
   D. **planning, development, and implementation stages.**

   Rationale:
   Formative evaluation is "the gathering of data to make decisions during the planning, development, and implementation of the program" (Lowenstein & Bradshaw, 2013, p. 353).

5. Formative evaluation is viewed as:
   A. **the ongoing, periodic, and routine assessment of the progression of the course process.**
   B. a single episode of the progression of the course process.
   C. the final assessment of the progression of the course process.
   D. an evaluation of the faculty member only.

   Rationale:
   Formative evaluation is viewed as the ongoing, periodic, and routine assessment of the progression of the course process (Caputi, 2010; Lowenstein & Bradshaw, 2013). This type of evaluation can

take many different forms. Faculty members tend to use this type of assessment to determine the quality of the course.

6. When seeking formative evaluation information, faculty members need to carefully determine:
   A. the student cohort makeup.
   B. **the specific reasons for the evaluation.**
   C. which faculty member is to be evaluated.
   D. only how to collect the data.

Rationale:
When seeking formative evaluative information, the faculty member initially determines the impetus and stimulus for the data collection process. The questions and/or other data-collecting methods can then converge on gathering the appropriate material being sought.

7. Summative evaluations are set up to:
   A. cover the same materials as found in the formative evaluations.
   B. provide a summarization of the material identified in the formative evaluations.
   C. **uniformly evaluate all courses and all programs within the school and university.**
   D. carefully collect data on courses and programs within the school.

Rationale:
Summative evaluations are used to confirm the overall success of the course, not the individual aspects within the course. Frequently, this evaluation process is uniform for all courses and all programs within the school and university. As a result, the information gained from these summative (outcome) evaluations is based on the content that is general and applicable across courses, programs, and schools. The questions habitually are global in nature.

8. The guiding documents that provide the framework for the annual evaluation of faculty members are:
   A. course evaluations and job descriptions.
   B. summative evaluations, formative evaluations, and gap analysis.
   C. job descriptions and accreditation standards.
   D. **job descriptions, tenure/promotion criteria, and accreditation standards.**

Rationale:
The job descriptions, tenure/promotion criteria, and accreditation standards provide the framework that guides the faculty evaluation. Job descriptions are established by the institution to reflect

the overall teaching and clinical responsibilities in addition to the general faculty participatory expectations, such as committee work, scholarly endeavors, and research/practice undertakings. For most institutions, the faculty members are obliged to document their different activities reflective of the aspects listed on the job descriptions.

9. Faculty members often are expected to develop annual professional goals to strive to meet. These goals are validated by:
   A. the dean of the school of nursing.
   B. the faculty member only.
   C. **the chairperson, associate dean, or dean-appointed representative.**
   D. both the chairperson and the dean of the school of nursing.

   Rationale:
   The annual goals developed by the individual faculty member are usually reviewed and approved by some member of the administration within the school. That person could be a chairperson, associate dean, faculty development designee, or dean-appointed representative. The goals are reviewed to ensure that faculty members are continuing to grow and develop in the role of academician.

10. Regional accreditation differs from professional or national accreditation in that:
    A. regional accreditation is voluntary.
    B. professional or national accreditation is voluntary.
    C. **regional accreditation applies to an entire institution.**
    D. professional or national accreditation applies to an entire institution.

    Rationale:
    All accreditation is voluntary, and only regional accreditation is sought by the entire institution. Professional or national accreditation is sought by individual professional schools within the institution.

11. Program evaluation can be described as a(n):
    A. cyclic activity done before accreditation or reaffirmation.
    B. **continuous activity done to fulfill program purposes.**
    C. activity done in isolation of state standards.
    D. activity done in isolation of national standards.

    Rationale:
    Program evaluation is a continuous activity undertaken to fulfill the program purposes. If evaluation occurs only during a self-study, indicators occurring in the years between accreditation may not be

examined. All program evaluation occurs in light of current state and national standards set within the discipline or profession.

12. Five core components in the depiction of the logic model for evaluation are:
    A. **inputs, outputs, outcomes, assumptions, and external factors.**
    B. contractual agreements, context evaluation, input evaluation, process evaluation, and impact evaluation.
    C. impact evaluation, effectiveness evaluation, transportability evaluation, sustainability evaluation, and meta-evaluation.
    D. inputs, outputs, effectiveness, assumptions, and external factors.

    Rationale:
    The core components of the logic model are inputs, outputs, outcomes, assumptions, and external factors for program evaluation. Options B and C are components of Stufflebeam's CIPP model, and option D is a combination of the logic and CIPP models.

13. Gap analysis can facilitate the improvement process if the user understands that the "gap" is:
    A. seen following the analysis of "where you want to be" and "where you have been."
    B. a real-time picture of where you want to be in the future.
    C. the analysis of national indicators and where you are in comparison to these indicators.
    D. **following the analysis of "where you are" as compared to "where you want to be."**

    Rationale:
    The gap analysis can facilitate the improvement process if the users understand the dynamics involved in what created the gaps. Therefore, where you are as compared to where you want to be is the correct choice. Option A is not of importance, as the past will not aid in finding the gap. Options B and C are not plausible, as gap analysis is the gap in individual performance that is identified and the bridge to improve the gap is defined by performance improvement.

14. Schools of nursing may select to seek accreditation from the Commission on Collegiate Nursing Education (CCNE) rather than the National Council of Evaluation and Accreditation (CNEA) or Accreditation Commission for Education in Nursing (ACEN) because:
    A. the CCNE is accredited by the Department of Education.
    B. **the CCNE accredits residency programs.**

C. the ACEN does not accredit higher degree programs.

D. the ACEN is not accredited by the Department of Education.

Rationale:

Both the CCNE and the ACEN are accredited by the Department of Education. Both the CCNE and the ACEN accredit higher degree programs. Option B is correct, as the CCNE also accredits residency programs.

DISCUSSION QUESTIONS

1. What types of course evaluations have you been involved with in the past either as a student or as a faculty member? Think carefully about what you consider as the strengths and challenges of using those types of course evaluations to improve the delivery of a course. What would you change to improve the process?

   Considerations:

   Formative evaluation is "the gathering of data to make decisions during the planning, development, and implementation of the program" (Lowenstein & Bradshaw, 2013, p. 353). Other terms used for this type of evaluation are content or process evaluation. Formative evaluation is viewed as the ongoing, periodic, and routine assessment of the progression of the course process (Caputi, 2010; Lowenstein & Bradshaw, 2013). This type of evaluation can take many different venues. Faculty members tend to use this form to get at the essences of quality of the course. Summative evaluations (also called outcome evaluations) are performed at the end of a course to determine if the student has achieved the course outcomes, in effect determining if the student's practice meets established standards of safety and competence (Oermann & Gaberson, 2013). Summative evaluations are used to confirm the overall success of the course, not the individual aspects within the course. Frequently, this evaluation process is uniform for all courses and all programs within the school and university. As a result, the information gained from these summative (outcome) evaluations is based on the content that is general and applicable across courses, programs, and schools.

2. Do you think schools should seek both professional program accreditation and regional accreditation? Please provide a rationale for your answer.

   Considerations:

Graduation from an accredited program fully recognized by a national professional association such as the NLN CNEA, ACEN, or the CCNE is required for students to progress to military service and graduate education. Additionally, professional accreditation is required by some state boards of nursing and many state higher education coordinating boards. There is a trend currently for state boards of nursing to waive campus visits in states where this is required if the school of nursing has full professional accreditation from the ACEN or the CCNE. While the institution seeks overall university or college quality recognition through regional accrediting agencies such as the SACS, professional accreditation for any practice discipline assures the public of the quality of individual school, college, or departmental educational practices.

3. Because performance evaluations are key to helping each of us to improve, what aspects would seem best to evaluate? How does a department and/or faculty member reflect these areas to demonstrate competency of the skills?

Considerations:

See Tables 10-1 and 10-2 for areas to consider for improving personal performance aspects. The job descriptions, tenure/promotion criteria, and accreditation standards provide the framework that guides the faculty evaluation. Job descriptions are established by the institution to reflect the overall teaching and clinical responsibilities in addition to the general faculty participatory expectations, such as committee work, scholarly endeavors, and research/practice undertakings. For most institutions, the faculty members are obliged to document their different activities reflective of the aspects listed on the job descriptions.

TEACHING SCENARIO

1. Invite the students to perform a brief mock accreditation review of a nursing program, either the program where they are currently enrolled or a neighboring program. Refer the students to the following website, where they may explore the components evaluated in the accreditation process: www.aacn.nche.edu/Accreditation/pdf/standards09.pdf.

2. Explore the current evaluation plan used in your program. The students may decide what type of evaluation plan is being used and how the feedback loop in this program works to enhance program

delivery. The students may want to attend school of nursing evaluation committee meetings or interview the faculty member who leads evaluation in this program.

References

Accreditation Commission for Education in Nursing. (2013). *Accreditation manual.* Atlanta, GA: Author.

American Association of Colleges of Nursing/Educational Benchmarking, Inc. (n.d.) EBI assessment surveys. Retrieved June 30, 2014, from http://www.aacn.nche.edu/research-data/ebi

Bastable, S. B. (2014). *Nurse as educator: Principles of teaching and learning for nursing practice* (2nd ed.). Burlington, MA: Jones and Bartlett Learning.

Bruce, B. C., & Rubin, A. (1993). *Electronic quills: A situated evaluation of using computers for writing in classrooms.* Hillsdale, NJ: Lawrence Erlbaum Associates.

Caputi, L. (2010). An overview of the educational process. In L. Caputi (Ed.), *Teaching nursing: The art and science* (2nd ed., pp. 27–47). Glen Ellyn, IL: College of DuPage Press.

Centers for Disease Control and Prevention. (2004). CDC evaluation working group. Retrieved July 15, 2014, from http://www.cdc.gov/EVAL/framework/

Commission on Collegiate Nursing Education (CCNE). (2009). CCNE mission statement and goals. Retrieved July 15, 2014, from http://www.aacn.nche.edu/ccne-accreditation/about/mission-values-history

Council on Higher Education Accreditation. (2012). CHEA-at-a-glance. Retrieved July 15, 2014, from http://www.chea.org/pdf/chea-at-a-glance_2012.pdf

Dana, C. (2004, March 30). Gap analysis: Overview of identifying gaps process. Middle Level School Principal Seminar, Austin, Texas. Retrieved June 30, 2014, from http://www.utdanacenter.org/downloads/presentations/gapanalysis_march04.pdf

Eisener, E. W. (1976). Education connoisseurship and criticism: Their forms and functions in educational evaluation. *Journal of Aesthetic Education, 10*, 135–150.

Hessler, K., & Humphreys, J. (2008). Student evaluations: Advice for novice faculty. *Journal of Nursing Education, 47*(4), 187–189.

Kirkpatrick, D. L. (1998). *Evaluating training programs: The four levels* (2nd ed.). San Francisco, CA: Berrett-Koehler Publishers.

Lowenstein, A. J., & Bradshaw, M. J. (2013). *Fuszard's innovative teaching strategies in nursing* (3rd ed.). Burlington, MA: Jones and Bartlett Learning.

Newhouse, R. P., & Johnson, K. (2009). A case study in evaluating infrastructure for EBP and selecting a model. *Journal of Nursing Administration, 39*(10), 409–411.

Oermann, M. H., & Gaberson, K. B. (2013). Evaluation and testing in nursing education. New York, NY: Spring Publishing Company.

Quality Matters. (n.d.). Higher ed program—Rubric. Retrieved June 30, 2014, from https://www.qualitymatters.org/rubric

Scriven, M. (1972). Pros and cons of goal-free evaluation. *Evaluation Comment, 3*(4), 1–7.

Sewell, J., Culpa-Bondal, F., & Colvin, M. (2008). Nursing program assessment and evaluation: Evidence-based decision making improves outcomes. *CIN: Computers, Informatics, Nursing,* 98S–101S.

Sloan Consortium. (2014). Evaluating the online program with the Sloan-C Quality Scorecard. Retrieved June 30, 2014, from http://sloanconsortium.org/conference/2014/et4online/evaluating-online-program-sloan-c-quality-scorecard

Southern Association of Colleges and Schools (SACS). (2010). Accrediting standards. Retrieved June 30, 2014, from http://www.sacscoc.org/principles.asp

Spector, N. (2010). Evidence-based nursing regulation: A challenge for regulators. *Journal of Nursing Regulation, 1*(3), 30–36.

Stufflebeam, D. L. (2002). The CIPP model for evaluation. In D. L. Stufflebeam & T. Kellaghan (Eds.), *The international handbook of educational evaluation* (Chapter 2). Boston, MA: Kluwer Academic Publishers.

Stufflebeam, D. L., Madaus, G. F., & Kellaghan, T. (2000). *Evaluation models: Viewpoints on educational and human services evaluation* (2nd ed.). Boston, MA: Kluwer Academic Publishers.

Tyler, R. W. (1949). *Basic principles of curriculum and instruction.* Chicago, IL: The University of Chicago Press.

University of Wisconsin Extension. (2009). Program development and evaluation. Retrieved June 30, 2014, from http://www.uwex.edu/ces/pdande/evaluation/evallogicmodel.html

U.S. Department of Education. (2010). The U.S. Department of Education database of accredited postsecondary institutions and programs. Retrieved June 30, 2014, from http://ope.ed.gov/accreditation/index.aspx

Virginia Tech. (2009). Design shop: Lessons in effective teaching. Retrieved July 15, 2014, from http://www.tlos.vt.edu/

Welch, W., & Reineke, R. A. (2003). *National Visiting Committee (NVC) handbook.* Kalamazoo, MI: Western Michigan University, The Evaluation Center.

Wittman-Price, R. A., Godshall, M., & Wilson, L. (2013). *Certified nurse educator (CNE) review manual.* New York, NY: Springer Publishing Company.

Worthen, B. R., Sanders, J. R., & Fitzpatrick, J. (1997). *Program evaluation: Alternative approaches and practical guidelines* (2nd ed.). New York, NY: Longman.

Chapter 11

Competency and Certification

Linda Caputi

At the conclusion of the chapter, the learner will be able to:

1. Discuss the process used by the National League for Nursing to establish the Certified Nurse Educator (CNE) program.
2. State the items included within the CNE test blueprint.
3. Explain the different aspects involved in the determination of competencies.
4. List the steps needed to prepare to take the CNE examination.
5. Discuss the impact that certification has on a profession.

KEY TERMS

- Accreditation Commission for Education in Nursing (ACEN)
- American Nurses Credentialing Center (ANCC)
- Certification
- Certified Nurse Educator (CNE)
- Competency
- Feasibility study
- National Commission for Certifying Agencies (NCCA)
- National Council of State Boards of Nursing (NCSBN)
- Needs assessment
- Nurse educator competencies
- Practice analysis
- Scope of practice
- Staff development
- Test blueprint
- Think tank

INTRODUCTION

The notion of evidence-based teaching is influencing faculty from many vantage points. For example, the **National Council of State Boards of Nursing (NCSBN)** published a position paper titled "Evidence-Based Nursing Education for Regulation." The NCSBN looked at which teaching methodologies had the best student outcomes (Spector, 2006). The NCSBN's recommendations for evidence-based nursing education for regulation include teaching methods, assimilation of the students into the role of nursing, promoting faculty–student relationships, and other areas of teaching. More recently, a book by Benner, Sutphen, Leonard, and Day (2010), titled *Educating Nurses: A Call for Radical Transformation*, reports on research conducted in schools of nursing and offers recommendations for changing nursing education based on this research.

Dr. Cathleen Shultz, editor of a 2012 publication from the National League for Nursing (NLN), offers a theoretical framework for the science of nursing education. This framework provides the structure in which evidence about nursing education can be conceptualized. The book, *Building a Science of Nursing Education: Foundation for Evidence-Based Teaching–Learning*, provides the writings of experts in nursing education to offer a scientific approach to evidence-based teaching.

In addition to book publications, periodicals provide a platform for the publication of nursing education research. Two journals, *Journal of Nursing Education* and *Nursing Education Perspectives*, focus on publishing nursing education research. These journals provide a constant source of evidence that is based on research.

Furthermore, the 2013 standards for accreditation of nursing programs by the **Accreditation Commission for Education in Nursing (ACEN)** also address evidence-based teaching. Criterion 2.6 states, "Faculty (full- and part-time) maintain expertise in their areas of responsibility, and their performance reflects scholarship and evidence-based teaching and clinical practices" (ACEN, 2013). This is a criterion for all levels of nursing education. But if ACEN defines evidence-based as "actions, processes, or methodologies that are grounded in and flow from the translation of substantive and current research" (Glossary, p. 2), where is the evidence to support that the specific activities that faculty engage in while carrying out their teaching roles are "actions, processes, or methodologies that are grounded in and flow from the translation of substantive and current research"? Where is the evidence that directs us in what we should be doing in the role of an academic nurse educator? How do we know if what we are doing is what we should be doing? What competencies define who we are as nurse educators?

Additionally, the NLN supports nurse educators as practicing in a specialty role; that is, teaching in academia requires the knowledge of a specialized practice. In 2005, the NLN issued a position statement titled "Transforming Nursing Education." One of the recommendations in that position statement was, "Faculty identify themselves as advanced practice nurses since teaching is an advanced practice role that requires specialized knowledge and advanced education and since certification now exists as a way to recognize expertise in the role" (NLN, 2005a, p. 5).

Finally, there now exists a basis for the evidence for what we do as nurse educators—a certification exam that measures one's knowledge of the "specialized knowledge" of the role of a nurse educator. That is, the answer to the question, "What evidence guides the practice of the academic nurse educator?" is found in *The Scope of Practice for Academic Nurse Educators* (NLN, 2012) and is measured by the **Certified Nurse Educator (CNE)** examination. The CNE is based on the best practices that define who we are as nurse educators in academia. Evidence now exists for what we are to do in our role as a nurse educator. The value of certification is acknowledged by the NLN because it is viewed as a symbol of professionalism.

Within the NLN *CNE 2014 Candidate Handbook, June 2013 Revision* (2014), the mission for the Academic Nurse Educator Certification Program is designated as recognizing "excellence in the advanced specialty role of the academic nurse educator" (p. 2). The goals for the CNE certification are designated as follows:

- Distinguish academic nursing education as a specialty area of practice and an advanced practice role within professional nursing.
- Recognize the academic nurse educator's specialized knowledge, skills, and abilities and excellence in practice.
- Strengthen the use of core competencies of nurse educator practice.
- Contribute to nurse educators' professional development. (NLN, 2014, p. 2)

The concepts and expectations suggested by these goals hold the participants to a high level of quality and excellence. The certification is designed to address academic nurse educators from diverse settings. The process is established to allow faculty members to be successful without regard to the manner of educational delivery—traditional classroom-based environments and/or nontraditional environments (e.g., distance delivery via video, closed-circuit television, and the Internet).

This chapter discusses the role of the nurse educator as outlined by the CNE examination and explores the importance of establishing competencies to focus the profession. It provides an overview of the history of the CNE, discusses the test blueprint, gives ideas for preparing for the examination, and concludes with ways the CNE can influence nursing education. The process by which the CNE was conceptualized, studied, and eventually developed is an extraordinary example of an evidence-based activity in nursing education. At this time within nursing education, the CNE certification process is the only course of action available for demonstrating competency for nurse educators. None of the other national organizations and testing entities has developed a certification process for the academic nurse educator.

EXCELLENCE THROUGH COMPETENCIES

To better understand the process involved in the development of a certification exam, a clear appreciation of the term **competency** is needed. According to Norman (1985), competency is greater than knowledge alone. It embraces the awareness of knowledge; clinical, technical, and communication skills; and the capacity to decipher a problem by employing clinical and/or technical judgment. Competencies are utilized to generate distinctive standards within disciplines and specialties. The clarification of the competencies within a profession allows for the different roles and functions of that position to be effectively and completely addressed and managed by the members of that professional group.

According to Adams and Valiga (2009):

> Nurses of today and tomorrow need to possess the following qualities: know the principles that underlie their practice; know how to find, manage, and use information; be comfortable with ambiguity and uncertainty; be leaders and change agents; communicate effectively; think critically and from multiple perspectives; function effectively in the face of conflict; and manage constant change, including technological developments. (p. 2)

Just as the competencies of practicing nurses have been studied and delineated, so should the competencies of academic nurse educators. The NLN's work on the CNE examination provides the basis for these competencies.

THE MAKING OF THE CNE EXAMINATION

Certification in nursing is not a new concept. **Certification** for many nursing specialty practice areas has been available for over 50 years. There is currently a certification for **staff development** educators provided by the

National Nursing Staff Development Organization (NNSDO) and administered by the **American Nurses Credentialing Center (ANCC)**. The exam is the Nursing Professional Development exam. The audience for this examination is strictly nurse educators in healthcare settings, not in academia. Although the role of the staff development educator and the role of the academic nurse educator have much in common, there are also many differences.

A certification exam did not exist that specifically addressed the role of the academic nurse educator. In fact, until recently, the role of the academic nurse educator had not been formally studied and delineated. The NLN provided this valuable information with its research that culminated with the publication of *The Scope of Practice for Academic Nurse Educators* (2005b). This publication has recently been updated to the 2012 version. This was the first publication that delineated the scope of practice and core competencies of nurse educators.

So, how does an organization such as the NLN go about developing a certification exam for academic nurse educators? Because this is a book about evidence and evidence-based teaching, it would follow that the process used must involve evidence based on research, and that is just what occurred.

Think Tank

In 1999, the NLN conducted a Delphi survey that included two questions related to faculty certification. One question asked if the NLN should develop a certification program, and the other asked if members would be interested in seeking certification. The results indicated an extremely positive response to these questions (Ortelli, 2010). With the interest in a certification exam documented, in December 2001, the NLN convened the Think Tank on Graduate Education Preparation for the Nurse Educator Role. The **think tank** was composed of experts in nursing education, who were viewed as master nurse educators, and higher education, with a variety of institutions and backgrounds represented (Halsted, 2007). The think tank was charged to answer the question: What do educators need to know, or be able to do, to implement the role successfully and effectively?

To reflect a complete picture of the academic nurse educator, all levels of academic institutions were considered as well as the various responsibilities of all levels of the educator role, from novice educator to expert educator. From these data, the think tank produced the first draft of the competencies for academic nurse educators. The NLN issued a formal position statement, summarizing this work, when it published *The Preparation of Nurse*

Educators (2002). In this position statement, the NLN specifically recommended that "competence as an educator can be established, recognized, and expanded through master's and/or doctoral education, post-master's certificate programs, continuing professional development, mentoring activities and professional certification as a faculty member" (NLN, 2002, p. 3). This was a bold step for the NLN to take because starting in the late 1980s, most colleges and universities ceased to offer a nursing education track in their graduate nursing programs. This call from the NLN challenged the education community to offer graduate-level programs that would specifically prepare nursing educators and also opened the door for professional certification as an academic nurse educator.

Position Statements

In the early 2000s, the NLN was calling for a reform in nursing education. Two position statements addressed the need for reform. These were *The Preparation of Nurse Educators* (2002) and *Innovation in Nursing Education: A Call to Reform* (2003). Both position statements addressed the need for preparation for the nurse educator role. Preparation as a nurse with a practice specialty is not enough. The nurse also needs the specialized knowledge and skills of the educator. Certification would demonstrate that the nurse educator has the expertise necessary to engage in the role of an academician.

Feasibility Study/Needs Assessment

The need for faculty to attain the knowledge and skills to function in the role of the academician had been established by the think tank and elaborated through the NLN's position statements. However, before committing the human and financial resources required to develop a certification exam, it was necessary to ensure the target population of academic nurse educators was ready.

The NLN assembled various committees and task groups to study this issue. To start, the NLN administered a survey to study the feasibility of developing a certification for academic nurse educators. Over 3,000 respondents, including nurse administrators and nurse faculty, answered the electronic survey. The results indicated that 84% of deans and directors recognized the role of a nurse educator as a specialty and 80% believed certification would be beneficial to their nursing programs (Ortelli, 2010). Faculty respondents indicated an even higher percentage, with 92% considering the role of nurse educator as a specialty. Seventy-six percent of the faculty responding indicated an interest in becoming certified (Ortelli, 2010). The results of these surveys provided evidence of the need to pursue the idea of developing a certification exam for academic nurse educators. The **feasibility study** and **needs assessment** revealed a need for a certification exam for academic nurse educators. The NLN was ready to take the next steps.

Scope of Practice for Academic Nurse Educator: Nurse Educator Competencies

The work of the task group and the findings from the feasibility study set the stage for the NLN to continue its efforts that eventually resulted in the CNE examination. The question to be considered at this point was, "What is the **scope of practice** of an academic nurse educator?" That is, what activities, roles, and knowledge define what the educator does, or **nurse educator competencies**? The answer to this question would require an intense search of the literature to reveal research that provided evidence about the scope of practice of the academic nurse educator. The members of NLN's Task Group on Nurse Educator Competencies searched the literature published between 1992 and 2004 and produced an evidence-based report that characterized the knowledge, skills, and attitudes required of academic nurse educators. However, the report appeared to lack some important competencies the task group members knew were part of the educator's role. Therefore, the task group turned to nonresearch literature to derive a more complete picture of the scope of practice by drawing upon best practices and exemplars to complete the picture (Halstead, 2007). The task group then developed the initial draft of the core competencies with task statements that provided a comprehensive look at the scope of practice of academic nurse educators (NLN, 2005b). These competencies were subsequently reviewed, revised, and refined after perusal and feedback from nurse educators across the country. The initial competencies were:

- Facilitate learning
- Facilitate learner development and socialization
- Use assessment and evaluation strategies
- Participate in curriculum design and evaluation of program outcomes
- Function as a change agent and leader
- Pursue continuous quality improvement in the nurse educator role
- Engage in scholarship
- Function within the educational environment

The first draft of the core competencies represented the results of a tremendous evidence-based undertaking by the NLN task group. Within each of these areas delineated by the core competencies, specific standards and hallmarks were organized from the evidence.

These master nursing educators continued the presentation of their work by publishing *Nurse Educator Competencies: Creating an Evidence-Based Practice for Nurse Educators* (Halstead, 2007). This publication provides an explanation of the evidence used to develop the nurse educator competencies. The book presents a synthesis of the research, the gaps in research identified by the task group, and proposed questions that can be used by educators for future research on the many aspects of the role of the nurse academician.

Practice Analysis

The work of the NLN task group that produced the nurse educator competencies and task statements provided a foundation for the CNE **practice analysis**. To ensure the validity of an exam that provides certification or licensure, a practice analysis is used to reveal the activities of the professional engaged in that practice. That is, a practice analysis reveals the activities the professional undertakes while carrying out the functions and responsibilities within the scope of practice of that professional role. The certification exam then tests the candidate's knowledge of those activities.

The NLN assembled a Practice Analysis Committee (PAC) that consisted of eight nurse educators representing faculty in academic settings from diverse geographic, ethnic, and nursing education program types (Ortelli, 2010). Their tasks included:

- Developing a sampling plan
- Identifying tasks for a survey instrument
- Classifying core tasks
- Developing a rating scale with demographic variables relevant to those who might take the examination

A survey tool was developed to gather information about the tasks engaged in by academic nurse educators. To develop the survey tool, the committee members used the previously developed core competencies of nurse educators (NLN, 2005b) and examined position descriptions from a number of academic institutions. The resulting survey consisted of 25 demographic variables and a list of job responsibilities or task statements. Those surveyed were to rate the significance of each task statement using a six-point Likert-type scale ranging from "not part of my job" to "of maximum significance."

The practice analysis survey was administered to randomly selected academic nurse educators in all levels of nursing education (Ortelli, 2006). The resultant information gleaned from the survey was judged as adequately or completely addressing the responsibilities of the academic nurse educator. As a result of this practice analysis survey, the CNE exam addresses academic nurse educators who are teaching at any level—LPN, ADN, BSN, and graduate. The examination addresses the role of the academic nurse educator, not any specific educational level.

A second practice analysis was conducted in 2009. This analysis resulted in an update of the CNE test blueprint, the percentage of questions for the various content areas, and changes in eligibility requirements.

The CNE Test Blueprint

A final list of 119 tasks was developed and used as the basis for the detailed **test blueprint** that guides the composition of the questions on the CNE. Major categories for the CNE test blueprint developed by the PAC are similar to the major areas of the original nurse educator competencies, with a slight change in verbiage and some of the competencies becoming subconcepts. That is, "Function Within the Educational Environment" became "Engage in Scholarship, Service, and Leadership." "Function as a Change Agent and Leader" and "Engage in Scholarship of Teaching" became subcompetencies under "Engage in Scholarship, Service, and Leadership." **Table 11–1** aligns the core competencies as established by the task force with the major content areas of the CNE exam (NLN, 2014).

The final step in developing the test plan was to weight each of the content areas according to significance of the task and breadth of the content within each major area (Ortelli, 2010). Areas of content with higher significance ratings were assigned a greater number of questions. After considering the item distribution that spans the major and minor content areas, the PAC members agreed that 130 items would be sufficient to obtain an acceptable sampling of content to ensure the exam is reliable. The total number of items on the exam is 150 items, with 20 items not scored that are being tested for future use. The PAC members elected to restrict the cognitive levels for the test items to three different levels—recall, application, and analysis. The test items are provided as four-option, multiple-choice questions. Test questions are developed by individuals who have successfully completed the CNE examination. Each suggested test question is carefully and thoroughly reviewed to ensure it meets and addresses a major content area while also meeting an appropriate cognitive level (Ortelli, 2010).

The test blueprint was then completed and determined to represent current practice activities of an academic nurse educator in the United States.

Table 11-1   Core Competences and Major Content Areas

Core Competencies	Major Content Areas of the CNE Exam
Competency I: Facilitate Learning	Category 1: Facilitate Learning
Competency II: Facilitate Learner Development and Socialization	Category 2: Facilitate Learner Development and Socialization
Competency III: Use Assessment and Evaluation Strategies	Category 3: Use Assessment and Evaluation Strategies
Competency IV: Participate in Curriculum Design and Evaluation of Program Outcomes	Category 4: Participate in Curriculum Design and Evaluation of Program Outcomes
Competency V: Function as a Change Agent and Leader	Category 5: Pursue Systematic Self-Evaluation and Improvement in the Academic Nurse Educator Role
Competency VI: Pursue Continuous Quality Improvement in the Nurse Educator Role	Category 6: Engage in Scholarship, Service, and Leadership
	Subcategory 6A: Function as a Change Agent and Leader
	Subcategory 6B: Engage in Scholarship of Teaching
	Subcategory 6C: Function Effectively Within the Organizational Environment and the Academic Community

Source: National League for Nursing. (2012). *Certified Nurse Educator (CNE) 2012-2013 Candidate Handbook 2012 Revision.* Carbondale, IL: National League for Nursing Academic Nurse Educator Certification Program.

This practice analysis was repeated in 2010 through 2011 to ensure the test blue print still represented current practice for the academic nurse educator. The analysis indicated all areas on the test plan still represented current practice, but the weighting of some of the areas was slightly changed. The test plan was revised in 2012 and again in June, 2013 to represent these changes. **Table 11-2** presents the major content areas and percentage of questions for each area on the revised CNE test plan (NLN, 2014).

CNE EXAM ACCREDITED BY THE NATIONAL COMMISSION FOR CERTIFYING AGENCIES (NCCA)

A mark of excellence for nursing programs is accreditation by an outside organization, such as the National League for Nursing Accrediting Commission or the Commission on Collegiate Nursing Education. The **National**

Table 11–2   CNE Test Blueprint

Major Content Areas	Percentage of Examination
1. Facilitate Learning	22%
2. Facilitate Learner Development and Socialization	14%
3. Use Assessment and Evaluation Strategies	17%
4. Participate in Curriculum Design and Evaluation of Program Outcomes	17%
5. Pursue Continuous Quality Improvement in the Academic Nurse Educator Role	9%
6. Engage in Scholarship, Service, and Leadership	21%

Source: National League for Nursing. (2012). *Certified Nurse Educator (CNE) 2012-2013 Candidate Handbook 2012 Revision.* Carbondale, IL: National League for Nursing Academic Nurse Educator Certification Program. Used with permission.

Commission for Certifying Agencies (NCCA) has a parallel accreditation that indicates excellence. The NCCA evaluates certifying agencies using its established NCCA Standards for the Accreditation of Certification Programs. The NLN's CNE Commission was granted initial accreditation for the CNE Program on April 1, 2009, and was reaccredited in 2014, effective through 2019. This was the final step in ensuring that the CNE exam is evidence-based because the evidence documented by the NLN while establishing the CNE exam was further confirmed by an accreditation organization outside the NLN. This accreditation also ensures that certification programs adhere to the standards of practice of the certification industry. Therefore, the CNE exam is legitimatized both internally by the NLN and externally by the NCCA.

ELIGIBILITY FOR TAKING THE CNE EXAM

Faculty desiring to take the CNE exam must meet specific criteria. All faculty members must hold an active RN license. There are two options for eligibility criteria. These options are described as follows (NLN, 2014):

Option A: Must meet criteria 1 and 2

1. **Licensure:** A currently active, unencumbered, registered nurse license in the United States or its territories

2. **Education:** A master's or doctoral degree in nursing *with*:
   - · a major emphasis in nursing education,
   - · post-master's certificate in nursing education, or
   - · nine or more credit hours of graduate-level education courses*

   * Examples of acceptable graduate-level education courses include Curriculum Development and Evaluation; Instructional Design; Principles of Adult Learning; Assessment/Measurement and Evaluation; Principles of Teaching and Learning; Instructional Technology. Note: Graduate-level research or statistics courses do *not* count toward this requirement.

Option B: Must meet criteria 1, 2, and 3

1. **Licensure:** A currently active, unencumbered, registered nurse license in the United States or its territories
2. **Education:** A master's or doctoral degree in nursing (with a major emphasis in a role other than nursing education)
3. **Experience:** 2 years or more employment in a nursing program in an academic institution within the last 5 years

These eligibility requirements are presented in the *2014 Candidate Handbook*, which is reviewed annually and subject to change. Therefore, the nurse educator should always reference the most current handbook found at www.nln.org.

The certification designation is valid for a 5-year period. The NLN has developed a certification renewal process, which reflects that the CNE faculty holding the CNE credential has continued to demonstrate quality improvement in the academic nurse educator role.

PREPARING TO TAKE THE CNE EXAM

As with all national exams, it behooves the candidate to prepare for the CNE. There are a number of resources available for this preparation. The *CNE Candidate Handbook* can be accessed from the NLN's website. This handbook provides extensive information about the examination and the procedure for taking it. A detailed test plan is included, which is invaluable as a guide for study. The handbook also contains explanations about the testing center and the procedures implemented at the testing center. Also included is a list of suggested reading materials.

The handbook contains sample questions. Most of the questions are written at the recall, application, or analysis cognitive levels. However, for a more intensive practice experience, the NLN offers two online practice exams called self-assessment exams (SAEs). There are 65 items on each of the practice exams, covering all areas of the test blueprint in the same distribution as those of the actual exam. Taking these exams provides the candidate with a tool that diagnoses areas of strength and those that need to be studied to be successful on the actual exam. It also provides the candidate with experience in answering CNE-type questions. The candidate can view rationales for correct and incorrect answers.

As an additional study aid, the NLN has published the *Certified Nurse Educator Review Book: The Official NLN Guide to the CNE Exam* (Caputi, 2015). This book is available for purchase and is an invaluable resource as a comprehensive review for the exam.

The CNE examination has gained popularity over the years and is perceived as a mark of excellence for both the individual faculty and the nursing program in which the CNE is employed. Therefore, many schools are encouraging their entire faculty to take the CNE exam. In these cases, preparation can be a group affair. One approach to a group study plan includes the following steps:

- Obtain all the books on the recommended reading list, including the NLN's official review book and any other publications that faculty members believe can be helpful.
- Provide an on-site review session for the entire faculty.
- Schedule weekly meetings, such as a 2- to 3-hour time block on a specific day, when all faculty members can meet for study sessions.
- Each week one of the major areas of the CNE test blueprint is presented by assigned faculty followed by discussion of application of the content to practice.

As the faculty group develops strategies for addressing the different aspects covered within the examination, an individualized program of study can be developed. One key aspect when developing a group study plan is the commitment to the study process and the clarification of the time table. Each member of the group must accept and pledge to participate as the different aspects are managed.

Application of the content to one's own practice is an extremely valuable exercise that assists the individual faculty to work in-depth with the content, providing meaningful learning. It also provides evidence that the faculty member is indeed engaging in the activities of the nurse academician. This exercise raises one's awareness of one's role. A tool that is helpful with this exercise is found in **Table 11–3**. This tool can also be used for faculty when planning their personal or professional development activities and to document how they are carrying out their role as a nurse academician.

Table 11-3   Faculty Development Tool Related to the Roles of the Academic Nurse Educator

Competencies of the Academic Nurse Educator (Ortelli, 2010)	Examples of How This Competency Is Used in My Teaching	Identified Areas for Faculty Development	Source of Study and Projected Date of Study for Identified Areas for Development
Facilitate Learning			
Facilitate Learner Development and Socialization			
Use Assessment and Evaluation Strategies			
Participate in Curriculum Design and Evaluation of Program Outcomes			
Pursue Continuous Quality Improvement in the Academic Nurse Educator Role			
Engage in Scholarship, Service, and Leadership			
Function as a Change Agent and Leader			
Engage in Scholarship of Teaching			
Function Effectively Within the Institutional Environments and the Academic Community			

Source: © 2009, Linda Caputi, Inc. Used with permission.

IMPACT OF THE CNE ON NURSING EDUCATION

Holding the CNE credential is a mark of excellence. Those who have passed the CNE are viewed as leaders in nursing education. Those holding the CNE are called upon to contribute to the science of nursing education and to serve as role models in advancing the specialty area of nursing education.

Additionally, the core competencies that serve as the basis for the CNE test blueprint delineate the activities of the academic nurse educator.

Therefore, these provide the basis for developing curricula of MSN programs in nursing education, thus providing an evidence base for those programs. Currently, there is not a common core of knowledge from nursing education research that is evident in all of these programs. Many programs are based on general education practice. General education is important as core content; however, general education practice should provide a foundation that is then applied to nursing education. The following are some examples:

- As learning theories are discussed, those learning theories should be immediately applied to nursing students.
- Nursing students, as an aggregate, often have very specific characteristics that are different from those of the traditional college student.
- Students in graduate-level nursing education programs must learn to apply general education theory to their student population.

Ensuring that the core competencies of the academic nurse educator as operationalized in the CNE test blueprint are spiraled through graduate-level nursing education programs provides an evidence-based structure for those curricula. Table 11-3 provides a concrete tool nurse educators can use to demonstrate the use of the evidence-based characteristics of an academic nurse educator as provided by the NLN through the *CNE Handbook*.

SUMMARY THOUGHTS

When evidence is used to validate the work of academic nurse educators, the resulting documents are strong and effectively positioned to address the changing work of nursing education. Each and every step within the process of establishing and maintaining a certification examination to showcase the uniqueness of the specialty of nursing education is strengthened and championed by the work of the NLN. This group of individuals realized the importance of engaging in the discussion concerning the distinctiveness of the role of the academic nurse educator. As a result of progressing in a logical and organized manner from engaging experts to think about the role, developing position statements about the role of the academic nurse educator, engaging in feasibility study and needs assessment activities, establishing a scope of practice, to finally conducting a practice analysis that resulted in a test blueprint, the end product provides a complete and comprehensive look at the role of the nurse educator.

SUMMARY POINTS

1. The National Council of State Boards of Nursing's recommendations for evidence-based nursing education for regulation include teaching methods, assimilation of the students into the role of nursing, promoting faculty–student relationships, and other areas of teaching.

2. The National League for Nursing (NLN) supports nurse educators as practicing in a specialty role; that is, teaching in academia requires the knowledge of a specialized practice.

3. *The Scope of Practice for Academic Nurse Educators* (2005b) was the first publication that delineated the scope of practice and core competencies of nurse educators.

4. To reflect a complete picture of the academic nurse educator, all levels of academic institutions were considered as well as the various responsibilities of all levels of the educator role, from novice educator to expert educator.

5. The need for faculty to attain the knowledge and skills to function in the role of the academician had been established by the think tank and elaborated through the NLN's position statements.

6. The initial competencies were: facilitate learning, facilitate learner development and socialization, use assessment and evaluation strategies, participate in curriculum design and evaluation of program outcomes, function as a change agent and leader, pursue continuous quality improvement in the nurse educator role, engage in scholarship, and function within the educational environment.

7. A final list of 119 tasks was developed and used as the basis for the detailed test blueprint that guides the composition of the questions on the CNE.

8. The total number of items on the exam is 150 items, with 20 items not scored that are being tested for future use.

9. The PAC members elected to restrict the cognitive levels for the test items to three different levels—recall, application, and analysis.

10. The test items are provided as four-option, multiple-choice questions. Test questions are developed by CNE-certified individuals.

11. Each suggested test question is carefully and thoroughly reviewed to ensure it meets and addresses a major content area while also meeting an appropriate cognitive level.

12. The NLN's CNE Commission was granted accreditation for the CNE Program on April 1, 2009. This was the final step in assuring

the CNE exam is evidence-based, because the evidence documented by the NLN while establishing the CNE exam was further confirmed by an accreditation organization outside the NLN.

13. The CNE exam is legitimatized both internally by the NLN and externally by the NCCA.

14. Faculty desiring to take the CNE must meet specific criteria.

15. The NLN publishes the *Certified Nurse Educator Review Book: The Official NLN Guide to the CNE Exam*.

16. The NLN developed a certification renewal process, which reflects that the CNE has continued to demonstrate quality improvement in the academic nurse educator role.

17. The *CNE Candidate Handbook* can be accessed from the NLN's website. This handbook provides extensive information about the examination and the procedure for taking the exam. A detailed test plan is included, which is invaluable as a guide for study.

18. The NLN offers two online practice exams called self-assessment exams (SAEs). There are 65 items on each of the practice exams, covering all areas of the test blueprint in the same distribution as those of the actual exam. Taking these exams provides the candidate with a tool that diagnoses areas of strength and those that need to be studied to be successful on the actual exam.

19. As the NLN has moved forward to assure the CNE process maintains a high level of quality, the Certification Commission has been established.

TIPS FOR NURSE EDUCATORS

1. Taking the NLN's self-assessment exam provides the candidate with a tool that diagnoses areas of strength and those that need to be studied to be successful on the actual exam. It also provides the candidate with experience in answering CNE-type questions. The candidate can view rationales for correct and incorrect answers.

2. For group study in preparation for the exam:
   · Obtain all of the books on the recommended reading list and any other publications that faculty members believe can be helpful.
   · Provide an on-site review session for the entire faculty.
   · Schedule weekly meetings, such as a 2- to 3-hour time block on a specific day, when all faculty members can meet for study sessions.

- Each week one of the major areas of the CNE test blueprint should be presented by assigned faculty, followed by discussion of application of the content to practice.

3. Knowledgeable individuals and groups have developed and offer workshops to help individuals prepare for the examination.

MULTIPLE CHOICE QUESTIONS

1. Which organization offers the CNE examination?
   A. AACN
   B. ANCC
   C. NCSBN
   D. **NLN**

   Rationale:
   A certification exam did not exist that specifically addressed the role of the academic nurse educator. In fact, until recently, the role of the academic nurse educator had not been formally studied and delineated. The NLN recognized the need and developed the CNE examination.

2. What is the purpose of a task analysis?
   A. **Provide validity for the content of an exam.**
   B. Determine the feasibility of offering an exam.
   C. Determine if there is a market for a specific exam.
   D. Decide who the target audience of an exam will be.

   Rationale:
   To ensure validity of an exam that provides certification or licensure, a practice analysis is used to reveal the activities of the professional engaged in that practice. That is, a practice analysis reveals the activities the professional undertakes while carrying out the functions and responsibilities within the scope of practice of that professional role. The certification exam then tests the candidate's knowledge of those activities.

3. Which statement describes a reason for the need for a certification exam for academic nursing faculty?
   A. **Teaching nursing is a specialty area.**
   B. Faculty will earn a higher salary if they are certified.
   C. Nursing accrediting bodies require faculty to be certified.
   D. Graduates of MSN programs require their students to pass the exam.

Rationale:
Preparation as a nurse with a practice specialty is not enough. The nurse also needs the specialized knowledge and skills of the educator. Certification would demonstrate the nurse educator has the expertise necessary to engage in the role of an academician.

4. The CNE exam is written for academic nurse educators teaching at which level?
   A. LPN
   B. ADN
   C. BSN and graduate
   D. **All levels**

Rationale:
As a result of the practice analysis survey, the CNE exam addresses academic nurse educators who are teaching at any level—LPN, ADN, BSN, and graduate. The examination addresses the role of the academic nurse educator, not any specific educational level.

5. Which of the following is the primary reason for conducting a feasibility study prior to developing the CNE exam?
   A. Ensure the cost of development can be recovered.
   B. **Confirm the target population is ready for such an exam.**
   C. Determine a fair market price for the exam.
   D. Ensure schools will reimburse faculty for the cost of the exam.

Rationale:
The feasibility study revealed a need for a certification exam for academic nurse educators. NLN was ready to take the next steps.

6. During the development of the CNE exam, a practice analysis survey was administered. To whom was this survey administered?
   A. Nursing program administrators.
   B. Nursing students.
   C. Developers of graduate-level programs in nursing education.
   D. **Academic nurse educators.**

Rationale:
The practice analysis survey was administered to randomly selected academic nurse educators in all levels of nursing education (Ortelli, 2006). The resultant information gleaned from the survey was judged as adequately or completely addressing the responsibilities of the academic nurse educator.

7. How many questions compose the scored CNE exam?
   A. 75
   B. 100

C. **130**
D. 150

Rationale:
The total number of items on the exam is currently 150 items, with 20 items not scored that are being tested for future use. The PAC members elected to restrict the cognitive levels for the test items to three different levels—recall, application, and analysis. The test items are provided as four-option, multiple-choice questions. At this time, test questions are developed by CNE-certified individuals. Each suggested test question is carefully and thoroughly reviewed to ensure that it meets and addresses a major content area while also meeting an appropriate cognitive level.

8. What is the minimum number of years of experience required for candidates who hold a graduate degree with a major emphasis in a role other than nursing education?
   A. 1
   B. **2**
   C. 4
   D. 5

Rationale:
For those faculty with a master's or doctoral degree in nursing with a major emphasis on a role other than nursing education, the experience requirement is 2 years of employment in the academic faculty role. There is no experience requirement for candidates with a master's or doctoral degree in nursing with a major emphasis in nursing education or 9 or more credit hours of graduate-level education courses (not including graduate-level research or statistics courses).

9. Which content area is assigned the largest percentage of questions on the CNE exam?
   A. **Facilitate learning.**
   B. Use assessment and evaluation strategies.
   C. Participate in curriculum design and evaluation of program outcomes.
   D. The combined subcategories included under engage in scholarship, service, and leadership.

Rationale:
The major content area of facilitating learning accounts for 22% of the total questions provided.

10. What is the expectation for those who hold the CNE credential?
    A. Serve as leaders in nursing education.
    B. Contribute to the science of nursing education.
    C. Serve as a role model in moving forward the specialty area of nursing education.
    D. **All of the above.**

    Rationale:
    As one looks at the core competencies and major content areas, each of the components is evident in the material included within the role of the academic nurse educator.

Discussion Questions

1. The entire faculty in one nursing program would like to take the CNE exam. What kinds of activities might help prepare the faculty?
   Considerations:
   · Form study groups and plan set days/times to work through the content.
   · Review all the study materials on the reading list in the *CNE Candidate Handbook*.
   · Take the online self-assessment examination to identify areas that need to be studied.
   · Examine the CNE test blueprint to identify areas that need to be studied.
2. You would like to develop a certification examination for a specific area of practice. How would you go about such a task?
   Considerations:
   Lay out the tasks similar to what the NLN did to develop the CNE exam.

References

Accreditation Certification for Education in Nursing. (2013). *Accreditation manual.* Atlanta, GA: Author.

Adams, M. H., & Valiga, T. M. (2009). *Achieving excellence in nursing education.* New York, NY: National League for Nursing.

Benner, P., Sutphen, M., Leonard, V., & Day, L. (2010). *Educating nurses: A call for radical transformation.* San Francisco, CA: Jossey-Bass.

Caputi, L. (Ed.). (2015). *Certified nurse educator review book: The official NLN guide to the CNE exam.* Philadelphia, PA: Wolters Kluwer, Lippincott, Williams, & Wilkins.

Halstead, J. A. (Ed.). (2007). *Nurse educator competencies: Creating an evidence-based practice for nurse educators*. New York, NY: National League for Nursing.

National League for Nursing. (2002). *Position statement: The preparation of nurse educators*. New York, NY: Author.

National League for Nursing. (2003). *Position statement: Innovation in nursing education: A call to reform*. New York, NY: Author.

National League for Nursing. (2005a). *Position statement: Innovation in nursing education: Transforming nursing education*. New York, NY: Author.

National League for Nursing. (2005b). *The scope of practice for academic nurse educators*. New York, NY: Author.

National League for Nursing. (2012). *The scope of practice for academic nurse educators: 2012 revision*. New York, NY: Author.

National League for Nursing. (2014). *Certified Nurse Educator (CNE) 2014 candidate handbook, June 2013 revision*. Carbondale, IL: National League for Nursing Academic Nurse Educator Certification Program.

Norman, G. (1985). *Assessing clinical competence*. New York, NY: Springer.

Ortelli, T. (2006). Defining the professional responsibilities of academic nurse educators: The results of a national practice analysis. *Nursing Education Perspectives*, *27*(5), 242–246.

Ortelli, T. (2010). The Certified Nurse Educator credential. In L. Caputi (Ed.), *Teaching nursing: The art and science* (2nd ed., pp. 564–585). Glen Ellyn, IL: College of DuPage Press.

Shultz, C. (2012). *Building a science of nursing education: Foundation for evidence-based teaching–learning*. Philadelphia, PA: Wolters Kluwer, Lippincott, Williams, & Wilkins.

Spector, N. (2006). *Systematic review of students of nursing education outcomes: An evolving review*. Chicago, IL: National Council of State Boards of Nursing.

Chapter 12

Future Perspectives

Carol Boswell and Sharon Cannon

At the conclusion of this chapter, the learner will be able to:

1. Identify the emergence, impact, and connection of evidence-based teaching for current and future directions in nursing education.
2. Discuss the role of the nurse educator in evidence-based teaching.
3. Utilize teaching strategies/techniques in a variety of educational settings.
4. Identify the role of competencies and certification for nurse educators in the current and future nursing education venues.
5. Explore nursing education research.

KEY TERMS

- Coach
- Evidence-based teaching
- Institute of Medicine
- Mentorship
- Preceptor
- Robert Wood Johnson Foundation
- Translational research

INTRODUCTION

Nurse educators tend to teach as they were taught. According to Benner, Sutphen, Leonard, and Day (2010), "The central goal of nursing education is for the learner to develop an attuned, response-based practice and capacity to quickly recognize the nature of whole situations in terms of most pressing and least pressing concerns" (p. 43). With the emergence of evidence-based practice (EBP), the focus is on utilization of evidence to provide the best outcomes for nursing. This movement toward supported practices has prompted nurse educators to seek the best evidence for student learning outcomes. In addition, the nursing shortage has impacted nurse educators as demands for increased enrollments, recruitment, and retention of students require nurse educators to explore strategies and skills to accommodate those demands through unique and innovative approaches that are grounded in solid evidence. Compounding the problem resulting from the nursing shortage is the aging population of both the nursing workforce and nurse educators. Another strong challenge to nursing education is "The Future of Nursing," a report by the Institute of Medicine (IOM) in partnership with the Robert Wood Johnson Foundation (2011). This report recommends that 80% of all registered nurses (RNs) be educated at the BSN level by the year 2020. In addition to increasing the educational level of the practicing RN, the report challenges schools of nursing to prepare these individuals to function at the full extent of their education and training, to encourage nurses to seek opportunities to be at the decision-making tables of board and other elected positions, and to lead the charge in regard to advancing health care (IOM, 2011). With more than 3 million RNs, the potential impact on health care is tremendous. Nurses must be educated to embrace the political aspect of health care to help steer the direction of nursing and health care.

Aging of the workforce and nursing faculty resulted in a 2010 joint statement of the Tri-Council for Nursing, in which Dr. Peter Buerhaus indicated that prior to 2010 approximately 900,000 RNs (out of the estimated 2.6 million working RNs) were older than 50 years of age (American Association of Colleges of Nursing [AACN], 2010). The report continued to speculate that increasing numbers of these RNs were projected to retire in the coming years (AACN, 2010). Buerhaus (AACN, 2010) further noted that replacement of the aging RNs and increasing the supply of RNs will be needed. The Tri-Council also suggested that the capacity of nursing education programs must increase. Consequently, nurse educators will be challenged to not only manage larger classes, but also to increase graduation rates and success rates on the National Council Licensure Examination (NCLEX). On a regular basis, the NCLEX testing blueprint is reevaluated to confirm that it continues to address the current practices within professional nursing care. Each time these revisions are made, the pass rate by first-time testers on the NCLEX tends to demonstrate a negative trend for the initial two to three testing periods. Nurse educators must anticipate and be ready to modify the current curricula when the NCLEX updates the testing process. A big change that occurred recently with the NCLEX is the inclusion of questions with the potential for multiple answers.

Individuals taking the NCLEX are confronted by questions that request "all that apply" instead of holding to the previous format, which was to select the one best answer. Nurse educators must take these areas into consideration. As schools work to increase fiscal responsibility, faculty members are confronted with larger classes and more demands to ensure the success rate for the students.

While much of the news seems to be disheartening, Rosseter (2012) reflected on the latest information from the Bureau of Labor. RNs are currently the top occupation in terms of job advancement. According to Rosseter (2012), the statistics imply that the number of employed RNs will increase by approximately 26% to a level of 3.45 million by the year 2020. With this growth, along with the need to replace outgoing RNs, it is estimated that the total number of job openings for nurses will be approximately 1.2 million by the year 2020. This type of growth reflects the need for nursing faculty members to become increasingly proficient at moving students through educational programs while ensuring that each one is qualified to function at least at a minimum level of competency. More and more pressure is placed on the academic community to embrace best practices and efficient tactics to confirm that the nurses practicing can meet the demands resulting from the changing healthcare arena. Intrinsic in this process is the realization that enrollment numbers for entry-level baccalaureate programs increased by only 5.1%. The enrollment numbers are not growing in proportion to the job opening increase. Add to this complex discussion the passage of the Patient Protection and Affordable Care Act of 2010, which is projected to open healthcare services to an additional 32 million individuals. RNs are being expected to step up to the plate to offset the healthcare changes as they begin in 2014.

The other chapters of this text are designed to provide a foundation for both novice and experienced faculty to build their knowledge and skills in the nursing education arena on evidence rather than relying on a "gut feeling" or past educational experience. Agencies outside of nursing, such as the **Institute of Medicine** (IOM) and **Robert Wood Johnson Foundation**, have emphasized the need for **evidence-based teaching** (EBT) and nurse educators who have the skills and abilities to teach nursing education today and in the future to meet the demands for a well-prepared healthcare workforce. Another area discussed in the other chapters is the impact of the Affordable Care Act (ACA) on the role of nurses in the future. The ACA strives to provide health care to the entire U.S. population and strongly encourages preventive health care. Both of these aspects are areas directly impacted within the role of the professional nurse. Curricula cannot maintain the focus on acute care settings for educational experiences. The new role of the professional nurse reflects increased accountability and responsibilities as new health delivery methods are considered and implemented. Nurse educators must ensure that the new graduates are prepared to be that team member who is knowledgeable, determined, and professional.

Let's see how the other chapters fit with EBT for current and future directions. Fostering the EBT perspective begins with the development of the role of the academician regarding the provision of preceptors/coaches and mentors, the ethics of teaching, utilization of multiple settings, teaching methodologies in various settings, evaluation, current EBT research, and establishing the competency of the nurse educator.

PRECEPTOR/COACH

The definition for **preceptor** is "an expert or specialist, such as a physician, who gives practical experience and training to a student" (Preceptor, 2009). Preceptors are frequently utilized to support and expand the learning environment for students. In contrast, the definition for **coach** is "a private tutor employed to prepare a student for an examination" (Coach, 2009). Within the nursing field, a coach is a private expert or specialist who works directly with one or two students to aid the acquisition of knowledge. Clinically competent nurses are called upon in many settings to provide the support and practical experience for students to allow for the advancement of the knowledge base. Didactic teaching settings are established to accentuate the cognitive domain of learning. Clinical instructors, preceptors, and coaches are required to translate the cognitive knowledge to the psychomotor and affective domains through application. From the evidence, Modic and Schoessler (2010) pinpointed four themes that preceptors identified as key areas needing to be strengthened: "(1) learning how to capitalize on teaching moments, (2) applying evidence-based teaching, (3) providing constructive performance feedback, and (4) adapting teaching strategies to match the different learning needs of students" (p. 134). Each of these areas is essential as orientation programs for preceptors and coaches are established, and as preceptors/coaches are supported and developed. Individuals who agree to serve as preceptors and coaches for the next generation of students want to support and develop the novice nurses in a positive and encouraging manner. The idea of "eating our young" is not the feedback that most nurses desire. In reality, the strengthening and championing of the next generation of nurses is the ultimate goal for individuals who accept the responsibility of precepting and coaching student nurses.

Manion (2010) wrote that "generational diversity was widely popularized in the early nineties when the advent of large numbers of GenXers into our workforce caused many Baby Boomers to shake their heads in bewilderment" (p. 8). The idea of groups of individuals precepting each other while holding differing values, attitudes, and work goals caused increased anxiety within the workplace. Multiple studies have been done to help validate the differences between the values, interests, and tactics to best use with the different groupings. Manion (2010) notes that little evidence was located related to specific leadership strategies that are effective based upon generational differences alone. In reality, the challenges and rewards confronted within the precepting/coaching experience are based upon the complexity of the workforce resulting from geographic, cultural, ethnic, generational, and professional diversity. No one aspect is the primary driver, but instead the intricacy of each individual as multiple forces come to bear on the development of that individual must be considered. From the research completed by Manion (2010), five basic human intrinsic motivators were identified as contributing to the creation of a dynamic work environment. Preceptors and coaches can utilize these five motivators as they strive to usher the learners toward their educational goals. The five motivators are healthy relationships (positive, healthy working interactions), meaningful work (perceived by the individual as worthwhile and fulfilling), competence (building on strengths to advance self), autonomy (having authority to make decisions and implement actions), and progress (realizing that activities completed have had an impact).

MENTORSHIP

A **mentor** is defined as "a wise and trusted counselor or teacher, to serve as a trusted counselor or teacher, especially in occupational settings, and/or to serve as a trusted counselor or teacher to (another person)" (Mentor, 2009). The concept of mentor differs from the role of preceptor/coach. A mentorship is considered to be a long-term commitment to the development of an individual. Preceptors and coaches are selected and appointed for a specific time period or grouping of objectives. Mentors are usually mutually selected by the individuals involved instead of being appointed. Within the mentoring process utilized by Latimer and Kimbell (2010), the recommendation was made to allow the mentoring process to have one-on-one consultation time rather than requiring mentoring activities to be done as a group action. The relationship established within a mentorship can be viewed as either a protégé–mentor or fellow–mentor pairing. Within each of these relationships, the custom is a one-on-one process directed toward one primary goal. Mentors can be outside the nursing discipline. A mentor is selected because the individual is an expert in that area. As the goal is established, the nurse needs to carefully consider who is the best individual to provide this expertise. To limit oneself to only nurses restricts the individual's growth. Individuals also should not limit themselves to only one mentor. A mentor is selected for the expertise. So a person could have several mentors if his or her goal reflects the need for multiple objectives. The protégé–mentor or fellow–mentor pairing can identify further goals as the relationship develops, but initially the pair is connected by a single ambition. As the rapport develops, further aspects may be ascertained that will allow the relationship to mature in a different way.

Barnsteiner, Reeder, Palma, Preston, and Walton (2010) discuss the use of a mentor program to promote EBP and **translational research**. Within this project, five clinical educators accepted the task of serving as mentors for staff nurses related to EBP and translational research. Over the course of a 1-year fellowship, these mentors provided support and instruction to the fellows as they moved from novice researchers toward a firmer understanding of the interconnectedness of EBP and translational research. The mentors served as EBP champions and resource individuals as the designated fellow initiated a project. According to Barnsteiner et al. (2010), the goal was "to fuel a love of knowledge, enthusiasm for questioning the status quo, and interest in exploring new approaches to practice based on emerging science and national standards" (p. 225). Within the mentor process, the love of learning was supported and encouraged.

Another example of the use of mentorship to transform an organizational EBP culture is presented by Ogiehor-Enoma, Taqueban, and Anosike (2010), who note, "A commitment to EBP begins with establishing a culture in which nurses are mentored in developing skills for defining problems and improving clinical decision making in their work environment" (p. 14). Within this example, six steps were used: (1) conducting an organizational inventory, (2) constructing a strong infrastructure for EBP, (3) valuing the EBP process while embracing the different parts, (4) augmenting internal resources via educational venues, (5) embedding the aspects into day-to-day practice, and (6) sustaining the culture change. Ogiehor-Enoma et al. (2010) note the expectation that direct care nurses should acquire an internal consultant, mentors, and coaches to facilitate the complex EBP activities. The use of consultants, mentors, and coaches was viewed as an integral aspect of the success of the transformation. Utilizing the expertise of champions to support and advance the other staff was viewed as a major strength within this process. The culture developed into one of support and encouragement, not competition.

Since mentoring is viewed as longer term than precepting/coaching, career mapping programs can be an EBT model for the advancement of the protégé-fellow relationship. Shermont, Krepcio, and Murphy (2009) stated that "meeting the demands of complex care environments requires a nursing workforce that is committed to continued learning and to advancing clinical as well as leadership skills" (p. 432). The process of career mapping involves the pairing of a mentor/clinical advisor with an individual to assist the individual to define distinct professional aspirations, cultivate a plan for achieving those goals, and collaborate as the plan is implemented. From the evidence, career planning has been found to empower individuals to chart their own professional path and take responsibility for that journey. Through the use of the mentor/clinical advisor process to validate the individual's attempts to chart his or her own course, a sense of confidence can be forthcoming and corroborated. The mentor/clinical advisor can assist the individual to set realistic goals. Once those goals are in place and the individual is committed to strive for them, the mentor/clinical advisor is used to access resources and act as a cheerleader. This cheerleading/championing of the individual's own plan provides further self-confidence and security. The individual can then develop skills to use in future career growth efforts. In summation of their work, Shermont et al. (2009) claim that by "revitalizing nurses' interest in their careers, the program enhanced nurse satisfaction as well as retention and reduces staff turnover and the attendant nurse replacement costs" (p. 437). By supporting individuals to strive for their own career goals, the agency received the benefit of satisfied employees who were invigorated to strive for quality and recognition. The benefits of this mentoring program resulted in a true "win–win" result for the employer and employee.

IMPACT OF CONTINUED NURSING

Just as nurses at the bedside need to be cognizant of new technologies and the need to keep current on EBP, so too does the nurse educator need to maintain competence and expertise in the realm of being a nurse educator. As efforts to produce more evidence for teaching nursing education occur, faculty will need to continue to add to their knowledge the best practices for obtaining learning outcomes of students and for overall evaluation of themselves, courses, and programs. Institutes for immersion in the faculty role, new technology, workshops/conferences (local, state, and national), postgraduate courses, and journal articles provide a wide array of choices to keep current and up-to-date on new evidence.

As mentioned previously, the RN workforce is aging. The current projections are that 260,000 new nurses will be needed by 2025 (AACN, 2010), and 1.2 million total nurses are projected to be needed by 2020 to meet the needs of growth and replacement (Rosseter, 2012). In 2011, 75,587 qualified applicants for nursing programs were turned away due to an insufficient number of nursing faculty members (Rosseter, 2012). Barriers to increasing enrollments are lack of faculty, clinical sites, and classroom space, as well as economic budgetary restraints. Unfortunately, compounding this issue is the aging of faculty, which will result in even fewer faculty members to teach future programs. However, before predicting doom and gloom, new technology and research in nursing education may offer a ray of hope. Faculty members will be challenged to seek innovative, creative EBT methods to address the pressures that will inevitably be present. Legislative efforts from national and state nursing organizations are working, and will continue to work, to improve the likelihood of increasing undergraduate and graduate funding for nursing education for scholarships, research, new program start-ups, and faculty salaries. In addition, the IOM and the Robert Wood Johnson Foundation conducted three forums across the United States to obtain feedback from recognized leaders in nursing education and clinical agencies to examine the future direction for nursing education. Their 2011 report recommends four key nursing initiatives to advance the profession of nursing. According to the report, nurses should (1) practice to the comprehensive scope of their education and training, (2) attain the highest levels of education and training possible by means of an enhanced education structure that endorses seamless academic progression, (3) be inclusive associates with physicians and other health professionals to work toward redesigned healthcare management, and (4) engage in operational workforce development and policy making demanding enhanced data collection and a first-class information infrastructure (IOM, 2011). Each of the areas mandates that nursing education carefully and thoroughly consider how the skills and execution of nursing care must be impacted to meet these goals. The Carnegie Foundation for the Advancement of Teaching has also stepped forward though the efforts of Benner et al. (2010), who call for a radical transformation for educating nurses. All of these combined efforts are designed to ensure that the 32 million more citizens of the future will be able to access health care and subsequently nursing care in a variety of settings.

RESEARCH IN NURSING EDUCATION

As described in other chapters, research endeavors within nursing education have ebbed and flowed. At times within our history, federal monies have been available to fund the research projects related to validating educational strategies. At other times, the monies have been scarce. In the current funding environment, some revenue streams are available. Funding sources for nursing education tend to be small grant amounts provided by nursing professional organizations, such as the National League for Nursing (NLN), Sigma Theta Tau International (STTI), and the American Nurses Association (ANA). Federal grant monies continue to be few and far between but primarily can be located within the U.S. Health Resources and Services Administration (HRSA). Projects that combine nursing education and clinical practice seem to be areas where federal monies can be sought. Funding sources for research endeavors related to simulation projects are available through the private sector. Private-sector companies such as Johnson and Johnson and the Robert Wood Johnson Foundation are opening selected funding streams related to specific focal points within each company's strategic plan.

SHORTAGE OF HEALTHCARE WORKERS

Mason (2010) states, "The new law (Patient Protection and Affordable Care Act—PL111.148) includes federal support for developing the healthcare workforce, including nurses, with a particular emphasis on expanding the number and preparation of primary care providers" (p. 24). Though the media has repeatedly discussed the growing concerns related to the shortages of healthcare workers, this law adds to the opportunities for change. The ACA opened healthcare benefits for uninsured individuals and advanced the coverage provided to many who did have insurance at some level. Some of the areas covered by this law addressed ambulatory patient services, prescription drugs, emergency care, mental health services, hospitalization, rehabilitative and habilitative services, and preventive and wellness services. While these services have been available for many people, this law opens the services to all Americans. The number of individuals who can access health care has grown considerably while the number of healthcare providers continues to be a grave concern. RN programs are changing the focus from inpatient management of health care to outpatient provision. Many of these outpatient services related to prevention, wellness, and rehabilitation mandate that the academic community develop a different scope of skills and expertise. The primary idea within this law focuses on reducing healthcare costs while providing improved opportunities for healthcare access. Improvements in the approaches and tactics used to meet the increasing demands placed on the educational community must be carefully and appropriately considered. Shortages of physicians, pharmacists, and nurses, to name a few key players, will lead to a greater demand. These groups will be called on to accommodate the increased population seeking to access the healthcare services when mandatory health insurance becomes a reality. These demands will stretch the limits for all healthcare practitioners. Each group will be required to provide the resources to address the changes within the healthcare field based upon the federal regulations.

APPLICATION TO SETTINGS OTHER THAN ACADEMIA

EBT will be essential for the preparation of nurses entering the workforce and for continuing competence of nurses. Thus, EBT has a major impact for nurse educators in clinics, hospitals, schools, home health, and hospice agencies. Nursing staff development personnel must also utilize EBT and, just as importantly, conduct research for the best evidence to teach in areas outside of academia. Keeping abreast of EBT advancements in nursing will assist those nurse educators in the preparation, implementation, and evaluation of programs for nursing staff. Clinical/Career Ladders, Magnet, and Pathway to Excellence status and accreditation agencies such as The Joint Commission will continue to urge education of staff to be a major priority. As a result, nurse educators outside of academia will also use evidence to demonstrate competency outcomes, which in turn impact patient outcomes.

CREATING A VISION FOR EVIDENCE-BASED TEACHING

As stated by Senthuran (2010):

> The journey to gain understanding and meaning is part of the evolution of nursing as a discipline. It is necessary for a group of people, a culture, to understand what and why they do things to gain a sense of themselves so that they can determine how they fit into the world and how to evolve. (p. 245)

As the profession begins to transition toward an EBT affiliation, care should be given to considering a model for the transition from student to competent nursing professional. Faculty members engaged in advancing the success of the educational process must promote the successful transition of students into the actual workplace setting. Another focus for the transition is related to moving novice faculty members toward a confident educator role.

Bahouth and Esposito-Herr (2009) embraced the Brown and Olshansky stages for transition from student to competent nurse practitioner. The four stages can be easily incorporated as a means for moving students of any level toward competent healthcare delivery. These same four stages can be applied to advancing the novice faculty member from initial role performance toward a level of secure management of the educational process. The four stages are (1) laying the foundation, (2) launching, (3) meeting the challenge, and (4) broadening the perspectives. According to Bahouth and Esposito-Herr (2009), the initial period provides the venue for students to move out of the educational process and into the workplace setting. The interlude results in stress for the individuals as they endeavor to determine appropriate work settings. The second stage includes the process of getting involved in the actual work of the job—moving from being that student who is waiting to break into the process to being that individual who assumes a place at the worktable with confidence and integrity. The next stage of meeting the challenges allows the individual to build and develop confidence and competence within the work setting selected. The final phase takes place as the student has moved from the learner on the side to a member of the team.

These same four stages can be readily applied to the novice educator. Novice faculty members must be provided the time and resources to lay a firm foundation for the effective management of the learning process. Opportunities for the faculty member to try out these different strategies with diverse student populations are mandatory. The novice faculty member needs to confront the challenges of the diverse student population while having the tools needed to be successful. These individuals should not be thrown out into the raging rapids to sink or swim without having a lifeguard (seasoned faculty member) to help them acquire the different skills and strategies needed to be successful in this different venue of practice. Clinically competent nurses can successfully transition into the educator role but do need to have the opportunities and resources to productively and effectively manage the education environment of the 21st century and beyond.

Within EBT, faculty members need to help the students to understand that this movement from the student role toward a competent member of the team takes time and energy. Just because a student acquires pieces of paper (diploma and licenses) does not mean the person is ready to take on all aspects of the workplace. Faculty members must acknowledge that it is a process and discover ways to help the student transition toward that exciting new role. Part of understanding EBT is knowing that even within the teaching/education role, evidence is key for helping each member progress toward his or her educational goals.

Benner et al. (2010) assert that four essential shifts are needed to actively engage students in a positive manner:

1. Shift from a focus on covering decontextualized knowledge to an emphasis on teaching for a sense of salience, situated cognition, and action in particular situations
2. Shift from a sharp separation of clinical and classroom teaching to integration of classroom and clinical teaching
3. Shift from an emphasis on critical thinking to an emphasis on clinical reasoning and multiple ways of thinking that include critical thinking
4. Shift from an emphasis on socialization and role taking to an emphasis on formation (pp. 82–86)

With each of these areas, faculty members move from a passive delivery to an active engagement of the students. Engaging the student within the learning process should result in a love for learning. Too frequently, individuals perceive that taking time to seek knowledge is too burdensome. By using these shifts, individuals become adept at seeking knowledge and excited about bringing in new and innovative ideas. By accepting the challenge of striving for new levels of health care founded on the latest knowledge, they become dependent on their own ability to confirm and validate information, instead of just accepting what others tend to say and do.

Another crucial aspect of utilizing EBT during the transition into practice relates to generational issues. Hudspeth (2009) states that consideration must be given "to having four generations, and sometimes five, in the same clinical setting at one time" (p. 352). As discussed elsewhere in this text, the concerns related to harmonizing the work expectations for each of these generations require that faculty carefully consider the needs, attitudes, and expectations for each of the generations. Forethought should be given to how best to engage each of the generations so that a smoother balancing of the opportunities can be ensured. Each of these generations embraces different lifestyles, educational types, and learning styles. Faculty members who are willing to investigate potential approaches for engaging the different groups should meet with a more positive outcome for the learning process. Stereotyping is not appropriate, but realizing the uniqueness of each group can be used to improve the learning process. As faculty members consider the generational issues, attention should be directed to the faculty group makeup, teaching team composition, and committee groups. It is not just about the student population, but all aspects within the teaching environment. Care should be given to understanding our peers, colleagues, and students.

In addition to the generational issues, cultural issues can go hand in hand with this need to welcome the uniqueness and distinctiveness of the different individuals encountered during the learning process. Sherman (2010) refers to this imperative as "building generational synergy" (p. 4). Determining a generational profile of the student cohort can aid the instructor to carefully consider the distinct needs that may be present. By establishing this blueprint of the cohort's composition, faculty can build the synergetic environment that allows the group to develop a strong foundation to foster future learning opportunities. While Sherman (2010) acknowledges that the nurse leader is principal in the environment, the idea can be translated to reflect that the educator holds the strategic position for setting the tone and culture within the learning environment. The faculty member who endeavors to use EBT realizes that the establishment of a culture of inclusion and respect is important and must include generational and cultural beliefs and biases. Sherman (2010) relates that "points of conflict can often be turned into teachable moments" (p. 5). Through the embracing of EBT, faculty members will understand the necessity for utilizing all knowledge to best present and advance the profession of nursing. As areas that can result in "pull back" from positive results are encountered, EBT champions will demand that evidence be sought to ensure that the learning environment is not negatively impacted. An example of this can be seen in the work being done by Gary Small at the University of California Los Angeles (UCLA) (Sherman, 2010). This work is suggesting that the "changes we see in the classroom with students today such as shortened attention spans and skimming of reading material may be a biological adaptation to new technology" (Sherman, 2010, p. 5). Diversity within the learning community allows for the strengths and limitations of each generation to be supported by others within the group. A diverse learning community can better handle the complexity and challenges encountered within the rapidly changing healthcare arena.

Creating a vision of EBT mandates the utilization of technology. The Technology Informatics Guiding Education Reform (TIGER) initiative is an exemplar of EBT. According to Hebda and Calderone (2010):

> The 2003 Institute of Medicine report, *Health Professions Education: A Bridge to Quality*, identified five core competencies for healthcare professionals: the ability to deliver patient-centered care, the ability to work as members of an interdisciplinary team, the use of evidence-based practice, quality improvement approaches, and informatics. (p. 56)

This project embraced the concepts of EBP (thus EBT) to identify the vision/mission/goals, develop informatics competencies, and implement these competencies into nursing education. Through the TIGER initiative, nurse educators have been provided with strategies for integrating technology-enhanced experiences into the lesson plans and curricula. The informatics competencies are divided into the following groups: all nurses, beginning nurses, and experienced nurses. The evidence has been assembled and harvested from multiple resources to ensure that the TIGER initiative project has the current core competencies that are needed. EBT can and does work to bring together important and needed information to advance the science of nursing and nursing education.

As agencies, groups, and educators begin to carefully and logically consider the idea of EBT, awareness grows that each individual has something to offer. Evidence can and does come from many different directions. Nursing must stay vigilant for its individual body of knowledge while embracing knowledge from other disciplines. Krom, Batten, and Bautista (2010) incorporated collaboration with a clinical nurse specialist, health science librarian, and staff nurse to advance the EBP process at their institution. Utilizing multiple individuals allowed for an effective collaborative effort that resulted in successful modification of the work environment at an academic medical center. It was found that "each brought an important perspective that would help the staff nurse become familiar with the concept and overcome any personal barrier" (Krom et al., 2010, p. 56). Realizing the expertise that is available through the engagement with other disciplines, departments, and resources opens the opportunities for advancement of the agenda toward EBT and EBP.

SUMMARY THOUGHTS

According to Ogiehor-Enoma et al. (2010), "In today's era of knowledgeable healthcare consumers, evidence-based practice has become the gold standard as consumers demand quality care that's proven to be effective and safe" (p. 14). If within health care and nursing care, EBP is the gold standard, then can nursing education require anything less than EBT? Just as EBP requires the best evidence, EBT must also accept the challenge to integrate the best-known teaching/educational strategies with clinical expertise and students' values to ensure that the knowledge level is appropriate and of high standards. Senthuran (2010) spoke of the evolution toward the next level. EBT is that process of evolving toward an improved delivery of the art of learning. Ensuring that the different processes used to augment knowledge acquisition are based upon the best evidence is sensible and logical. As each aspect of EBP and EBT is incorporated into the day-to-day delivery of health care, the outcomes will be improved and validated.

Benner et al. (2010) stated that "high-stakes learning is a necessity; only experiential learning can yield the complex, open-ended, skilled knowledge required for learning to recognize the nature of the particular resources and constraints in equally open-ended and underdetermined clinical situations" (p. 42). Nurse educators must accept the challenge to move nursing education toward an evidence-based delivery process that encompasses experiential learning. The time for passive learning strategies has passed. Active learning strategies are required in the fast-paced healthcare arena. With the challenges of an aging faculty, nursing shortage, and changing healthcare agendas, the educational process must pull from the evidence to actively engage the students to confirm that they are capable of meeting the future challenges to come within nursing and health care.

Valiga (2010) stated that "excellence in teaching involves challenging ourselves and trying to do things beyond what we have already mastered, so that we continue to grow and so that our students' educational experiences are powerful and inspiring" (p. 1). Within EBT, the call and challenge is for each of us as faculty members to strive for the excellence within the educational experience. If we do not reach for the stars and expect the striving for distinction from ourselves and students, where will the nursing profession be in the future? Each of us must pursue the ultimatum to not accept mediocrity, but rather to strive for the highest level within each and every activity in which we engage.

SUMMARY POINTS

1. The nursing shortage is a result of the aging of the workforce, the aging of faculty, and a lack of financial support, clinical sites, and classroom space.

2. Regardless of the clinical setting, continued nursing education of nurse educators is vital for the provision of health care.

3. Research in nursing education has ebbed and flowed but is currently being conducted due to new streams of funding.

4. EBT has a major impact for nurse educators in clinics, hospitals, schools, home health, and hospice agencies.

5. A preceptor is an expert or authority who provides realistic experience and instruction to a student.

6. A coach is an expert or specialist who works with one student directly to help disseminate knowledge.

7. Individuals who agree to serve as preceptors and coaches for the next generation of students want to support and develop the novice nurses in a positive and encouraging manner.

8. The challenges and rewards confronted within the precepting/coaching experience are based upon the complexity of the workforce resulting from geographic, cultural, ethnic, generational, and professional diversity.

9. Five motivators that can be used by preceptors and coaches are healthy relationship, meaningful work, competence, autonomy, and progress.

10. A mentor is considered to hold a long-term commitment to the development of an individual.

11. The process of career mapping involves the pairing of a mentor/clinical advisor with an individual to assist the individual to define distinct professional aspirations, cultivate a plan for achieving those goals, and collaborate as the plan is implemented.

12. Faculty members engaged in advancing the success of the educational process must embrace the idea of promoting the successful transition of students into the actual workforce setting.

13. Part of understanding EBT is knowing that even within the teaching/education role, evidence is key for helping each member progress toward his or her education goals.

14. In addition to the generational issues, cultural issues can go hand-in-hand with the need to welcome the uniqueness and distinctiveness of the different individuals encountered during the learning process.

15. By establishing a blueprint of the cohort's composition, faculty members can build the synergetic environment that allows the group to develop a strong foundation to foster future learning opportunities.

16. The faculty member who endeavors to use EBT realizes that the establishment of a culture of inclusion and respect is essential and must include consideration of generational and cultural beliefs and biases.
17. Nursing must stay vigilant for its individual body of knowledge while embracing knowledge from other disciplines.
18. Evidence-based teaching must accept the challenge to integrate the best-known teaching/educational strategies with clinical expertise and students' values to ensure that the knowledge level is appropriate and of high standards.

TIPS FOR NURSE EDUCATORS

1. When selecting preceptors and coaches, care should be given to ensure that the individual has the desire to engage with the student to develop the student's knowledge base and skills.
2. Preceptors and coaches strive to impart knowledge and skills for a directed period of time, whereas a mentor works to develop an individual's professional goals over a longer time.
3. Didactic teaching settings are established to accentuate the cognitive domain of learning.
4. Clinical instructors, preceptors, and coaches are depended upon to translate the cognitive knowledge to the psychomotor and affective domains through application.
5. Continuing nursing education opportunities abound to assist nurse educators in their teaching role.
6. EBT activities designed to improve student learning outcomes are essential to add to the body of nursing education knowledge.
7. EBT is not restricted to the academic setting but rather should be actively sought by nursing staff development personnel.

MULTIPLE CHOICE QUESTIONS

1. A preceptor is an expert or specialist who provides:
   A. **practical experience and training for a student.**
   B. day-to-day support to a clinical instructor.
   C. one-on-one interaction with a physician.
   D. long-term support to a student.

Rationale:

The definition for preceptor is "an expert or specialist, such as a physician, who gives practical experience and training to a student" (Mentor, 2009). Preceptors are frequently utilized to support and expand the learning environment for students.

2. A coach is an expert or specialist who provides:
   A. cognitive experience and training for a student.
   B. day-to-day support to a clinical instructor related to affective knowledge.
   C. **one-on-one interaction with a student related to practical experience.**
   D. long-term support to a student.

Rationale:

The definition for coach is "a private tutor employed to prepare a student for an examination" (Coach, 2009). Within the nursing field, a coach is a private expert or specialist who does work directly with a student to aid in the acquisition of knowledge.

3. Within the clinical setting, the primary knowledge domains addressed are:
   A. cognitive and psychomotor.
   B. **psychomotor and affective.**
   C. affective and cognitive.
   D. cognitive and psychomotor.

Rationale:

Didactic teaching settings are established to accentuate the cognitive domain of learning. Clinical instructors, preceptors, and coaches are depended upon to translate the cognitive knowledge to the psychomotor and affective domains through application.

4. Modic and Schoessler (2010) identified four themes that preceptors acknowledged as needing to be strengthened to be successful at clinical instruction. One of those themes is to:
   A. **develop the ability to find the teachable moment.**
   B. stick with tried-and-true teaching methods.
   C. utilize negative feedback to make a strong point.
   D. not worry about evidence when trying to make a clinical point.

Rationale:

From the evidence, Modic and Schoessler (2010) identified four themes that preceptors noted as key areas needing to be strengthened: "(1) learning how to capitalize on teaching moments, (2) applying evidence-based teaching, (3) providing constructive performance feedback, and (4) adapting teaching strategies to match the different learning needs of students" (p. 134). Each of these areas is essential as orientation programs for preceptors and coaches are established and as preceptors/coaches are supported and developed.

5. Career mapping is a process in which a mentor/clinical advisor and an individual strive to:

   A. define organization goals, determine a plan for the unit, and implement that plan.

   B. define agency goals, cultivate a plan to achieve those goals, and work to implement it.

   C. **define distinct professional aspirations, cultivate a plan for achieving those goals, and collaborate as the plan is implemented.**

   D. define distinct personal aspirations, cultivate a plan for achieving agency goals, and collaborate as the plan is implemented.

Rationale:

The process of career mapping involves the pairing of a mentor/clinical advisor with an individual to assist the individual to define distinct professional aspirations, cultivate a plan for achieving those goals, and collaborate as the plan is implemented. From the evidence, career planning has been found to empower individuals to chart their own professional path and take responsibility for that journey.

6. Faculty members who want to build a synergetic environment need to:

   A. ignore generational issues, as they are not important.

   B. set the agenda for all classes to reduce stress.

   C. determine the required aspects to ensure that all areas are covered.

   D. **set the tone and culture within the learning environment.**

Rationale:

Determining a generational profile of the student cohort can aid the instructor to carefully consider the distinct needs that may be present. By establishing this blueprint of the cohort's composition, faculty can build the synergetic environment that allows the group to develop a strong foundation to foster future learning opportunities. While Sherman (2010) acknowledges that the nurse leader is principal in the environment, the idea can be translated to reflect that the educator holds the strategic position for setting the tone and culture within the learning environment.

7. A key aspect identified by the 2003 Institute of Medicine report is that students need to have developed competencies in:
   A. managed care.
   B. generalist skills.
   C. medication administration.
   D. **informatics.**

Rationale:

This project embraced the concepts of EBP (and thus EBT) to identify the vision/mission/goals, develop informatics competencies, and implement these competencies into nursing education. Through the TIGER initiative, nurse educators have been provided with strategies for integrating technology-enhanced experiences into lesson plans and curricula. The informatics competencies are divided into the following categories: all nurses, beginning nurses, and experienced nurses.

8. The current nursing shortage is most impacted by:
   A. lack of interest in nursing.
   B. **aging of the workforce and faculty.**
   C. little support from national nursing organizations.
   D. too many other professions from which to choose.

Rationale:

Aging of the workforce and nursing faculty resulted in a 2010 joint statement of the Tri-Council for Nursing, in which Dr. Peter Buerhaus indicated that prior to 2010 approximately 900,000 RNs (out of the estimated 2.6 million working RNs) were older than 50 years of age (AACN, 2010). The report continued to speculate that increasing numbers of these RNs were projected to retire in the coming years (AACN, 2010).

9. Nurse educators must rely on:
   A. their own "gut feelings" about teaching.
   B. teaching as they were taught by others.
   C. **EBT to provide a foundation for novice and experienced faculty.**
   D. other healthcare professionals to design educational activities/programs to produce a better nursing workforce.

Rationale:

EBT provides a foundation for both novice and experienced faculty to build their knowledge and skills in the nursing education arena on evidence rather than relying on a "gut feeling" or past educational experiences.

10. Competence and expertise are:
    A. **needed in the realm of being a nurse educator.**
    B. not essential for nursing education.
    C. a nice approach for nurses at the bedside.
    D. expected but seldom applied to nursing education.

Rationale:
Just as nurses at the bedside need to be cognizant of new technologies and the need to keep current on EBP, so too does the nurse educator need to maintain competence and expertise in the realm of being a nurse educator.

11. Barriers to increasing enrollments are:
    A. too many programs from which to choose.
    B. too many novice faculty who are young in age.
    C. **lack of faculty, clinical sites, and classroom space, as well as budgetary restraints.**
    D. aging of faculty, lack of scholarships, program requirements, and living accommodations.

Rationale:
Barriers to increasing enrollments are lack of faculty, clinical sites, and classroom space, as well as economic budgetary restraints.

12. Research in nursing education has:
    A. abounded over the years.
    B. decreased every year.
    C. little impact on EBT.
    D. **ebbed and flowed in the past.**

Rationale:
Research endeavors within nursing education have ebbed and flowed over the last decade. At this time, funding sources and/or streams seem to be opening up for nursing educational research projects.

13. Evidence-based teaching can be utilized:
    A. only in universities.
    B. only in community colleges.
    C. **in multiple settings.**
    D. in hospitals only.

Rationale:
Evidence-based teaching has a major impact for nurse educators in clinics, hospitals, schools, home health agencies, and hospice agencies.

DISCUSSION QUESTIONS

1. Over the last few semesters, faculty members have investigated the idea of using preceptors for all of the different students. What aspects do the faculty members need to carefully consider in regard to developing an orientation program for the preceptors?

   Considerations:

   Clinically competent nurses are called upon in many settings to provide the support and practical experience for students to allow for the advancement of the knowledge base. Didactic teaching settings are established to accentuate the cognitive domain of learning. Clinical instructors, preceptors, and coaches are depended upon to translate the cognitive knowledge to the psychomotor and affective domains through application. From the evidence, Modic and Schoessler (2010) pinpointed fours themes that preceptors identified as key areas needing to be strengthened: "(1) learning how to capitalize on teaching moments, (2) applying evidence-based teaching, (3) providing constructive performance feedback, and (4) adapting teaching strategies to match the different learning needs of students" (p. 134). Each of these areas is essential as orientation programs for preceptors and coaches are established and as preceptors/coaches are supported and developed. Individuals who agree to serve as preceptors and coaches for the next generation of students want to support and develop the novice nurses in a positive and encouraging manner. The idea of "eating our young" is not the feedback that most nurses desire. In reality, the strengthening and championing of the next generation of nurses is the ultimate goal for individuals who accept the responsibility of precepting and coaching student nurses.

2. Nursing faculty members need to consider and experiment with methods of advancing excellence in teaching. Within Valiga's (2010) article, she suggested several ways to accomplish this, such as:
   - Constructing open, adaptable curricula that embrace students' learning needs and ignore faculty biases and "sacred cows"
   - Engaging the learner in ascertaining at least some of the learning objectives for a course or module
   - Embracing the affective domain of learning, rather than ignoring it to concentrate on the cognitive domain of learning only
   - Launching teaching practices based on evidence instead of depending on tradition and/or past experiences

What other suggestions can you identify that could be used to advance excellence in teaching?

Considerations:

The guest editorial provided by Valiga (2010) in the *Journal of Nursing Education* identifies 15 different tactics that could be considered by a faculty member as excellence is sought. Within this editorial, Valiga challenges each of us to strive for the next level of nursing education. Each faculty member is encouraged to reach for the stars and break out of the box of traditional nursing education. As the old rules are tested and questioned, new and innovative evidence will be determined that can be used to advance the practice of nursing education to the next level of learning.

REFERENCES

American Association of Colleges of Nursing. (2010). Joint statement from the Tri-Council for Nursing on recent registered nurse supply and demand projections. Retrieved December 30, 2013, from http://www.aacn.nche.edu/Education/pdf/Tricouncilrnsupply.pdf

Bahouth, M. N., & Esposito-Herr, M. B. (2009). Orientation program for hospital-based nurse practitioners. *AACN Advanced Critical Care, 20*(1), 82–90.

Barnsteiner, J. H., Reeder, V. C., Palma, W. H., Preston, A. M., & Walton, M. K. (2010). Promoting evidence-based practice and translational research. *Nursing Administrative Quarterly, 34*(3), 217–225.

Benner, P., Sutphen, M., Leonard, V., & Day, L. (2010). *Educating nurses: A call for radical transformation.* San Francisco, CA: Jossey-Bass Higher and Adult Education Series.

Coach. (2009). In *American Heritage Dictionary of the English Language* (4th ed.). Houghton Mifflin Company. Retrieved July 1, 2014, from http://www.thefree-dictionary.com/coach

Hebda, T., & Calderone, T. L. (2010). What nurse educators need to know about the TIGER initiative. *Nurse Educator, 35*(2), 56–60.

Hudspeth, R. (2009). Regulation's burden regarding transition to practice. *Nursing Administrative Quarterly, 33*(4), 352–354.

Institute of Medicine. (2011). *The future of nursing: Leading change, advancing health.* Washington, DC: The National Academies Press.

Krom, Z. R., Batten, J., & Bautista, C. (2010). A unique collaborative nursing evidence-based practice initiative using the Iowa model: A clinical nurse specialist, a health science librarian, and a staff nurse's success story. *Clinical Nurse Specialist, 24*(2), 54–59.

Latimer, R., & Kimbell, J. (2010). Nursing research fellowship: Building nursing research infrastructure in a hospital. *Journal of Nursing Administration, 40*(2), 92–98.

Manion, J. (2010). The challenges and rewards of an intergenerational workforce. *Voice of Nursing Leadership: The American Organization of Nurse Executives, 3*(4), 8–10.

Mason, D. J. (2010). Health care reform: What's in it for nursing? *American Journal of Nursing, 110*(7), 24–26.

Mentor. (2009). In *American Heritage Dictionary of the English Language* (4th ed.). Houghton Mifflin Company. Retrieved July 1, 2014, from http://www .thefreedictionary.com/mentor

Modic, M. B., & Schoessler, M. (2010). Preceptorship. *Journal for Nurses in Staff Development,* 134–136.

Ogiehor-Enoma, G., Taqueban, L., & Anosike, A. (2010). 6 steps for transforming organizational EBP culture. *Nursing Management,* 14–17.

Preceptor. (2009). In *American Heritage Dictionary of the English Language* (4th ed.). Houghton Mifflin Company. Retrieved December 30, 2013, from http://www .thefreedictionary.com/preceptors

Rosseter, R. J. (2012). Nursing shortage fact sheet. Retrieved December 30, 2013, from http://www.aacn.nche.edu/media-relations/NrsgShortageFS.pdf

Senthuran, R. A. (2010). Why ask why? *Nursing Science Quarterly, 23*(3), 245–247.

Sherman, R. (2010). Creating synergy on multigenerational nursing teams. *Voice of Nursing Leadership: The American Organization of Nurse Executives, 3*(4), 4–6.

Shermont, H., Krepcio, D., & Murphy, J. M. (2009). Career mapping: Developing nurse leaders, reinvigorating careers. *Journal of Nursing Administration, 39*(10), 432–437.

Valiga, T. (2010). Excellence: Does the word mean anything anymore? *Journal of Nursing Education.* Guest Editorial.

Glossary

ACESTAR model A research model that represents how to interpret the sequences, description, and features of knowledge that are used in different phases of evidence-based practice. The model is depicted as a star with the five points embracing knowledge discovery, evidence summary, translation into practice recommendations, integration into practice, and evaluation.

Academician A person devoted not just to teaching but more generally to the pursuit of knowledge and to the values of an academic institution.

Accreditation Commission for Education in Nursing (ACEN) The agency through which the National League for Nursing accredits all levels of nursing programs. It was formerly called the National League for Nursing Accrediting Commission (NLNAC).

Adult learning principle A characteristic of the adult learner that must be attended to if learning is to be successful.

American Nurses Credentialing Center (ANCC) A subsidiary of the American Nurses Association (ANA) committed to promoting excellence in nursing and health care globally through credentialing programs.

Andragogy The education of adults. Knowles asserted that the andragogical approach is learner-directed, focused on "the tasks of life," immediately applicable, and focused on learning how to learn.

ARCC model A research model created to (1) advance EBP among advanced practice nurses, (2) establish a network of clinicians to act as EBP mentors, and (3) disseminate the best evidence.

Asynchronous activity An online class activity that is completed by each student independently of the other class members.

Baby Boomer The generation of individuals born between 1946 and 1964.

Behavioral objective A specific action required of a student in meeting the goals of a course.

Behavioral learning theory The theory that learning is little more than a response to a stimulus.

Benner's model A research model intended for nurses to develop patient care skills and knowledge through education and experience and to advance from novice to expert level.

Blog An online forum in which a person publishes his or her thoughts in an informal manner, usually on an ongoing basis.

Bloom's taxonomy The gold standard and hallmark of behavioral objectives. It is divided into six levels of learning: recall, grasp, apply, analyze, synthesize, and judge.

Brain-based learning An educational approach that considers how our brains work and how that influences how we learn, the environments that enhance our learning, the extent to which we retain or lose bits of information, and the ways in which we are able to make connections among what we know.

Care ethics An approach to ethical decision making that centers on the interaction of the specific nurse and the individual patient or family. Participants are expected to contemplate the milieu of the circumstances, preserve the interactions involving the individuals, and ensure that everyone is supported and strengthened.

Case study An educational exercise in which a scenario is provided and students must apply critical-thinking skills to explain how the situation should be handled.

Certification The confirmation of one's knowledge and skills by passing a designated testing process.

Certified Nurse Educator (CNE) An educator who has passed the CNE examination, which is administered by the National League for Nursing as a measure of the educator's understanding of best practices within nursing education.

Classroom assessment An assessment method that continuously and unobtrusively measures students' understanding of the lessons being taught in class.

Classroom management The effort of achieving an ideal learning environment in which course objectives can be met. Two primary considerations must be addressed: (1) managing the size of the class and (2) considering the number of faculty needed to teach the course.

Clicker A remote control device that allows students to respond to a specific question posed by faculty during a polling.

Clinical decision making The process of using critical thinking along with nursing knowledge, proficiency, and viewpoints to ascertain an appropriate action and/or response.

Clinical judgment Identification of the dynamic transitions by individuals across time as they react to health concerns and associated treatment.

Clinical reasoning The process of combining critical thinking, clinical decision making, and additional cognitive elements to see beyond the obvious solutions to innovative management of the clinical situation.

Coach A private expert or specialist who works directly with one or two students to aid the acquisition of knowledge. Coaches usually work with their students over a relatively long period (e.g., an entire semester or even an entire education program), with increased attention to learning opportunities.

Cochrane Collaboration An international, not-for-profit network established in 1993 to help healthcare providers and others make well-informed healthcare decisions.

Cognitive knowledge acquisition Learning that incorporates listening to, watching, touching, and experiencing the world around us.

Cognitive learning theory The theory that learning is stimulated by an environment that presents the learner with disequilibrium, imbalance, and tension. It argues that rewards and punishment are not necessary to facilitate learning.

Collaborative and cooperative learning An educational approach in which students work together to gain an understanding of a subject.

Commission for Nursing Education Accreditation An innovative accreditation commission being developed by the National League for Nursing.

Commission on Collegiate Nursing Education The agency through which the American Association of Colleges of Nursing provides accreditation for baccalaureate and graduate nursing programs.

Committee In nursing education, faculty members who are elected or appointed to accomplish the mission and goals of the school.

Competency In nursing, the awareness of knowledge; clinical, technical, and communication skills; and the capacity to decipher a problem by employing clinical and/or technical judgment.

Compliance Acceptance of a rule or responsibility.

Computer-based instruction The dissemination of course content through a computer.

Concept-based The selection, organization and sequence of an idea/notion/set of consequences.

Concept-based learning An approach to curriculum design that suggests that concepts are a way to organize knowledge such as categories or themes. In regard to classroom exercises, it refers to an activity to which students must respond by applying critical-thinking skills.

Concept-based thinking A cognitive process identifying patterns and connections.

Constructivist theory of learning The theory that knowledge is acquired through discovery and experimentation.

Contextual learning A type of learning that includes cultural aspects to frame the provision of care. It incorporates symbols, political aspects, power, relationships, values, aesthetic aspects, ethical perspectives, and philosophical facets as a transition into compassionate and positive care.

Critical thinking Disciplined clinical inquiry that provides nurses with alternatives that allow learning and engagement with the knowledge available.

Curriculum The educational plan that leads a student to the desired outcome. It takes into consideration the learning institution's philosophy, program objectives, and educational activities.

Debriefing An activity following a clinical simulation during which faculty challenge students to "think like a nurse" by critically reflecting on the events that just occurred.

Deep-dive brainstorming An online class activity that allows students to suggest ideas, concepts, and thoughts within a short time via a discussion board, blog area, or other medium.

Deontology The ethical theory that the correct course in any situation originates from rules and duty.

Directive learning A type of learning concerned with the ascertainment of regulations, restrictions, and omissions. It involves systems of directions that provide the "do's" and "don'ts" for everyday jobs.

Distance learner A student who engages in the educational process from a distance, frequently due to time, geographic, financial, or other constraints that restrict the student from attending traditional classes.

E-book A book that is accessed through an electronic device such as a tablet or smart phone rather than the traditional print format.

Educator A professional whose responsibility and major contribution to society relates to enhancing the total development of learners—their minds, their values, their skills—and to advancing knowledge and understanding in their field.

Email A means of sending or receiving a message electronically.

Emoticon A symbol that conveys a particular feeling, allowing some aspects of nonverbal communication to come into play during an online interaction or when text messaging.

Engaged learning Learning focused on the student, requiring the student to become directly involved in the entire learning process.

Ethics From the Greek word *ethos*, standards of conduct and social values.

Evaluation model A method of deriving the evidence needed for delivering effective teaching methodologies, curricula, and program development.

Evidence-based practice A process of using confirmed evidence (research and quality improvement), decision making, and nursing expertise to guide the delivery of holistic patient care.

Evidence-based teaching Current scholarship along with faculty expertise and student preferences.

Experiential learning Learning that relies on active participation by all members involved.

Facebook A social media service that allows individuals to share information with a personally selected network of fellow Facebook users.

Face-to-face The term applied to traditional classroom experiences in which all class participants are physically present.

Faculty incivility Faculty behavior that creates a stressful, hostile learning environment. It may result from faculty demeaning and belittling students, setting unrealistic expectations for performance, being overly critical, evaluating subjectively and showing favoritism, and targeting students for failure.

Feasibility study A detailed review of the likelihood of a proposed initiative's success.

FERPA An abbreviation for the Family Educational Rights and Privacy Act, which was enacted in 1974 to protect the privacy of student education records. It applies to all schools receiving federal funds. It is commonly known as the Buckley Amendment.

Flipped classroom A teaching approach in which content is delivered online, then reinforced through in-class exercises.

Formative evaluation An assessment method applied on an ongoing, periodic, and routine basis to measures students' understanding of the course materials.

Gap analysis A tool that educators can use to compare where they are to where they want to be.

Generation X The generation of individuals born between 1965 and 1976.

Generational cohort A group of people who were born near the same time and who have shared defining life experiences.

Hard skill A skill learned through classroom experience.

High-fidelity simulation A learning opportunity that offers a realistic clinical experience that may involve advanced interactive equipment.

HIPAA An abbreviation for the Health Insurance Portability and Accountability Act, which was enacted in 1996 to protect health information through a "privacy rule" to establish standards about the use and disclosure of health information.

Humanistic An educational approach that is attentive to learners' feelings, draws on their life experiences, and strives to help them grow personally and be fulfilled as individuals.

Hybrid course An educational process that combines face-to-face delivery with online delivery.

Incivility A violation of socially accepted norms of communication or behavior.

Inquiry learning A type of learning that encourages resourcefulness, exploration, theorizing, strategizing, ascertaining, illuminating, and categorizing challenges and approaches to understand aspects of care. It involves questioning processes and demanding validation for information provided.

Institute of Medicine A nongovernmental organization committed to providing healthcare-related research and advice.

Interprofessional education An educational approach in which students in various health disciplines learn with and from one another.

Iowa model A research model established to help guide bedside nursing staff members toward the use of research findings to improve the care provided. This model emphasizes the organization, primarily acute care settings.

Item learning A type of learning focused on facts, pieces of information, individual aspects, and straightforward associations. It is involuntary, automatic, and predictable.

Joanna Briggs Institute An organization committed to improving healthcare research and education.

Johns Hopkins model A problem-solving approach intended to help answer questions relating to clinical, administrative, and educational practice.

Learning style/preference A unique way in which an individual perceives, interacts with, processes, and responds to information and learning situations.

Legislative policy The laws embedded in nursing practice and nursing education.

Low-fidelity simulation A learning opportunity that engages students in case studies, role playing, or group activities that are specific to a narrow skill process.

Mentorship A long-term commitment that an experienced professional makes to the development of a less experienced individual.

Millennial The generation of individuals born between 1977 and 1997.

Mission In nursing education, the objective that an institution sets for itself to ensure that healthcare providers are properly educated and trained to meet patients' needs.

Mobile learning Any type of online class activity that allows students to acquire course material by using a mobile device such as a smart phone.

Model According to the *Encarta World English Dictionary* (2009), a simplified version of the complex analysis and problem solving related to a topic and/or an explanation of a theory and/or the concepts related to that theory.

Moderate-fidelity simulation A learning opportunity that is two-dimensional in its focus on the experience being learned. This level encourages problem solving.

Motivation The force that drives an individual to achieve a given objective.

Muddiest point A classroom assessment technique, often done as a 1-minute paper, that asks students to respond to the most confusing point of a lesson.

1-minute paper A classroom assessment technique that requires students to write a maximum of a half a page in 5 minutes to answer one question.

National Commission for Certifying Agencies (NCCA) An agency that evaluates certifying agencies using its established NCCA Standards for the Accreditation of Certification Programs.

National Council of State Boards of Nursing (NCSBN) An organization committed to providing a forum for boards of nursing to collaborate on matters of common interest relating to the public health, safety, and welfare, including the development of licensing examinations in nursing.

Needs assessment A review of the resources required to accomplish a given task.

Netiquette rule A concept or method for engaging in proper online communication.

Nurse educator competencies The activities, roles, and knowledge required of the educator.

Objective structured clinical examination A simulated clinical scenario that can be used to build skills and competencies, and for evaluation.

Online course Any activity or course that is provided via the Internet.

PDA An abbreviation for personal digital assistant, a handheld electronic device used for organizing and accessing information.

Pedagogy The education of children. A pedagogical approach calls for the learner to be passive, the subject matter to be central, motivation to come from external rewards, and learning to be focused on the future.

Philosophy The foundation for the entire educational experience at an institution.

Podcast lecture An online class activity in which media files (e.g., MP3 files) are provided for individuals to access as needed for playback on a diverse group of mobile instruments such as computers and portable media players.

Policy A course of action—a plan.

Practice analysis An evaluative process that reveals the activities of a professional engaged in a particular practice to determine the validity of an exam that provides certification or licensure.

Preceptor A subject expert used to support and expand the learning environment for students. Preceptors usually work with their assigned students during a specific period (usually 1 day or 1 week).

Problem-based Exploring solutions of situations or health issues which are unclear.

Problem-based learning An approach to curriculum design that focuses heavily on clinical situations, which may be based in the classroom, in simulation, or both. In regard to classroom exercises, it refers to an activity to which students must respond by applying critical-thinking skills.

Procedure The means to carry out an action or plan.

Professional formation The process of understanding and adopting the behavioral norms of a professional community.

Professional or national accreditation A means of defining a quality unit or discipline within a community college, college, and/or university.

Program evaluation An ongoing process in nursing education that focuses on review and improvement. The need for curriculum revision, resources, and faculty and staff may become apparent during this process.

Promotion An elevation in professional status, often to a position of greater responsibility and often involving a pay increase.

PSCOT format A guide to answering questions posed during evidence-based practice. PSCOT stands for population, strategy, comparison, outcome, time period.

Quality improvement In nursing, an effort to improve nursing care at the point of care.

Rational learning A type of learning that introduces theory and the "why's" for doing things into the logical management of tasks. It introduces the use of logic to influence judgment and decision making.

Reflective journaling An educational activity in which students document their responses to or feelings about a given prompt.

Regional accreditation A continuous improvement process involving the entire university or college to maintain the standards required by the regional accrediting agency.

Regulatory agency A review body that ensures that nursing programs are meeting educational standards and benchmarks. This agency is generally the state nursing board.

Regulatory policy The regulations embedded in nursing practice and nursing education.

Rights ethical theory An approach to ethical decision making in which rights established by society and endorsed by the larger, ruling population are used as the foundation for the decisions made.

Robert Wood Johnson Foundation An organization committed to improving health care in the United States through health promotion efforts and research funding.

Role play An educational activity in which students are assigned roles and must act out a given scenario in anticipation of how they will react to a similar situation in practice.

Rosswurm-Larrabee model A research model established for use in primary care settings with advanced practitioners. It strives to guide the individual through the entire process of evidence-based practice.

Rubric An evaluation tool that outlines the requirements and expectations of an assignment.

Scaffolding The process of breaking down the key concepts into chunks to allow for the comprehension of each chunk as it relates to the whole.

Scope of practice The activities, roles, and knowledge required of the educator, or nurse educator competencies.

Self-confidence An individual's certainty of his or her own capacity, credibility, or dependability.

Self-efficacy An individual's conviction in his or her capacity to thrive in a given situation.

Social learning theory The theory that individuals learn from observing others and paying attention to what happens to them.

Social media Internet-based networks that allow individuals to quickly and easily exchange information with one another.

Socialization In nursing, the process whereby students acquire nursing knowledge, skills, and attitudes.

Soft skill A skill learned through hands-on work.

Staff development The process of improving nursing educators' ability to conduct a classroom and prepare their students.

Static manikin A partial task trainer used to practice specific skills. Examples include ear or prostate manikins.

Stetler/Marran model A model of research utilization that assimilates the individual nurse while promoting the use of both internal and external data/evidence. It was developed in 1976 and revised in 1994 with the addition of conceptual underpinnings and a set of assumptions.

Stress An unwelcome and potentially debilitating emotional response to a challenging situation, such as that faced by an overwhelmed student.

Student evaluation A means for students to voice their opinions of the effectiveness of the course and its instructor.

Student incivility Student behavior that is inappropriate and disruptive to the learning community.

Summative evaluation A final comprehensive examination.

Synchronous activity An online class activity that requires all of the members to be online and/or connected at the same time.

Syntactical learning A type of learning that involves investigation into the understanding of the whole. In it, relationships and patterns are sought to guide unique client care. It encourages individuals to make intuitive efforts as theory is meshed into practice.

Teacher In the broadest sense, anyone who communicates knowledge to someone else. For example, parents teach their children values, skills, and ways of interacting with others.

Technology In nursing education, the audiovisual and communications (including Internet) tools that enhance the educational process.

Tenure A status earned by educators that ensures greater job permanence.

Test blueprint A guide for the composition of the questions on the Certified Nurse Educator examination.

The Joint Commission An agency that accredits healthcare organizations and sets standards required for consumers of health care, especially hospitals and clinics where nurses are employed.

Theory According to the *Encarta World English Dictionary* (2009), (1) a set of rules and/or techniques that can be applied to a subject and/or abstract thoughts and (2) the ideas that form the underpinning that is used to move a distinct practice into reality.

Think tank A group of experts convened to resolve a given issue.

Traditionalist/Veteran The generation of individuals born before 1945.

Translational research Research conducted with the intent of making scientific findings applicable to practice.

Twitter A social media service that allows individuals to share (or "tweet") information in an immediate and concise form.

Utilitarianism An approach to ethical decision making that endeavors to envision the consequences of each action possible. As a result of considering all of the possible outcomes, the best decision for the most individuals can be selected.

Virtue ethical theory An approach to ethical decision making that is founded on character rather than actions or rules. The character of a person in normal behavior is used as the groundwork for determining the plan for managing an ethical situation.

Web-based instruction Any activity or course that is provided via the Internet.

Index

Note: Page numbers followed by *f* or *t* indicate material in figures or tables respectively.